Titles of related interest

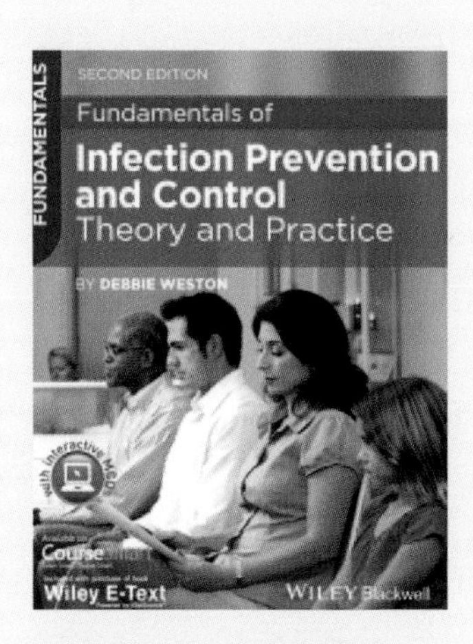

ISBN: 978-1-118-30665-9
Review of the first edition: “Interesting and readable . . . the most important book any healthcare professional or healthcare student can own.” (Amazon reviewer)

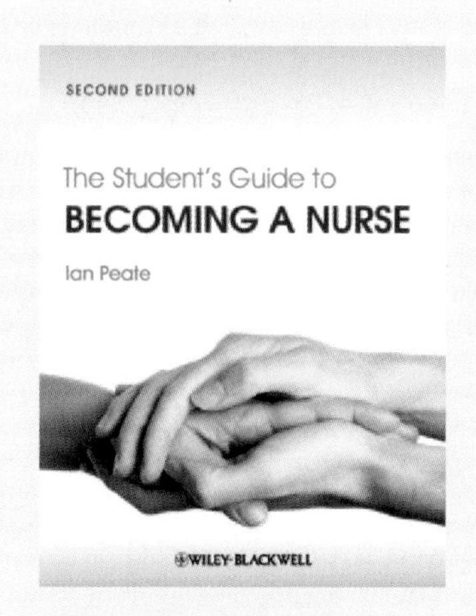

ISBN: 978-0-470-67270-9
“This comprehensive book will be indispensable throughout a student’s education.” (Nursing Standard by Sarah Lovie, nursing student, Royal Cornhill Hospital)

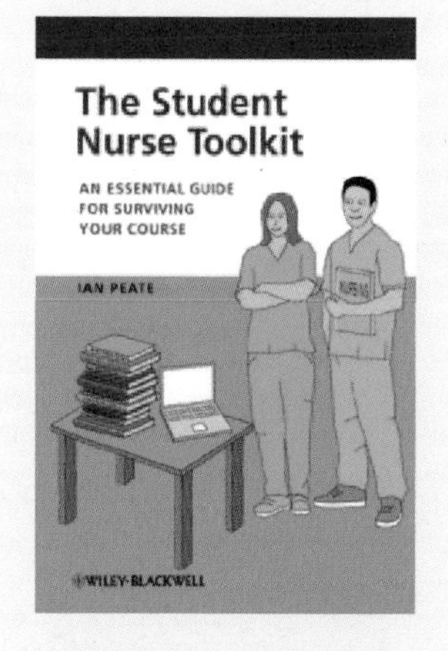

ISBN: 978-1-1183-9378-9
“I instantly felt like I could relate to the book and to the ideas of the author in a way that really built trust between me as the reader and what the book was teaching me.” (Second year adult nursing student, University of Nottingham)

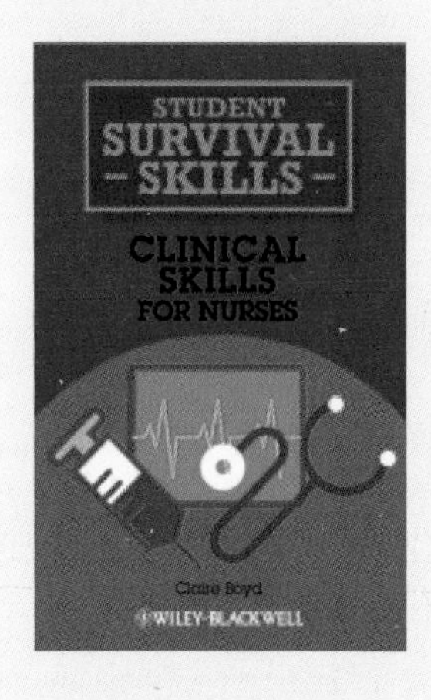

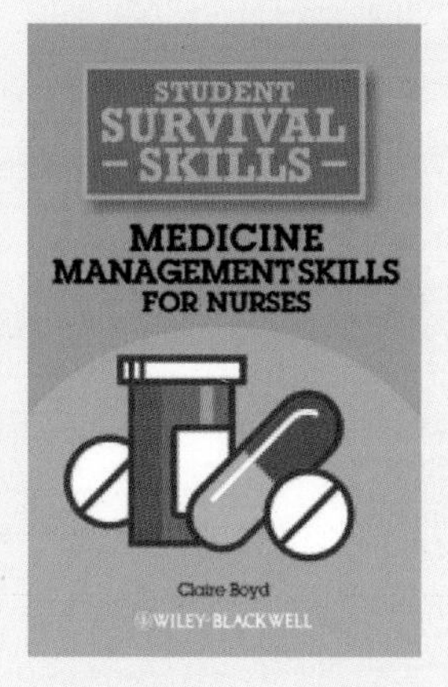

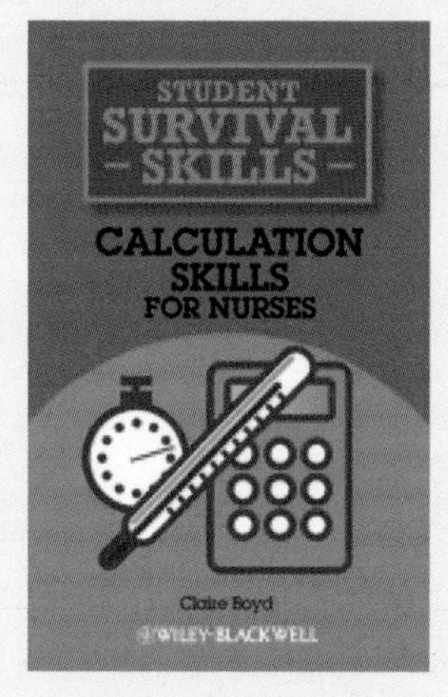

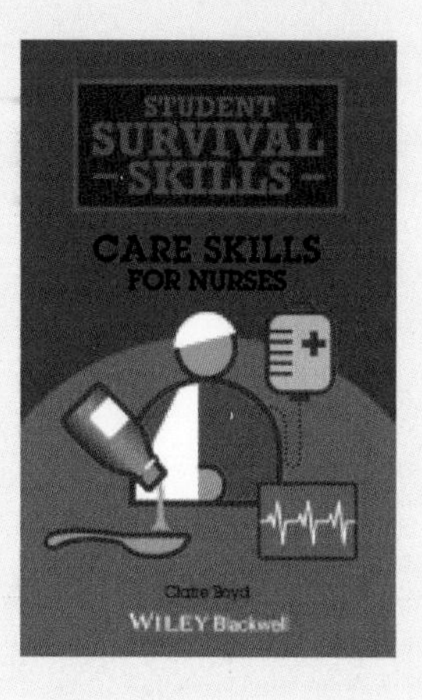

ISBN: 978-1-1184-4877-9 ISBN: 978-1-1184-4885-4 ISBN: 978-1-1184-4889-2 ISBN: 978-1-118-65738-6
“I love this series. . . . I am truly looking forward to them being published as I can’t wait to get my hands on them.” (Second year nursing student, University of Abertay, Dundee)

Fundamentals of

Health Promotion for Nurses

SECOND EDITION

Fundamentals of Health Promotion for Nurses

EDITED BY

JANE WILLS

Professor, Health Promotion
London South Bank University, London, UK

WILEY Blackwell

This edition first published 2014 © John Wiley & Sons Ltd

Registered Office
John Wiley & Sons Ltd, The Atrium, Southern Gate, Chichester, West Sussex, PO19 8SQ, UK

Editorial Offices
350 Main Street, Malden, MA 02148-5020, USA
9600 Garsington Road, Oxford, OX4 2DQ, UK
The Atrium, Southern Gate, Chichester, West Sussex, PO19 8SQ, UK

For details of our global editorial offices, for customer services, and for information about how to apply for permission to reuse the copyright material in this book please see our website at www.wiley.com/wiley-blackwell.

Library of Congress Cataloging-in-Publication Data

Promoting health (Wills)
Fundamentals of health promotion for nurses / edited by Jane Wills. -- 2nd edition.
p. ; cm.
Preceded by Promoting health / edited by Jane Wills. 2007.
Includes bibliographical references and index.
ISBN 978-1-118-51577-8 (pbk.)
I. Wills, Jane, 1954- editor. II. Title.
[DNLM: 1. Health Promotion--Nurses' Instruction. 2. Public Health Nursing--methods--Nurses' Instruction. 3. Nurse's Role--Nurses' Instruction. 4. Nurse-Patient Relations--Nurses' Instruction. 5. Patient Education as Topic--Nurses' Instruction. WY 108]
RT97
613--dc23

2014005312

A catalogue record for this book is available from the British Library.

Cover image: Reproduced from iStock © alengo
Cover design by Grounded Design

Set in 10/12pt Myriad Pro by Laserwords Private Limited, Chennai, India
Printed and bound in Malaysia by Vivar Printing Sdn Bhd

1 2014

Contents

About the series

Wiley's *Fundamentals* series are a wide-ranging selection of textbooks written to support pre-registration nursing and other health care students throughout their course. Packed full of useful features such as learning objectives, activities to test knowledge and understanding, and clinical scenarios, the titles are also highly illustrated and fully supported by interactive MCQs, and each one includes access to a **Wiley E-Text: powered by VitalSource** – an interactive digital version of the book including downloadable text and images and highlighting and note-taking facilities. Accessible on your laptop, mobile phone or tablet device, the *Fundamentals* series is *the* most flexible, supportive textbook series available for nursing and health care students today.

Preface

This book is intended to clarify for new nurses the importance of developing public health and health promotion skills. The Nursing and Midwifery Council (NMC) has established standards of competence and specific skills that student nurses must be able to perform (NMC, 2010). One of the NMC standards for pre-registration education states that:

> *All nurses must understand public health principles, priorities and practice in order to recognise and respond to the major causes and social determinants of health, illness and health inequalities. They must use. health screening, health promotion, and promote social inclusion.*
>
> (NMC, 2010)

Part of the reason why health promotion and public health have assumed increasing importance in nursing is a consequence of changing understandings of medicine and health care and the importance of reducing preventable illness and deaths. Infection-control measures, the modification of unhealthy lifestyles and the appropriate use of health services can offer a cheaper solution to demands for health care and threats to individual health. Health promotion and public health can seem a vast area of new knowledge and skills that may also be difficult to put into practice. The nurse needs to use a range of information and data to assess needs, promote access to services and identify effective ways to promote health. It is also expected that all nurses will use their communication and interpersonal skills to encourage patients to adopt healthier behaviours. Changing behaviour is a challenge for patients and may also be so for the nurse and this requires an understanding of the social and psychological dimensions of lifestyle change.

Developing such skills demands a wide range of knowledge, drawing from the scientific knowledge of epidemiology to communication skills. Such knowledge must then be applied to the needs of the individual, family, group, community or population and because the National Health Service (NHS) is not the only sector that affects and is concerned with health, the nurse must work in partnership with other professions and groups in public, private and voluntary sectors who have an impact on people's health and well-being.

This book is written for new student nurses whose placements may include working with children, adults, people with mental health issues or a learning disability and the community and who may in the future, work in many different contexts including health centres, primary care, walk-in centres, and specialist clinics such as Genitourinary Medicine and Sure Start areas as well as the acute hospital setting. While specialist community public health nurses are recognized as making a specific contribution to the promotion of health and are registered on Part 3 of the Nursing and Midwifery Council (NMC) register, many other nurses have an interest in, and responsibility for, enabling people to achieve optimum health.

The terms health promotion and public health are often used interchangeably. In this book we see these as complementary and overlapping areas of practice in which health promotion refers to efforts to prevent ill health and promote positive health, a central aim being to enable people to take control over their own health. This may range from a relatively narrow focus on changing people's behaviour to community action or public policy change reflective of tackling the wider determinants of health. Public health has traditionally been associated with public health medicine and its efforts to prevent disease. It takes a collective view of the health needs and health care of a population rather than an individual perspective. Its strategies thus include the assessment of the health of populations, formulating policies to prevent or manage health problems and signi¬ficant disease conditions such as immunization programmes and the promotion of healthy living environments and sustainable development.

Health promotion is a difficult concept because there are many different perspectives on health that underpin current approaches. For the nurse, promoting health means much more than the traditional role of addressing symptoms, experiences of pain, distress or discomfort. It means enabling people to increase control over their health though this may be at odds with the medical approach to care which may too often dismiss the patient's perspective and cast the patient's role as one which involves passivity, trust and a willingness to wait for medical help. This book tries to help the nurse understand health promotion activities by suggesting that these may relate to the following:

- developing personal skills through health education;
- strengthening community links and networks;
- reorienting services to promote health;
- creating environments that make the healthy choice easier;
- working towards policies that support the public's health.

This book is a substantially revised second edition of a textbook published in 2007, *Promoting Health: Vital Notes for Nurses*. Many of the same authors have contributed to this volume but we have adopted a different structure for the book to enable new nurses to better orientate themselves to how they can be health promoting in practice. Part One is therefore a discussion of some of the core concepts in health promotion. Part Two outlines some of the major public health priorities and how they may be addressed by the nurse. Part Three is an introduction to some of the core skills of public health and health promotion including epidemiology, communication and health education, evidence-based practice and health protection and infection control. Part Four is a completely new addition to this book in which practising nurse educators explain how their branch of nursing can be health promoting. Although health promotion and/or public health are central aspects of the nurse's job description, part of their training and a core dimension in the NHS knowledge and skills framework for the competent nurse, these aspects of a nurse's role are not well understood and so this section is to make real health promotion as an approach and set of activities.

The book is organized consistently throughout to enable you to find your way. Each chapter has learning outcomes and a chapter summary. At the end of each chapter there are some suggestions to follow up in further reading or web resources. Each chapter also contains an 'on placement: checklist' of practice points for the new student nurse to take note of and assess whether health promotion is visible on placement.

Acknowledgements

Textbooks are an important but sometimes unrecognized part of the work of academics and I am grateful to my colleagues who have found time in their busy workloads to contribute their expertise to this book. Also to my family who had to forego their summer holiday to its production. Finally, I want to acknowledge the enormous assistance provided by Katrina Rimmer, the Development Editor in the Health Sciences team at Wiley, who was both patient and meticulous in preparing the manuscript.

Jane Wills

Glossary of key terms

You can download these key terms by visiting the companion website at:
www.wileyfundamentalseries.com/healthpromotion

Chapter 1

Empowerment Developing the capacity of people to make informed decisions by building self-efficacy and understanding.

Health education Facilitating learning and behaviour change.

Health promotion A range of activities to enable people to take greater control over their health that may be directed at individuals, families and communities or whole populations.

Holistic Taking all the elements of a person's life into account – including physical, emotional, mental and spiritual elements.

Primary prevention Interventions to avoid occurrence of a disease. Secondary prevention includes measures to diagnose before a disease causes morbidity.

Public health The science and art of preventing disease and prolonging life through the identification of need and population actions such as screening

Chapter 2

Health inequality The avoidable and unfair differences in health status between groups of people.

Social determinants The economic and social conditions in which a person lives that influence their health.

Social exclusion A term used to describe those who are unable to participate fully in life due to social and economic factors.

Chapter 3

Model While the definition of health promotion has been universally adopted, there have been a number of different approaches to promoting health and these are described or analysed in models.

Preventative medical Sometimes called biomedical approach which focuses on addressing risk behaviours and healthy lifestyles as the means by which health can be improved.

Social model Acknowledges the social determinants of health and the reciprocal relationship between health-related behaviours and the environments in which people live and work.

Chapter 4

Setting A setting is the term used to describe environments which influence a person's health. Settings such as a school or workplace can also be used to promote health as they are vehicles to reach individuals.

Supportive environment An environment that offers people protection from the factors that can threaten good health and makes healthy choices easier. It will also foster participation in health and enable people to control their health.

Chapter 5

Cessation Also called quitting in relation to smoking. Four-week quit rates are taken as the measure of success and these are validated by testing smokers' carbon monoxide (CO) level.

Harm reduction Strategies to reduce harm caused by continued tobacco/nicotine use, such as reducing the number of cigarettes smoked, or switching to different brands or products, e.g. e-cigarettes.

Pharmacotherapy A treatment using pharmaceutical drugs, e.g. Nicotine Replacement Therapy (NRT), bupropion.

Second-hand smoke Also called passive smoking or environmental tobacco smoke (ETS). A mixture of smoke exhaled by smokers and smoke released from smouldering cigarettes, cigars, pipes, bidis, etc. The smoke mixture contains gases and particulates, including nicotine, carcinogens and toxins.

Chapter 6

Binge drinking The consumption of five or more alcoholic drinks on at least one occasion.

Dependent drinking Dependent drinking means that a person feels that they are unable to function without alcohol. Withdrawal symptoms can be both physical and psychological and include a compulsion to drink. Sweating, shakiness, and anxiety occur when alcohol use is stopped after a period of heavy drinking.

Harmful drinking When a person drinks over the recommended weekly amount of alcohol and experiences health problems that are directly related to alcohol, e.g. depression, pancreatitis, cirrhosis, some types of cancer, such as mouth cancer and bowel cancer.

Hazardous drinking When a person drinks over the recommended weekly limit of alcohol (21 units for men and 14 units for women). It is also possible to drink hazardously by binge drinking.

Low risk drinking Is called "lower-risk" rather than "safe" because drinking alcohol is never completely safe but there is lower risk of causing future harm. Low risk is men who drink less than 3–4 units a day and women who drink less than 2–3 units a day.

Chapter 7

Sexual rights The basic right of all couples and individuals to decide freely and responsibly the number, spacing and timing of their children and to have the information and means to do so. The right to make decisions concerning reproduction and sexual activity free of discrimination, coercion and violence.

Sexual risk Behaviours which can increase the chance of contracting or transmitting disease, or increase the chance of the occurrence of unwanted pregnancy.

Sexuality Encompasses sex, gender identities and roles, sexual orientation, eroticism, pleasure, intimacy and reproduction.

Chapter 8

Bariatric surgery Surgery on the stomach and/or intestines to help the patient with extreme obesity lose weight. Bariatric surgery is a weight-loss method used for people who have a body mass index (BMI) above 40.

Body mass index (BMI) A measure of body weight relative to height. BMI can be used to determine if people are at a healthy weight, overweight, or obese.

Obesity A person is considered obese if he or she has a body mass index (BMI) of 30 kg/m^2 or greater.

Overweight Being too heavy for one's height: having a body mass index (BMI) of 25–30 kg/m^2.

Chapter 9

Care pathway The steps in the treatment and care of a patient with a particular condition. Care pathways set out the expected progress of the individual as their condition progresses.

Chronic condition A disease, illness or injury which has one or more of the following characteristics: it needs ongoing or long-term monitoring; it needs ongoing or long-term control or relief of symptoms; it requires rehabilitation ; it continues indefinitely; it has no known cure; it comes back or is likely to come back.

Long-term condition Those conditions that cannot, at present, be cured but can be controlled by medication and other therapies.

Self-management Encouraging a patient to take responsibility for managing a condition.

Chapter 10

Epidemiology The study of the distribution and determinants of disease and conditions in particular populations.

Incidence Number of new cases of disease in a given time period.

Measures of deprivation Ways of assessing levels of disadvantage in a population.

Prevalence The total number of people in a given population with a disease at any given point in time.

Rate The frequency with which an event occurs in a defined population. In whole populations, usually expressed as number per 100000.

Risk factor An aspect of personal behaviour or lifestyle, an environmental exposure, that is associated with an increased occurrence of disease or other health-related event or condition.

Surveillance The systematic collection and analysis of health data on an ongoing basis, in order to control and prevent disease or outbreaks in the community.

Chapter 11

Causality is "*the relating of causes to the effects they produce*".

Critical appraisal standards that are used to evaluate research evidence.

Evidence Facts or information to prove whether or not something is true.

Intervention An action or programme that aims to bring about identifiable outcomes.

National Institute for Health and Clinical Excellence (NICE) An independent organization responsible for providing national evidence-based guidance on the promotion of good health and the prevention and treatment of ill health.

RCT Randomized controlled trial is an experimental research design.

Systematic review A synthesis of available evidence usually collected from RCTs.

Chapter 12

Advocacy Activities such as lobbying aimed at changing the policy of organizations or government.

Health literacy The skills needed to function in a health care environment which includes basic reading and numerical skills.

Lifestyle The behaviours that make up how we live.

Motivation Internal factors within a person that influence their actions.

Motivational interviewing A discussion focusing on a key issues that encourages the patient to change by exploring cost and benefits.

Self efficacy Feeling able to do or change something and having confidence and control.

Victim blaming Blaming or judging someone for unhealthy behaviours without acknowledging the social factors that influence that behaviour.

Chapter 13

Communicable disease A disease that can be communicated or transmitted from one person to another.

Health protection Part of the Public Health function that includes safety and quality of food, water, air and the general environment; preventing the transmission of communicable diseases; managing outbreaks.

Non-communicable disease (NCD) Disease or conditions that are non-infectious and non-transmissible among people. NCDs may be chronic diseases or they may result in more rapid death. Risk factors such as a person's lifestyle and socio-economic environment are known to increase the likelihood of certain NCDs.

Screening Screening is a process of identifying apparently healthy people who may be at increased risk of a disease or condition. They can then be offered information, further tests and appropriate treatment to reduce their risk and/or any complications arising from the disease or condition.

Chapter 14

Complex needs A person who has a range of "layered" issues that may include learning disability and other difficulties such as physical and sensory impairment, mental health problems or behavioural difficulties.

Learning disability Everyone is individual, and will have individual needs, preferences and ambitions. Learning disabilities are a significant, lifelong experience in which there is a reduced ability to understand or learn new or complex information, a reduced ability to cope independently, and starts before adulthood with a lasting effect on the individual's development.

Chapter 15

Advocacy Independent help to enable people to take control of their lives, explore and express their own needs and access the services and support they need to meet their needs.

Mental health Mental health is a state of well-being in which an individual realizes their own abilities, can cope with the normal stresses of life, can work productively and is able to make a contribution to their community.

Mental health promotion Mental health promotion aims to promote mental health and well-being for all; prevent mental health problems for at-risk groups through increasing protective factors and reducing risk factors; promote mental health for people with mental health problems.

Mental illness Severe and enduring mental health problems.

Well-being A multidimensional concept that includes happiness, positive affect, low negative affect, and satisfaction with life as well as psychological functioning.

Chapter 16

Activities of Daily Living Tasks that people carry out to look after their home, themselves, and their participation in work, social and leisure activities.

Carer Someone, usually unpaid, and often a friend or family member who supports a person with social care needs, either full-time or part-time.

Older adult In the developed world, the age of 60 or 65, roughly equivalent to retirement ages in most developed countries, is said to be the beginning of old age. In other countries, chronological age has less meaning and an elder is associated with wisdom and possibly accompanying physical decline.

Chapter 17

Community People who share a set of characteristics that may relate to geography, interest, culture or family.

Community development Problem solving approach whereby the community is empowered with knowledge and skills to identify and prioritize its needs and problems, harness its resources to deal with the problems and take action.

Community nurses Registered nurses who work in the community: in people's homes, in schools and in local surgeries and health centres. Also called public health nurses.

Chapter 18

Children's nurses Nurses who care for sick or injured children and young people in hospital or in the home.

Child Health Profile These provide a snapshot of child health and well-being for each Local Authority in England using indicators such as infant death, dental health, immunisation rates.

Safeguarding The responsibilities and actions taken to protect children from maltreatment and to prevent impairment of their health.

Contributors

Thomas J. Currid
Course Director, Mental Health
London South Bank University, London, UK

Joanne Delrée
Senior Lecturer, Learning Disability Nursing
London South Bank University, London, UK

Pat England
Faculty Information Adviser, Health and Social Care
London South Bank University, London, UK

Renee Francis
Senior Lecturer, Learning Disability Nursing
London South Bank University, London, UK

Amanda Hesman
Senior Lecturer, Adult Nursing
London South Bank University, London, UK

Sandra Horner
Senior Lecturer, Specialist Community Public Health Nursing
London South Bank University, London, UK

Jenny Husbands
Senior Lecturer, Adult Nursing
London South Bank University, London, UK

Linda Jackson
Senior Lecturer, Public Health and Health Promotion
London South Bank University, London, UK

Maxine Jameson
Senior Lecturer, Specialist Community Public Health Nursing
London South Bank University, London, UK

Muireann Kelly
Research Assistant
London South Bank University, London, UK

Matthew Lester
Senior Lecturer, Child Nursing
London South Bank University, London, UK

Susie Sykes
Senior Lecturer, Public Health and Health Promotion
London South Bank University, London, UK

Jane Wills
Professor, Health Promotion
London South Bank University, London, UK

Sandie Woods
Senior Lecturer, Occupational Therapy
London South Bank University,
London, UK

How to use your textbook

Features contained within your textbook

The overview page gives a summary of the topics covered in each part.

Part One

Health Promotion and Public Health

Learning outcome boxes give a summary of what a student can expect to know and understand in a chapter.

Learning outcomes

By the end of this chapter you will be able to:

1. Define health and well-being
2. Analyse the difference between a medical and social model of health and identify how these apply to nursing practice
3. Define and discuss the concepts of public health and health promotion and how they apply to nursing practice

On placement: checklists give key points to note when on placement.

On placement: checklist

- Are all dimensions of health considered in care plans?
- Are health promotion materials available for patients and families? Are these kept up to date?
- Is health promotion included in care plans? What is included?
- Is information personalized?
- Is information on patients' social circumstances recorded or known e.g. who they live with, education levels, socio-economic status?
- Is health behaviour information recorded, e.g. smoking status including ever smoked, alcohol consumption including drinking behaviour, BMI, physical activity?

Key learning point boxes provide key points from each chapter to aid revision.

Key learning points

1. Health is not just the absence of disease but includes social, emotional, psychological, and spiritual elements.
2. Promoting health is about activities that enable a person to live well, even with a diagnosed condition.
3. Promoting health is also about a way of working that is empowering and participatory. It is not about persuasion or coercion to get people to adopt particular health behaviours.
4. Public health usually means actions to protect from disease and knowledge work to identify where and how resources should be used to best meet needs.
5. Health promotion includes many different activities at different levels of intervention: individuals, families and communities and populations. It is sometimes called health improvement.

Chapter summaries provide a brief statement of the chapter's content.

Chapter summary

This chapter has discussed the concept of health and why it is central to the practice of all health care professionals. There are many ways that the concept of health can be understood. Students were encouraged to look beyond the traditional medical model of health to a social model of health. In the medical model, health is seen as the absence of disease and illness, which has led to the perception that health is an individual phenomenon where each person is responsible solely for their health. A social model of health focuses on social and political determinants and the unequal access that people may have to health. It looks at social interactions, socio-economic factors and their interaction with people's lives. This relates to nursing practice in encouraging nurses to look beyond the disease or illness that a patient may present with to the causes of that disease or illness and to include the patient in the treatment process.

Activity, evidence, scenario and case studies give further insight into topics and opportunities for self-test.

Activity 1.1

For me, being healthy means …

Tick whichever apply:

- ❑ Taking regular exercise.
- ❑ Getting enough sleep.
- ❑ Eating fruit and vegetables.
- ❑ Enjoying life.
- ❑ Bouncing back when things are tough.
- ❑ Being safe.
- ❑ Having plenty of friends.
- ❑ Being the right weight for my height.
- ❑ Having a job.
- ❑ Feeling at peace with myself.
- ❑ Not smoking.
- ❑ Not getting sick.
- ❑ Drinking in moderation.
- ❑ Enjoying work and study with not too much stress.

Scenario 1.1

Patient on ward following an intra-cerebral haemorrhage

Mr C is 58 and has been transferred to a rehabilitation unit following a stroke which has caused right-sided weakness. Mr C can walk a few steps with sticks and can transfer from the bed to the chair with assistance. He has no swallowing problems though his appetite is poor. He is uncommunicative and repeats certain phrases such as "What's the time?"

- ❑ What would be the likely health needs of the patient?
- ❑ What is the health promotion role of the nurse?

Case Study 15.1

Evaluation of a Well-being Support Programme

A Cochrane review of physical health monitoring for patients with SMI has concluded that there was no evidence from RCTs to support current practice (Tosh *et al*., 2010) but many areas have adopted the model of a Well-being Support Programme (Ohlsen *et al*., 2005). This is a health promotion initiative for people with SMI in which nurses are trained to do the following:

- ❑ Identify physical health problems.
- ❑ Promote treatment adherence.
- ❑ Encourage positive lifestyle change.
- ❑ Strengthen links between primary and secondary care.
- ❑ Provide support and advice to carers.
- ❑ Direct patients to appropriate primary and secondary care services.

The website icon indicates that you can find accompanying resources on the book's companion website.

The anytime, anywhere textbook

Wiley E-Text

For the first time, your textbook comes with free access to a **Wiley E-Text: Powered by VitalSource** version – a digital, interactive version of this textbook which you own as soon as you download it. Your **Wiley E-Text** allows you to:

Search: Save time by finding terms and topics instantly in your book, your notes, even your whole library (once you've downloaded more textbooks)
Note and Highlight: Colour code, highlight and make digital notes right in the text so you can find them quickly and easily
Organize: Keep books, notes and class materials organized in folders inside the application
Share: Exchange notes and highlights with friends, classmates and study groups
Upgrade: Your textbook can be transferred when you need to change or upgrade computers
Link: Link directly from the page of your interactive textbook to all of the material contained on the companion website

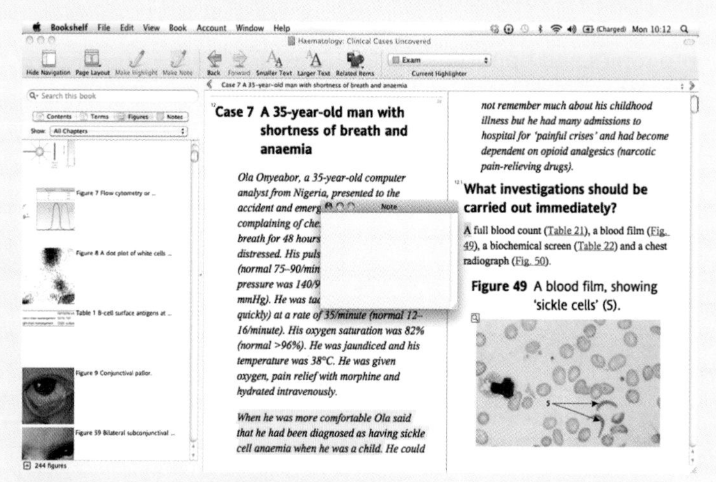

The Wiley E-Text version will also allow you to copy and paste any photograph or illustration into assignments, presentations and your own notes.

To access your Wiley E-Text

- Find the redemption code on the inside front cover of this book and carefully scratch away the top coating of the label. Visit **www.vitalsource.com/software/bookshelf/downloads** to download the Bookshelf application to your computer, laptop, tablet or mobile device.
- If you have purchased this title as an e-book, access to your **Wiley E-Text** is available with proof of purchase within 90 days. Visit **http://support.wiley.com** to request a redemption code via the 'Live Chat' or 'Ask A Question' tabs.
- Open the Bookshelf application on your computer and register for an account.
- Follow the registration process and enter your redemption code to download your digital book.
- For full access instructions, visit www.wileyfundamentalseries.com/healthpromotion.

The VitalSource Bookshelf can now be used to view your Wiley E-Text on iOS, Android and Kindle Fire!

- **For iOS:** Visit the app store to download the VitalSource Bookshelf: **http://bit.ly/17ib3XS**
- **For Android:** Visit the Google Play Market to download the VitalSource Bookshelf: **http://bit.ly/ZMEGvo**
- **For Kindle Fire, Kindle Fire 2 or Kindle Fire HD:** Simply install the VitalSource Bookshelf onto your Fire (see how at **http://bit.ly/11BVFn9**). You can now sign in with the email address and password you used when you created your VitalSource Bookshelf Account

Full E-Text support for mobile devices is available at: **http://support.vitalsource.com**

CourseSmart

CourseSmart gives you instant access (via computer or mobile device) to this Wiley-Blackwell e-book and its extra electronic functionality, at 40% off the recommended retail print price. See all the benefits at **www.coursesmart.com/students.**

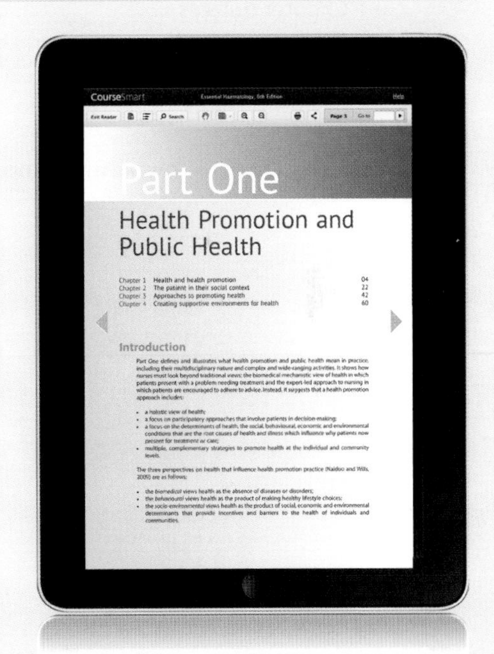

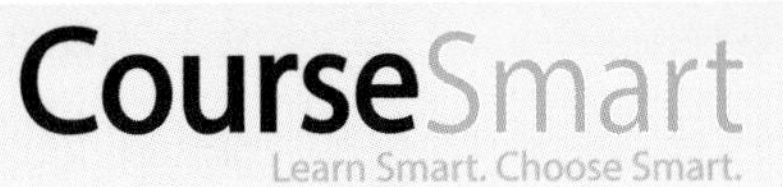

Instructors … receive your own digital desk copies!

CourseSmart also offers instructors an immediate, efficient, and environmentally-friendly way to review this textbook for your course.

For more information visit **www.coursesmart.com/instructors**.

With **CourseSmart**, you can create lecture notes quickly with copy and paste, and share pages and notes with your students. Access your **CourseSmart** digital textbook from your computer or mobile device instantly for evaluation, class preparation, and as a teaching tool in the classroom.

Simply sign in at **http://instructors.coursesmart.com/bookshelf** to download your Bookshelf and get started. To request your desk copy, hit 'Request Online Copy' on your search results or book product page.

We hope you enjoy using your new textbook. Good luck with your studies!

About the companion website

Don't forget to visit the companion website for this book:

www.wileyfundamentalseries.com/healthpromotion 

There you will find valuable material designed to enhance your learning, including:

- Chapter quizzes
- Interactive case-based scenario questions
- Glossary of key terms
- References and further reading

Scan this QR code to visit the companion website:

Part One

Health Promotion and Public Health

Introduction

Part One defines and illustrates what health promotion and public health mean in practice, including their multidisciplinary nature and complex and wide-ranging activities. It shows how nurses must look beyond traditional views: the biomedical mechanistic view of health in which patients present with a problem needing treatment and the expert-led approach to nursing in which patients are encouraged to adhere to advice. Instead, it suggests that a health promotion approach includes:

- a holistic view of health;
- a focus on participatory approaches that involve patients in decision-making;
- a focus on the determinants of health, the social, behavioural, economic and environmental conditions that are the root causes of health and illness which influence why patients now present for treatment or care;
- multiple, complementary strategies to promote health at the individual and community levels.

The three perspectives on health that influence health promotion practice (Naidoo and Wills, 2009) are as follows:

- the *biomedical* views health as the absence of diseases or disorders;
- the *behavioural* views health as the product of making healthy lifestyle choices;
- the *socio-environmental* views health as the product of social, economic and environmental determinants that provide incentives and barriers to the health of individuals and communities.

These perspectives represent three different ways of looking at health and influence the ways in which health issues are defined. They also influence the choice of strategies and actions for addressing health issues. If health is viewed simply as the absence of disease, then health promotion is seen as preventing disease principally through treatment and drug regimes. If health is viewed as the consequence of healthy lifestyles, then health promotion is seen as education, communication of health messages, giving information and facilitating self help and mutual aid programmes. If, on the other hand, health is seen as a consequence of the socio-economic and environmental circumstances in which people live, then health promotion becomes a matter of tackling these issues to make healthy choices easier. The first two perspectives are much in evidence in nursing practice. A socio-economic and environmental perspective is more challenging for a setting which still emphasizes one-to-one care.

Chapter 1 introduces the fundamental features of health promotion and details the broad range of activities that can come under the umbrella of health promotion, and describes the health promotion role of the individual nurse.

Chapter 2 summarizes some of the evidence showing how social factors can affect health. Inequalities in health status exist across geographical areas, social class, ethnicity and gender. People may also not have equal access to health services and often those most in need have least access or the worst services. The delivery of care may be discriminatory, making it harder for individuals because of their language, race, age or disability. Material disadvantage has been shown to be a major factor not only directly in restricting opportunities for a healthy life but also indirectly in educational attainment and employment options. There is also emerging evidence of psychosocial risk factors for poor health especially weak social networks and stress in early life.

Current health policy (DH, 2010) is committed to tackling inequalities in health and a raft of government legislation is designed to: address areas of deprivation, increase the opportunities for disadvantaged and marginalized groups, and take children out of poverty. Public health thus reflects ideological debates about the rights and responsibilities of individuals and the state for the nation's health. Throughout this book we challenge the individualistic model which focuses on the presenting patient's problems alone and encourage the nurse to be aware of significant economic or social circumstances that might make it difficult for individuals, families and communities to adopt or experience healthier lifestyles despite being informed and offered advice. We urge the nurse to avoid victim blaming in which individuals are encouraged to feel responsible and guilty for their own health status. This sort of approach runs the risk of increasing inequalities by which only the most educated, articulate and confident individuals will be able to accept and adopt health messages.

Chapter 3 discusses the various models of health promotion which have attempted to describe approaches to a health issue. Many practitioners do not use theory when planning health promotion and work far more from intuition or existing practice wisdom, which is often rooted in a traditional health education approach. Health promotion models are not, by and large, planning models but attempts to 'scope' the broad field of health promotion. Nevertheless an awareness of health promotion models and models of behaviour change encourages much more rigour in planning, making the practitioner be more explicit about what they are trying to do and articulating those determinants that are thought to influence behavioural or clinical outcomes and which they think can be changed. An effective project or intervention, even if it is simply a one-to-one education session, will benefit from explicitly stated goals, methods and means of evaluation showing how any change following the intervention can be demonstrated.

The task-oriented culture of hospitals and little time for extended patient contact mean health promotion is often a peripheral activity, even though episodes of acute illness or injury can be seen as windows of opportunity for advice and education on disease self-management, rehabilitation and to empower patients to make better use of health services. Chapter 4 discusses how the hospital can be a more health-promoting setting. As the hospital is part of the community, so creating supportive environments for health means integrating the hospital with wider health concerns such as sustainable development and environmental management. Within the hospital itself, promoting health would mean closer relationships of different disciplines such as occupational health, infection control, catering managers and new structures for patient and public involvement. The chapter describes the World Health Organization Health Promoting Hospital movement and its call for hospitals to be at the heart of their communities and part of a seamless service that addresses health services across the whole health and social care continuum. The modern nurse, whatever their context, recognizes that they work in partnership with others in a multi-agency, multi-professional team to improve health and well-being.

Most hospital nurses have close and continuous contact with patients and at a time when they have a heightened awareness of their health. In the past, many nurses would employ a prescriptive approach to their practice, reassuring patients but intent on giving information usually about minor events such as the type of medication or a procedure. In order to be fulfilling their role, many felt they needed to be doing something to patients. Health promotion then was often characterized as "nannying", due to the nurse assuming an expert role and telling patients what to do, ignoring the knowledge and experience that patients may already have about their own condition or lifestyle. Yet many nurses are taught that a basic principle underpinning practice should be to "empower" patients. So what does it mean to foster empowerment? Empowerment in health promotion can be defined as a process through which people gain greater control over decisions and actions affecting their health (Nutbeam, 1998). To do this, the nurse needs to be able to clarify the individual's beliefs and values about health, health risks and health behaviours and help the patient to become aware of the factors that negatively and positively contribute to their health. Activities and interactions are characterized by participation – starting from the patient's health situation, to setting realistic goals and increasing their motivation and confidence, to taking action to improve their health. We see this as a health-promoting way of working. But health promotion is far more than just developed interpersonal or counselling skills of active listening and open questioning.

References

DH (Department of Health) (2010) *Healthy Lives, Healthy People: Our Strategy for Public Health in England.* DH, London.

Naidoo, J. and Wills, J. (2009) *Health Promotion: Foundations for Practice,* 3rd edn. Baillière Tindall, London.

Nutbeam, D. (1998) Health promotion glossary. *Health Promotion International*, **13**, 349–364.

1

Health and health promotion

Jane Wills

Professor of Health Promotion, London South Bank University, London, UK

Linda Jackson

Previously Senior Lecturer, Public Health and Health Promotion, London South Bank University, London, UK

Learning outcomes

By the end of this chapter you will be able to:

1. Define health and well-being
2. Analyse the difference between a medical and social model of health and identify how these apply to nursing practice
3. Define and discuss the concepts of public health and health promotion and how they apply to nursing practice

Introduction

This chapter considers the concepts of health and well-being and why they are central to the practice of all health care professionals. There are many ways that the concept of health can be understood. The traditional medical model, where health is seen as the absence of disease and illness, has led to the perception that health is an individual phenomenon for which each person is responsible. A social model of health focuses on social and political determinants and the

Fundamentals of Health Promotion for Nurses, Second Edition. Edited by Jane Wills.

Companion website: www.wileyfundamentalseries.com/healthpromotion

unequal access that people may have to health. This chapter will look at the definitions for health, holistic health, health promotion, and public health, as well as describing the medical and social models of health. As these are basic and commonly used terms, it is important to clearly define and examine what is meant by them and how they are applied to nursing practice. By exploring these other concepts of health, it will challenge nursing students to consider whether, in addition to the more reactive nursing role of responding to disease and illness, they also will have a proactive role in promoting health.

What is health?

Health can be hard to define, as it is one of those words that can mean many different things to different people. It is often looked at in two main ways:

- a positive or wellness approach, where health is viewed as an asset or the ability to do something, or
- a more negative approach, which focuses on the absence of illness and diseases.

The medical model of health sees health as being about illness and disease and ill health pertains to the individual patient or person. The nurse's role is thus seen as treatment and cure.

Activity 1.1

For me, being healthy means …

Tick whichever apply:

- ❑ Taking regular exercise.
- ❑ Getting enough sleep.
- ❑ Eating fruit and vegetables.
- ❑ Enjoying life.
- ❑ Bouncing back when things are tough.
- ❑ Being safe.
- ❑ Having plenty of friends.
- ❑ Being the right weight for my height.
- ❑ Having a job.
- ❑ Feeling at peace with myself.
- ❑ Not smoking.
- ❑ Not getting sick.
- ❑ Drinking in moderation.
- ❑ Enjoying work and study with not too much stress.

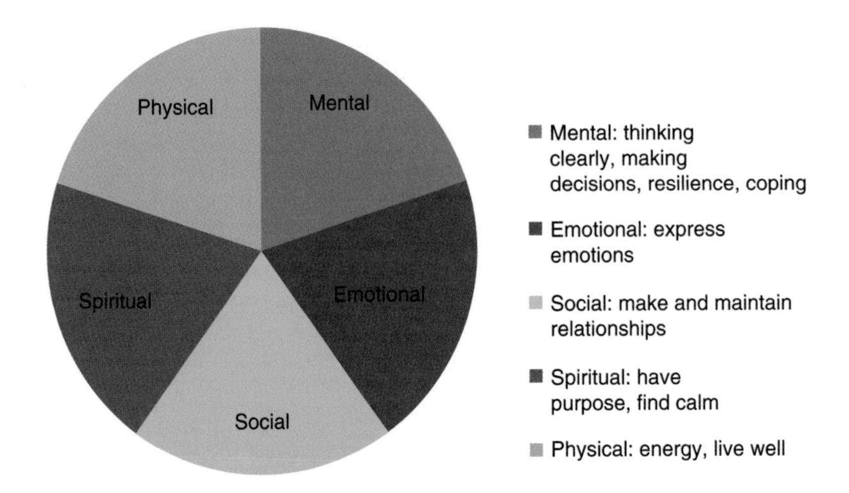

Figure 1.1 The dimensions of health.

Yet people interpret what "being healthy" means in different ways. For many people, it means not being sick or having any diagnosed condition, a view which can be described as a biomedical viewpoint. Others see health as having a lifestyle that contributes to health, such as not drinking too much and not smoking. But health may also be seen positively as a sense of well-being that includes a person's mental health and feeling of control over their life and their social relationships. The World Health Organization (WHO) defined health as a "*state of complete physical, mental and social well-being and not merely the absence of disease or infirmity*" (WHO, 1948). The WHO's definition of health is both holistic and positive and reflects more accurately how ordinary people view their health than the more medical perspective. Health encompasses many aspects, as shown in Figure 1.1.

- *Mental health*: being able to think clearly and adapt to different situations and have a resilience to cope.
- *Emotional health*: being able to recognize, express and manage emotions such as anger and fear
- *Social health*: being able to form and maintain relationships.
- *Physical health*: having energy and vitality and feeling well.
- *Spiritual health*: being able to be at peace with oneself and find calm.

Because health may be viewed differently, nurses need to recognize individual needs and priorities. Younger people, for example, tend to see being healthy as being fit while older people see health as being able to fulfil their daily activities such as getting to the shops.

Activity 1.2

Consider the following case studies – which of these patients would you regard as healthy?

- Mr A is 46 and has been living with HIV for 20 years, has a long-standing relationship and works for a computer company.
- Mrs B is a new widow, aged 80, who has been admitted following a fall.

Discussion

While individuals may regard themselves as healthy even when having a diagnosed condition such as Mr A, health care professionals tend to view health as the absence of disease or illness and that this is essential to fulfil life's functions.The nurse might be looking more at his physical health in terms of his medication and viral load counts. It would be important to first ask the patient how he is coping and what he considers to be the most important aspect of living with his disease as opposed to focusing on monitoring physical signs and symptoms and getting blood work done.

The nurse might take a functional view of Mrs B's health and may focus on her ability to perform selected duties of everyday life, e.g. dressing, cooking, climbing stairs and moving about unaided. Her mental health may or may not be assessed, however, though this may be the most important issue for this woman. Her major concern may be depression, social isolation and anxiety all of which impact on her health and well-being. The health promotion role could involve listening to the patient and trying to identify her needs as she sees them and offering emotional support.

The medical model of health is based on knowledge about the physical and biological causes of disease. It sees health as the absence of disease. It developed with the growth of the medical profession and tends to take a curative approach.

The social model of health focuses on the social distribution of health and illness between different groups (e.g. death rates vary between social classes). The social model is interested in the environmental and social causes of ill health. It tends to take a preventive approach.

Influences on health

A person's health is inextricably linked to everything around that person.

Activity 1.3

Would you describe yourself as healthy?

Write down a list of factors, e.g. personal, medical, external, that you think have a bearing on your health.

____

____

Discussion

Many things affect your health – your family history, where you live, where you work, what you can afford to eat, whether your friends are active, and so on.

Poor health, illness, disease and early death have many causes. Some are genetic, some may be the consequence of age and degeneration and some may be due to people's lifestyle choices but it is also known that some social groups have much higher rates of illness and early death than others. The causes of these inequalities lie in wider structures in society. These factors are termed the social determinants of health and include:

- living conditions;
- employment (or unemployment);
- education;
- housing.

These influences are well illustrated in the model in Figure 1.2 by Barton and Grant (2006), that adapts an earlier model by Dahlgren and Whitehead (1991). It clearly shows the difference between individual and social factors, with an onion likeness, where each layer can be peeled away. The core consists of inherited factors that are fixed. The inner layer suggests that health is partly determined by lifestyle factors such as smoking, physical activity and diet. Moving outwards, Figure 1.2 draws attention to relationships with family, friends and others in the community. The next layer focuses on living and working conditions – housing, transport, workplaces among other factors. The outer layers show the importance of the built, natural and global environment and their impact on health. Chapter 2 discusses how the social context of a patient affects their health.

Many people live with chronic conditions such as diabetes or heart disease (see Chapter 9). The factors that predispose to these conditions are often seen as related to lifestyle choices such as obesity or smoking. The links between a chronic health condition like coronary heart disease and social and environmental factors that impact on the condition may be less recognized.

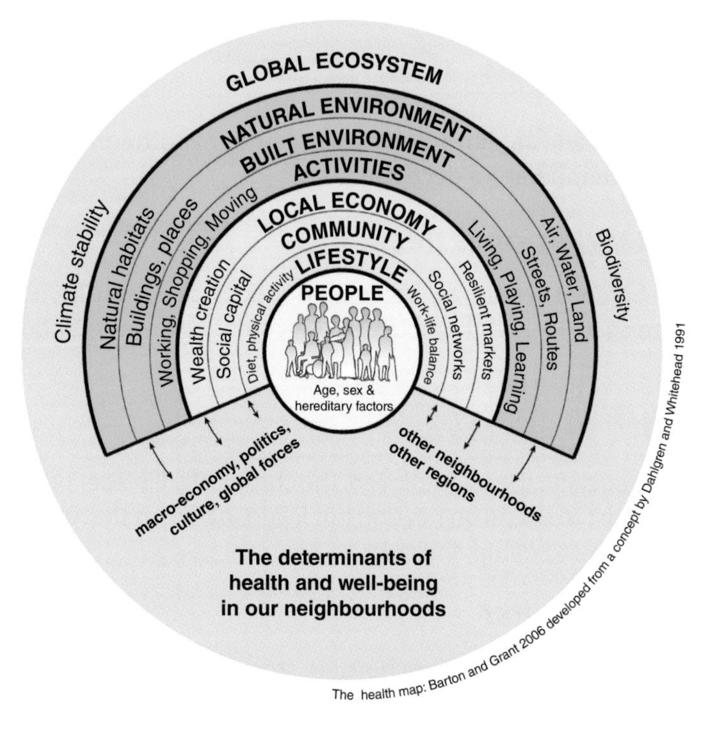

Figure 1.2 The social determinants of health. Source: Barton, H. and Grant, Figure 1.

Evidence 1.1

Housing and coronary heart disease (Hicks and Crowther, 2000)

Why is housing relevant to health?

When room temperatures fall below 12 °C, cardiovascular changes can be seen that increase the risk of myocardial infarction and stroke.

There is excess mortality in Britain in the winter. Approximately 40 000 more people die in Britain in winter than in summer, and most of these are older people. These excess deaths are

(Continued)

Evidence 1.1 *(Continued)*

mostly due to respiratory and cardiovascular diseases, not hypothermia. Therefore, the risk to health increases as the temperature decreases.

What action/intervention is needed?

Standards need to be set so than an acceptable indoor temperature, e.g. 20 °C, can be achieved at no more than 10% of the household income. Any excess should be paid for by social benefits.

Who will benefit?

The poorest people in society: the unemployed, the chronically ill, older people. "Fuel poverty" describes those with least to spend on heating but living in houses that are hard to heat. Many low-cost houses are prone to damp and cold.

What are the key targets?

The indoor temperature of local authority housing stock to be kept to a minimum of 20 °C.

While a medical model of health works towards the absence of disease and is focused on diagnosis and treatment, the social model of health acknowledges the wide range of factors (determinants) that influence health, and focuses on empowering people and communities and influencing policy so that people can have greater control of their health.

What is health promotion?

Much of nursing is about treatment and restoring a patient to health. Sometimes this is referred to as "downstream" actions as they do not address why a person has become ill in the first place. Health promotion is principally about "going upstream" and initiating care to prevent people becoming ill in the first place. Nurses have a key role in minimising the impact of illness, promoting health and function (capabilities), and helping people maintain their roles at home, at work, at leisure and in their communities. Figure 1.3 shows the key areas for nurse involvement in public health and health promotion: promotion of health and health education; protection from harm; and the prevention of ill health underpinned by the assessment of health needs (RCN, 2012).

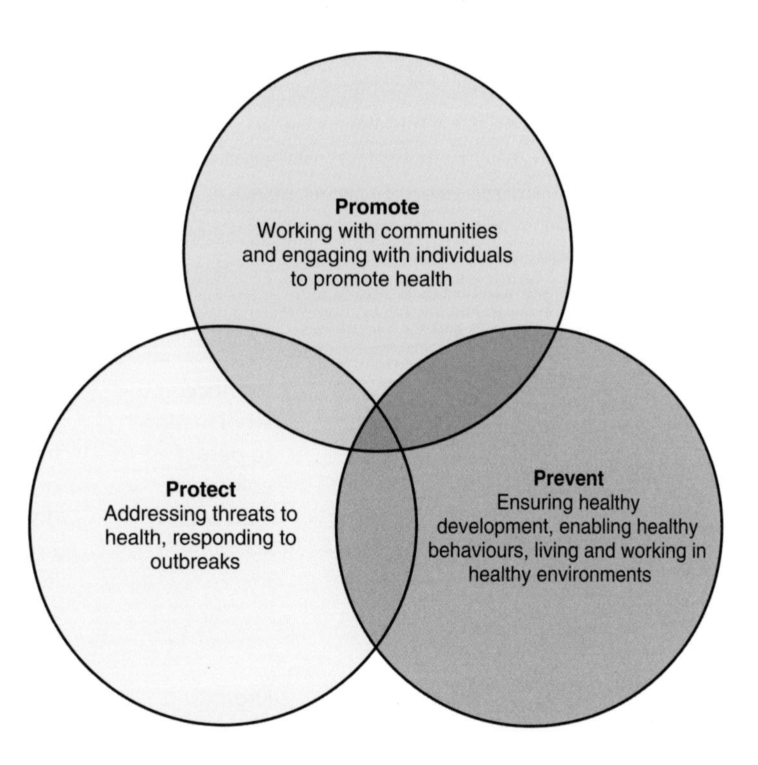

Figure 1.3 A framework for nursing and public health and health promotion. Source: adapted from Royal College of Nursing, 2012, Figure 3, p. 14. Reproduced under the Open Government Licence.

Part of the nursing role is to promote the health of patients and clients. This can take place at three different levels: primary, secondary or tertiary prevention:

- *Primary prevention* seeks to prevent the onset of specific diseases via risk reduction: by altering behaviours or exposure that can lead to disease through education or protection. For example, respiratory disease might be reduced through smoking cessation and through state actions to restrict smoking in public places.
- *Secondary prevention* includes procedures that detect and treat pre-clinical pathological changes and thereby control disease progression. Screening procedures (such as mammography to detect early stage breast cancer) or routine blood sugar testing for people over 45 can lead to early interventions.
- *Tertiary prevention* seeks to reduce the disability or complications arising from a condition and improve a patient's function, longevity, and quality of life. Cardiac rehabilitation following a myocardial infarction can seek to alter behaviours to reduce the likelihood of a re-infarction by encouraging a patient to lose weight.

Activity 1.4

Table 1.1 shows the levels of prevention applied to bowel cancer. Fill in the same table to show the activities at each level relevant to coronary heart disease.

Table 1.1 Levels of prevention.

Disease	Intervention level	Primary prevention	Secondary	Tertiary
Colorectal cancer	Individual	Health education advice on healthy diet, smoking cessation and alcohol reduction	Hemoccult stool testing to detect colorectal cancer early	Follow-up exams to identify recurrence or metastatic disease: physical examination, liver enzyme tests, chest X-rays, etc.
	Population	Publicity campaigns alerting the public to the early warning signs; health education promoting high fibre diets, exercise and non-smoking; subsidies to help people access exercise programmes	Organised screening prorgramme: Making testing easier by the provision of home screening kits for those over 60	Implementation of health services organisational models that improve access to high-quality care

A very broad range of activities can thus be considered health promotion. It is a broad term that can be visualized like an umbrella that has under its cover:

- Education and marketing.
- Social, environmental, political and economic actions to improve and promote health.
- Protection actions that control risks to population health.

Often the word "promotion", when used in the context of health promotion is associated with the idea of media and even propaganda. This is a misunderstanding of the term. Promotion, in this context, is about improving health at all levels from individuals to society to worldwide policy and supporting and encouraging it to be higher on personal and public agendas.

A landmark international WHO conference on health promotion was held in Ottawa, in Canada, in 1986 and it published the key document, the *Ottawa Charter for Health Promotion*, which continues to guide health promotion practice today. The following WHO (1986) definition was part of that document and combines these two elements of improving health and having more control over it: "*Health promotion is the process of enabling people to increase control over and to improve their health (including the determinants of health).*" The Ottawa Charter provides five action areas that are central to the conceptual framework of health promotion:

1. Build healthy public policy.
2. Create supportive environments.
3. Develop personal skills.
4. Reorient health services.
5. Strengthen community action (WHO, 1986; Nutbeam, 1998).

These five areas suggest that for the health of the population to be improved, it is important not only to help individuals to lead healthier lives but also make it easier for them to do so, e.g. encouraging healthy workplaces and supporting a physical environment that is more conducive to health with "green" public transport and locally grown fresh food.

Activity 1.5

Examples of the action areas identified in the Ottawa Charter are listed in Table 1.2. Can you think of any others?

Table 1.2 Action areas of the Ottawa Charter.

Ottawa Charter action areas	Examples of interventions
Build healthy public policy	• No smoking policy in public buildings including all NHS buildings • Breastfeeding policy in hospitals • Motorcycle helmet laws • Drink driving policies and laws
Create supportive environments	• Healthy food choices for staff in workplaces (including hospital canteens) • Healthy school meals for children • Easy access to condoms (including reasonable prices) • Safe and well-lit play and walking areas
Develop personal skills	• Smoking cessation skills • Information on health issues • Food product label reading • Parenting skills

(*Continued*)

Table 1.2 (*Continued*)

Ottawa Charter action areas	Examples of interventions
Reorient health services	• Blood pressure screening at chemists • Breastfeeding support services in the community • Immunization clinics at neighbourhood clinics or surgeries • Chlamydia screening on mobile buses in areas where young people can access them
Strengthen community action	• Housing estate action group to clean up and increase safety in children's play area • Community Drug Action Teams including schools, parents, churches and shop owners • Anti-graffiti action groups in neighbourhoods

Source: Adapted from WHO (1986).

The health promotion role of most nurses will be to:

- provide health information and advice about healthy lifestyles;
- promote every encounter between a nurse and a patient or client as a health promotion encounter;
- develop personal skills for their clients and patients that are empowering and enable people to feel more confident and competent in managing their health;
- enable access and use of the health care system;
- encourage social change and addressing inequalities.

Scenario 1.1

Patient on ward following an intra-cerebral haemorrhage

Mr C is 58 and has been transferred to a rehabilitation unit following a stroke which has caused right-sided weakness. Mr C can walk a few steps with sticks and can transfer from the bed to the chair with assistance. He has no swallowing problems though his appetite is poor. He is uncommunicative and repeats certain phrases such as "What's the time?"

- ❑ What would be the likely health needs of the patient?
- ❑ What is the health promotion role of the nurse?

Discussion

Patient priorities are likely to be to resume daily activities and be able to go home quickly. The nurse's health promotion role would include:

- *listening to the patient's and family's concerns and identifying needs in his daily activities such as returning to work and driving;*
- *involving the patient/client in their health care plan, including, e.g. how to use a dosset box so he can remember to take his medication;*
- *offering a short focused intervention to Mr C and his family and skills to decrease risk factors on safe drinking levels and the importance of weight control;*
- *providing information to Mr C and his family about support organizations such as the Stroke Association and its health promotion material;*
- *awareness of patient's living situation when returning home (e.g. cooking facilities, transport, support in the home, as well as hobbies and social life);*
- *benefits advice;*
- *referral information to community programmes on patient's needs (e.g. smoking, walking, cooking, hobby groups that may aid communication).*

Health promotion and public health

The term health promotion is not always used in the UK and instead, public health is often used to describe this aspect of the nurse's role. Traditionally, the term public health meant efforts to improve the health of communities by providing protection from environmental hazards and responding to the health needs. Its broadest definition is *"the science and art of preventing disease, prolonging life and promoting health through organised efforts of society"* (Acheson, 1988). However, most policy discourse refers to nurses delivering public health and health promotion is one aspect of this, e.g. *"Nurses delivering public health are working to create the opportunities for people to live positive healthy lives, by influencing public policy and by health promotion"* (RCN, 2007). Confusingly, the term "health improvement" may also be used to describe health promotion activities, as seen in Table 1.3 which illustrates the Public Health Outcomes Framework and the actions expected at national, local and community levels.

Table 1.3 Public Health Outcomes Framework.

Domain 1 Health Protection and resilience	Domain 2 Tackling the wider determinants of health	Domain 3 Health improvement	Domain 4 Prevention of ill health	Domain 5 Healthy life expectancy and preventable mortality
Protecting the population from major emergencies and remaining resilient to harm	Tackling factors which affect well-being and health inequalities	Helping people to live healthy lifestyles, make healthy choices	Reducing the number of people living with preventable ill health	Preventing people from dying prematurely

Health promotion and nursing practice

Health promotion is increasingly important to nursing practice. It enhances the way in which health care and services are viewed, looking beyond the medical model to consider the broader influences on health. It can be seen from previous discussions in this chapter that health promotion shares many of the characteristics of good nursing practice:

- It is patient-centred, in that it is based on an assessment of the patient's individual needs and valuing the patient's own views.
- It includes spending time listening to and talking to the patient to identify their individual needs and using high-level communication skills and methods.
- It seeks to involve patients in their own health care decisions.

Table 1.4 illustrates some of the shared principles of nursing and health promotion.

New nurses are expected to do the following:

- Be able to identify patients' needs for health-promoting activity and include health promotion in a care plan.
- Be able to select an appropriate range of health promotion materials relevant to patients' care need.
- Be able to take account of patients' capacity, expressed preferences and social and cultural context.

Generally, nurses are enthusiastic about health promotion and are certain that they have a role to play. However, that role is not as well defined or as clear as may be presented in descriptions of the role. Although health promotion is being taught in the nursing curriculum, it has tended to focus on communication and therefore health education along with the principles of health promotion practice: empowerment, equity, collaboration, participation. Yet many studies of nurses and health promotion report that they felt health promotion was part of their work but they were unsure how to do it, e.g. (Cross, 2005). Many student nurses report a gap between what is taught as health promotion and what is "seen" and observed in practice. These included a lack of time that reduces health promotion activity to simple information-giving, and a predominantly behavioural and disease-focused view of the determinants of health that means practice is focused on the sick individual. For many nurses, health promotion work might be short-term or individually driven. This will be particularly true for hospital nurses. Community nurses may have more opportunities for family and community intervention.

Table 1.4 Nursing and health promotion.

Nursing principle	Example of how health promotion practice (HPP) may complement or evidence the principle
Dignity and humanity	HPP involves valuing the person, offering hope for health improvement, investing time and energy in meeting health promotion needs in a sensitive, non-judgmental and respectful manner.
Taking responsibility for care	HPP involves working in partnership with the patient to ensure that health promotion is embedded and relates to all nursing practice, e.g. health promotion is recognized as an essential need in the current episode of care rather than seeing it as an activity that happens after the patient has been discharged.
Managing risk	HPP understands that a range of factors can increase and predispose to health risks. Health promotion takes a promotional approach and seeks to reduce risk or prevent illness occurring.
Patient-centred care	HPP also puts patients at the centre of care and nurses work in partnership to ensure that the interventions employed are understood, chosen and tailored to meet individual needs.
Communication	HPP requires sensitive communication, particularly if it relates to making changes that can be anxiety-provoking or is trying to motivate a patient to change. In addition, health promotion uses a range of communication approaches (e.g. written, verbal, role modelling) to convey and communicate interventions.
Up-to-date knowledge and skills	HPP recognizes and requires nurses to keep abreast of evidence-based interventions that are proven to be effective. In addition, HPP requires nurses to update their knowledge to ensure that their practices are current.
Co-ordinated care	HPP requires co-ordination among health and social care professionals as health is influenced by many factors not just NHS services.
Leadership	HPP requires nurses to demonstrate leadership skills, to be visionary and to ensure that health promotion is a demonstrable part of practice. In doing so, leading by example is key; this may include appropriate self-disclosure or role modelling.

On placement: checklist

- ❑ Are all dimensions of health considered in care plans?
- ❑ Are health promotion materials available for patients and families? Are these kept up to date?
- ❑ Is health promotion included in care plans? What is included?
- ❑ Is information personalized?
- ❑ Is information on patients' social circumstances recorded or known, e.g. who they live with, education levels, socio-economic status?
- ❑ Is health behaviour information recorded, e.g. smoking status including ever smoked, alcohol consumption including drinking behaviour, BMI, physical activity?

Key learning points

1. Health is not just the absence of disease but includes social, emotional, psychological, and spiritual elements.
2. Promoting health is about activities that enable a person to live well, even with a diagnosed condition.
3. Promoting health is also about a way of working that is empowering and participatory. It is not about persuasion or coercion to get people to adopt particular health behaviours.
4. Public health usually means actions to protect from disease and knowledge work to identify where and how resources should be used to best meet needs.
5. Health promotion includes many different activities at different levels of intervention: individuals, families and communities and populations. It is sometimes called health improvement.

Chapter summary

This chapter has discussed the concept of health and why it is central to the practice of all health care professionals. There are many ways that the concept of health can be understood. Students were encouraged to look beyond the traditional medical model of health to a social model of health. In the medical model, health is seen as the absence of disease and illness, which has led to the perception that health is an individual phenomenon where each person is responsible solely for their health. A social model of health focuses on social and political determinants and the unequal access that people may have to health. It looks at social interactions, socio-economic factors and their interaction with people's lives. This relates to nursing practice in encouraging nurses to look beyond the disease or illness that a patient may present with to the causes of that disease or illness and to include the patient in the treatment process.

The terms health education and health promotion are often thought to mean the same thing, however, they are not. Education is one of the means of improving health and is often the main one that is used by health professionals. Health education is concerned with communicating information and with building the motivation, skills and confidence necessary to take action to improve health. However, health promotion is about improving the health status of individuals and communities. It is a broader term that can be visualized like an umbrella that has under its cover, education, as well as social, environmental, political and economic components to improve and promote health. Health promotion is about improving health at all levels, from individuals to society to worldwide policy and supporting and encouraging it to be higher on personal and public agendas.

Nurses are encouraged to have a wider health promotion role. This might mean going beyond health education and helping clients: to access and use the health care system; to assess their own risks to health and decision-making about their health lifestyle; and to understand the economic, social and environmental influences on their health.

Further reading and resources

Department of Health (2004) *Choosing Health: Making Healthy Choices Easier*. TSO, London.
This White Paper sets out the key principles for supporting the public to make healthier and more informed choices in regards to health. It is followed by delivery and action plans which can be found on the same website. Available at:
http://webarchive.nationalarchives.gov.uk/+/dh.gov.uk/en/publicationsandstatistics/publications/publicationspolicyandguidance/dh_4094550.

Department of Health (2011) *Healthy Lives, Healthy People: Our Strategy for Public Health in England*. TSO, London.
This White Paper sets out a new structure for public health in England and identifies priorities through the life course. Available at:
https://www.gov.uk/government/uploads/system/uploads/attachment_data/file/216096/dh_127424.pdf.

Naidoo, J. and Wills, J. (2009) *Health Promotion: Foundations for Practice*, 3rd edn. Ballière Tindall, London.
This wide-ranging text provides a comprehensive and critical framework for promoting health. There are in-depth discussions, reflection points and case studies. It is reader-centred and an excellent resource for anyone interested in this field.

Scriven, A., Ewles, L. and Simnett, I. (2010) *Promoting Health: A Practical Guide*, 6th edn. Baillière Tindall, London.
This text is a popular basic text on health promotion and provides comprehensive and readable information on the theory and practice of health promotion. It includes questionnaires, practical exercises and case studies.

World Health Organization (WHO) (1986) *Ottawa Charter for Health Promotion*. WHO, Geneva.
The first International Conference on Health Promotion met in Ottawa, Canada, on the 21st day of November 1986 and developed this Charter for action to achieve Health for All by the year 2000 and beyond. This conference was primarily a response to growing expectations for a new public health movement around the world. Discussions focused on the needs in industrialised countries, but took into account

similar concerns in all other regions. It built on the progress made through the Declaration on Primary Health Care at Alma-Ata, the World Health Organization's Targets for Health for All document, and the recent debate at the World Health Assembly on intersectoral action for health. The Charter is still widely used today as framework for action in health promotion. See http://www.who.int/healthpromotion/conferences/previous/ottawa/en/.

References

Acheson, D. (1988) *Public Health in England: Report of the Committee of Inquiry into the Future of the Public Health Function*, Cm 289. HMSO, London.

Barton, H. and Grant, M. (2006) A health map for the local human habitat. *The Journal for the Royal Society for the Promotion of Health*, **126** (6), 252–253.

Cross, R. (2005) Accident and Emergency nurses' attitudes towards health promotion. *Journal of Advanced Nursing*, **51** (5), 474–483.

Dahlgren, G. and Whitehead, M. (1991a) *Policies and Strategies to Promote Social Equity in Health*. Institute for Future Studies, Stockholm.

Dahlgren, G. and Whitehead, M. (1991b) "The main determinants of health" model, version accessible, in *European Strategies for Tackling Social Inequities in Health: Levelling Up Part 2* (eds G. Dahlgren and M. Whitehead, 2007), WHO Regional Office for Europe, Copenhagen. Available at: http://www.euro.who.int/_data/assets/pdf_file/0018/103824/E89384.pdf.

Department of Health (2012) *The Public Health Outcomes Framework for England, 2012–2016*. The Department of Health, London.

Hicks, N.R. and Crowther, R. (2000) Coronary heart disease: a practical tool and structured approach to developing and implementing a HimP, in *Health Improvement Programmes* (eds S. Rawaf and P. Orton), Royal Society of Medicine, London.

Nutbeam, D. (1998) Health promotion glossary, *Health Promotion International*, **13**, 349–364.

RCN (Royal College of Nursing) (2007) *Nurses as Partners in Delivering Public Health*. RCN, London. Available at: http://www.rcn.org.uk/_data/assets/pdf_file/0011/78734/003114.pdf.

RCN (Royal College of Nursing) (2012) *Going Upstream: Nursing's Contribution to Public Health. RCN Guidance for Nurses*, RCN, London. Available at: http://www.rcn.org.uk/_data/assets/pdf_file/0007/433699/004203.pdf.

World Health Organization (1948) *Constitution*. WHO, Geneva.

World Health Organization (1986) *Ottawa Charter for Health Promotion*. WHO, Geneva.

Don't forget to visit the companion website for this book: www.wileyfundamentalseries.com/healthpromotion where you can find self-assessment tests to check your progress.

2

The patient in their social context

Jenny Husbands

Senior Lecturer, Adult Nursing, London South Bank University, London, UK

Jane Wills

Professor of Health Promotion, London South Bank University, London, UK

Learning outcomes

By the end of this chapter you will be able to:

1. Describe major social, economic and environmental influences on health;
2. Define health inequalities
3. Understand the challenges of addressing health inequalities
4. Describe the role of the nurse in tackling health inequalities

Introduction

Health and disease are determined by factors in the wider socio-economic and physical environment. Low income and inadequate housing, for example, may limit people's ability to take control or have any power to alter the conditions affecting their health. Understanding those factors that impact on a patient's health and their capacity to develop and maintain good health is a vital aspect of the nurse's role. The WHO Health Report each year, the health profiles

Fundamentals of Health Promotion for Nurses, Second Edition. Edited by Jane Wills.

Companion website: www.wileyfundamentalseries.com/healthpromotion

produced by the Public Health Observatories and the data produced by the Office of National Statistics (ONS) all provide a picture of the current health of populations locally, nationally and globally. Yet all these reports show that health and life chances vary.

Although health status is improving in the UK, with people living longer and early mortality from many diseases declining, these improvements have benefited those who are more affluent in society. At both the community and individual level, poor health is linked to social and economic disadvantage and deprivation. Differences in income, employment, education, housing, social environment and access to services all produce inequalities in health outcomes. Living in areas of low income, poor employment and poor infrastructure increase the risk of ill health above and beyond factors on an individual level. Health inequalities and the differences between population groups have received considerable interest from governments. This chapter will discuss the nature of health inequalities and the various explanations for their existence.

Inequalities in health

A health inequality is a term that describes an unjust disparity in health outcomes between individuals or groups. This may arise from differences in socio-economic status that may influence behaviour or lifestyle choices or access to resources, geographical area, ethnicity, age or gender, health status and access to and use of health services. Inequalities are not inevitable and so are deemed unfair.

There are three types of health inequalities:

1. inequalities in the determinants of health, e.g. education, employment and housing can all have an influence on health status;
2. inequalities in health outcomes, e.g. there is a six-year difference in life expectancy at birth across boroughs in London;
3. inequality of access to health care, e.g. refugees or homeless people often have difficulty in obtaining access to primary health care services, such as registering with a general practitioner (GP).

Figure 2.1 shows the many dimensions in which inequalities in health may be found. The social determinants of health are the collective set of conditions in which people are born, grow up, live and work. These layers of influence include individual lifestyles but also social support, working conditions, education, housing and the physical environment. These conditions are shaped by a powerful over-riding set of forces: economics, social policies and politics.

It is now widely accepted that these social determinants are responsible for significant levels of unfair health "inequities". So while some health inequalities are the result of natural biological differences or free choice, others are beyond the control of individuals or groups and could be avoided.

A wealth of research has shown the relationship between socio-economic status and health status in most Western countries. People from lower socio-economic groups have much poorer health than those in other groups. This is evident in relation to disease prevalence, life expectancy and infant mortality.

Figure 2.2 shows the step-wise increase in poor health. There is a social gradient in health whereby the most poor have the worst health. Across all countries, in general, the lower an individual's socio-economic position, the worse their health, and a social gradient in health runs

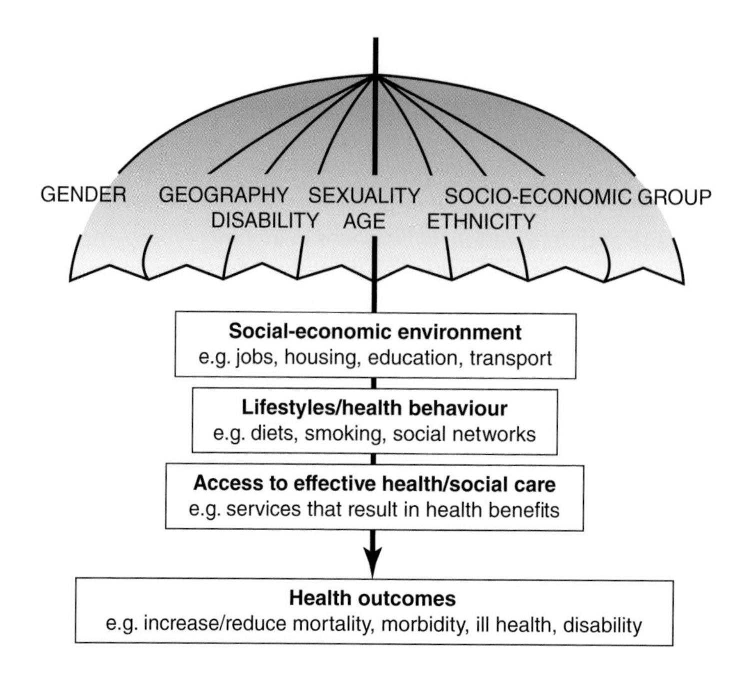

Figure 2.1 Dimensions of health inequalities. Source: London Health Observatory, Public Health England website, Figure 2. Reproduced under the Open Government Licence.

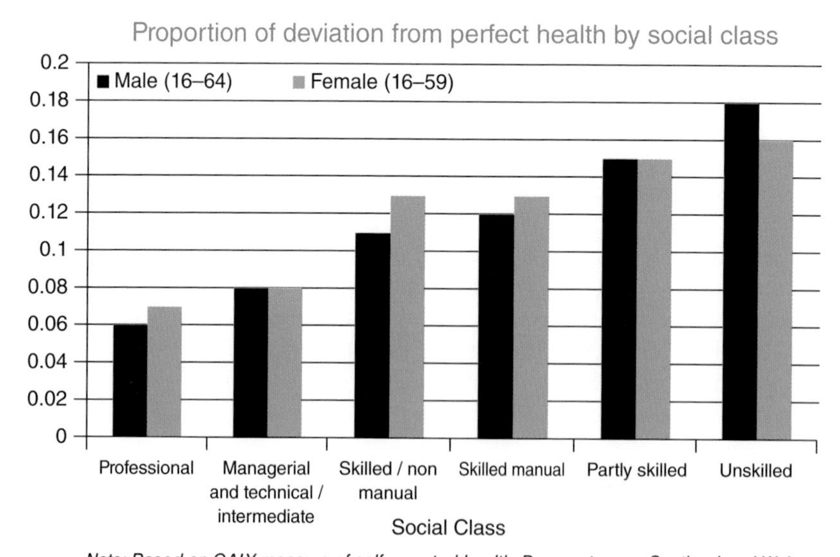

Figure 2.2 Proportion of deviation from perfect health by social class. Source: Department of Health, 2008, Figure 2.7, p. 36. Reproduced under the Open Government Licence.

Table 2.1 Examples of health inequalities.

Coronary heart disease	The death rate from CHD is three times higher among unskilled manual men of working age than among professional men
Obesity	28% of women in social class V (unskilled) are obese, compared to 14% in social class I (professional)
Accidents	Manual workers make up 42% of the workforce but account for 72% of reportable work-related injuries
	Children in social class V are five times more likely to suffer accidental death than children in social class I
Residential fire deaths	Residential fire deaths are 15 times more common for children in social class V compared to children in social class I
Mental health	Unskilled working men are almost four times more likely to commit suicide than their professional counterparts. Suicide rates in semi-skilled and manual unskilled workers are twice as high as the professional group

from top to bottom of the socio-economic spectrum. The EQ-5D QALY measure in Figure 2.2 is based on how people describe their health in surveys. It has a scale in which 1 represents perfect health, and 0 represents death. The scale shows the amount of deviation from 1 (health), and long-term illness or disability typically leads to a deviation from a QALY of 1.0 of between 0.2–0.4.

Table 2.1 illustrates how belonging to a lower socio-economic group may influence the health status of the individual. Major causes of death and illness in the UK – cancer, coronary heart disease (CHD), stroke, diabetes, accidents and deaths by suicide – are closely linked to socio-economic status and people's access to and the availability of health service provision. For example, there is an inverse correlation between socio-economic status and cancer incidence and mortality (particularly related to the impact of tobacco consumption), but there is also a socio-economic gradient at each stage of the patient pathway from knowledge of all the major risk factors relating to cancer to early presentation and diagnosis (Cancer Research UK, 2006).

As shown in Table 2.2, there are also inequalities that relate to the determinants of health. For example, poor housing is associated with a number of mortality and morbidity indicators: children living in cold homes are more than twice as likely to suffer from a variety of respiratory problems than children living in warm homes and 1 in 4 adolescents living in cold homes is at risk of multiple mental health problems compared to 1 in 20 living in warm homes (Shelter, 2006).

Unemployed individuals and individuals with low income and poor educational qualifications use services less relative to need than their employed, more affluent or better-educated counterparts. This may be due to difficulties with transport and lack of car ownership, ability to take time off to attend appointments, less developed communication skills and inability to navigate the system.

There are also inequalities in the health experienced by Black and minority ethnic groups. For example, Black British people are 30% more likely to rate their health as fair, poor or very poor.

Table 2.2 The impact of social factors on health.

London Health Strategy – high level indicators	Relevance to health inequalities
1. Unemployment	Associated with morbidity, injuries, poisoning and premature mortality, especially coronary heart disease. Also related to depression, anxiety, self-harm and suicide.
2. Unemployment among Black and Minority Ethnic (BME) population	As above
3. Educational attainment*	Education reduces risk of unemployment and poverty which have a negative effect on health
4. Proportion of homes judged to be unfit to live in	Can cause or contribute to ill health or injury and exacerbate existing conditions, e.g. through damp, cold, poor design or bad lighting
5. Burglary rate per 1000 population	The factors that affect the local crime rate also seem to affect health. Crime can also affect health indirectly through feeling unsafe
6. Air quality indicators – NO_2 and PM_{10}	Polluted air can damage health. The young, the elderly and those with respiratory difficulties are particularly vulnerable
7. Road traffic casualty rate per 1,000 population	Road traffic accidents are a major avoidable hazard to health, and there are large social class differences
8. Life expectancy at birth	A good summary indicator of the health status of the population
9. Infant mortality rate	The infant mortality rate is influenced by maternal health, social class and quality of care
10. Proportion of people with self-assessed good health	A good indicator of health status in adults

Note: *The percentage of pupils achieving five General Certificate of Secondary Education (GCSE) grades A*–C.
Source: Greater London Authority (2005), Table 1, p. 3. Reproduced with permission from the London Health Commission.

Pakistani and Bangladeshi people have the worst health of all the ethnic groups. South Asian people who live in the UK are up to six times more likely to have diabetes than the white population. The premature mortality rate for stroke in England is higher for those born outside the UK than for those born within, and people from South Asia are approximately 50% more likely to die prematurely from coronary heart disease (CHD) than the general population (see Figure 2.3). Furthermore, stroke mortality rates are falling more slowly in minority ethnic groups than in the rest of the population, thus widening inequality.

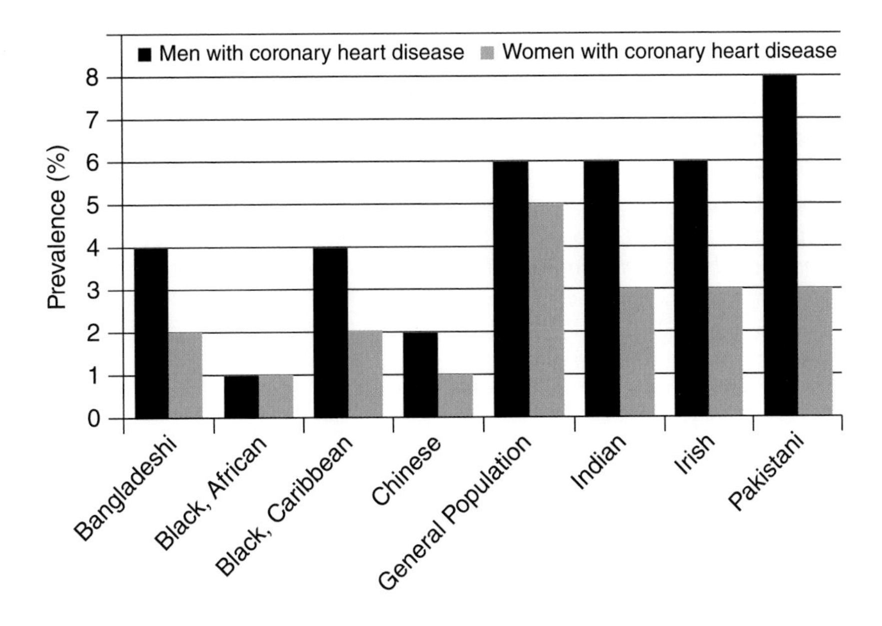

Figure 2.3 Prevalence of coronary heart disease in men and women by ethnic group in England. Source data: NHS Health and Social Care Information Centre, Public Health Statistics, 2005.

One major access barrier to health care for first-generation migrants is language difference. For some groups, cultural differences in the perception of ill health and lack of knowledge about the availability and range of health services can inhibit or delay their access to care until conditions become more serious. There is some evidence of this in relation to CHD in South Asian groups. "Cultural competence" is the term used to describe services perceived by Black and minority ethnic users as being in harmony with their cultural and religious beliefs. As a result, cultural competence training in nursing is becoming widespread.

Activity 2.1

Socio-economic status

- Why is it important for a nurse to know the socio-economic status of their patient?
- What information needs to be collected to determine the social conditions in which your patients live?

Discussion

Nurses need to be aware of the type of housing and the environment their patients live in, their means of social support, their income, employment status and their access to healthy, affordable food and leisure activities. This information will enable the nurse to plan care to meet the needs of their patients and address gaps in service provision. Information about a patient's social situation will enable the nurse not only to address their medical needs.

The RCN (2012, p. 7) states:

> *Nurses reach deep into the heart of families and communities. They are confronted daily with the consequences of social conditions on the health and well-being of the communities they are caring for … Because nurses witness the impact of social determinants on the health of both patients they are providing care to and the wider population, they have a clear stake in the direct and underlying causes of bad health. Nurses recognise that until the root causes of illness and poor health behaviours are tackled, the NHS will constantly be required to deal with the consequences.*

Explaining health inequalities

There have been many attempts to explain why ill health is socially patterned and there is no single answer. It is often claimed that people on low incomes are more likely to lead unhealthy lifestyles which results in poorer health status but there are many other explanations.

The life course explanation

This explanation for health inequalities suggests that there are cumulative effects over the life course of an individual of material and psychosocial hazards and that these effects explain observed differences in health and life expectancy. According to Kawachi *et al.* (2000), life course explanations are believed to have three pathways that are relevant to health status:

1. The underlying effect of the early life environment affects the health of the adult, irrespective of other health behaviour or influences on health. If, for example, the mother smoked during her pregnancy, or was exposed to passive smoking during her pregnancy, this may have a detrimental effect on the health of the foetus in utero. Foetal origins theories suggest that low birth-weight has been shown to be associated with health outcomes 50 years later in respect of CHD, stroke and respiratory disease mortality.
2. The early life environment of the individual will shape the individual's life course and in turn will affect their health status over time. A less advantaged family background is linked to worse education results, worse housing, job insecurity or unemployment and low work autonomy. Pre-school education programmes have been shown to be related to later health through educational achievement, adult income and home ownership.
3. The cumulative effects of being exposed to a health-damaging environment, as well as the intensity and duration of that exposure can adversely affect the health status of the individual. For example, if the adult had been exposed over the course of their lifetime to a hazardous or unhealthy environment, it could increase their likelihood of dying from cancer, CHD, strokes or respiratory illness.

Some conditions such as strokes, asthma and cancer of the stomach may be determined by early childhood circumstances, whereas conditions such as deaths from lung cancer, accidents and violent attacks are more likely to be determined by the life course of the adult. The 1958 birth cohort study provides information on a sample of individuals as they grow older. Analysis of the data reveals childhood factors such as low birth-weight and height are linked to socio-economic circumstances. Childhood is also important in determining the later health status of the individual, as this is a period of dynamic global development, i.e. physical, social, intellectual and psychological. Therefore, the individual will be more sensitive to environmental influences on health (Graham and Power, 2004).

Activity 2.2

Think of a patient that you have provided care for who has a long-term health condition, e.g. diabetes, hypertension or a stroke.

- Reflecting on their medical history, what life events or circumstances do you think may have contributed to their current health status?
- What actions could have been taken during their childhood to prevent their poor health status in adulthood?

Disscussion

The Marmot Review, Fair Society, Healthy Lives (Marmot, 2010) adopts a life course approach as depicted in Figure 2.4. The framework proposed by this review shows that influences accumulate across our lives. Some may be protective, e.g. breastfeeding to improve a baby's immune system or a supportive environment in early childhood to increase self-esteem and resilience. Some, on the other hand, may present a risk, e.g. low educational attainment limiting our ability to earn a living wage or smoking. Where risk outweighs protective factors, chronic disease, disability and mortality begin manifesting from around age 50.

The materialist/structural explanation

The materialist/structural explanation for health inequalities suggests that the health of the individual is determined by socio-economic and structural factors that contribute to the levels of poverty and deprivation experienced by the individual. Put simply, it is the situation in which the individual lives that will determine their health. Those who are materially deprived are more likely to be exposed to poor housing conditions, environmental and work hazards, accidents at home, at work and on the road and find it difficult to sustain a healthy life.

In order to understand the relationship between socio-economic status and health, we need to understand definitions of poverty, the scale of poverty, and how poverty affects health. Poverty can be defined as absolute poverty or relative poverty. Absolute poverty, for example, would be the inability to meet basic human needs such as access to food, shelter, warmth and safety. Relative poverty is determined by the standards of the rest of the society in which the individual lives. Although a person's basic needs may be met, they may be unable to afford any social participation. This inability to participate in the activities that enhance health such as

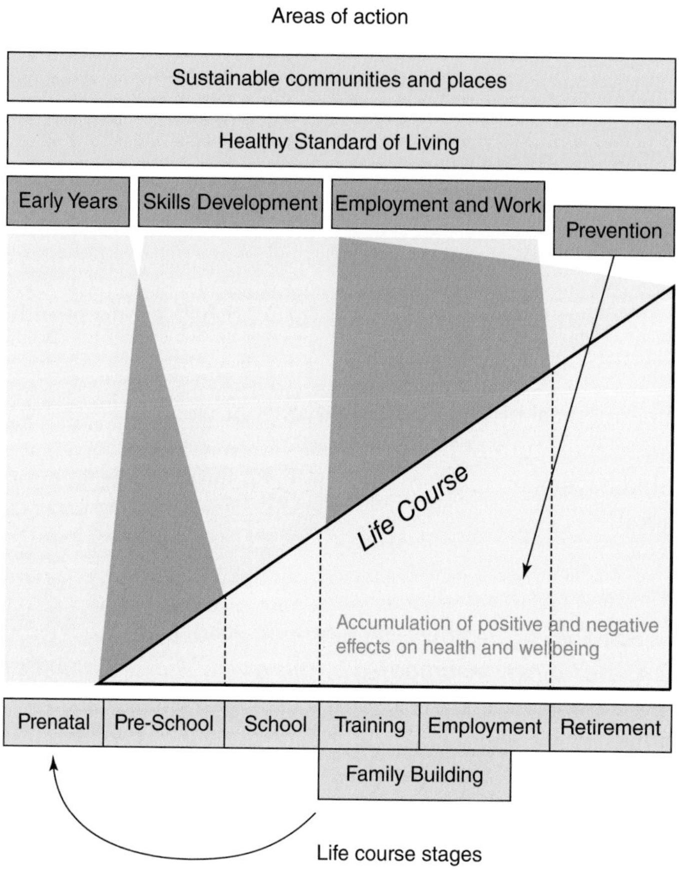

Areas of action
Sustainable communities and places
Healthy Standard of Living
Early Years
Skills Development
Employment and Work
Prevention
Life Course
Accumulation of positive and negative effects on health and wellbeing
Prenatal
Pre-School
School
Training
Employment
Retirement
Family Building
Life course stages

Figure 2.4 Life course model. Source: Marmot Review, 2008, Figure 5, p. 20. Reproduced with permission from the UCL Institute for Equity.

community activities or social events is called social exclusion and has been used to describe those excluded from typically normal society. If people are socially excluded for any length of time, they are more likely to suffer from a range of physical health problems, e.g. such as CHD, as well as social and emotional health stress and depression, marital breakdown and addiction to drugs and alcohol (WHO, 2003).

The individual's ability to socially engage with others and to make healthy choices will be determined by many factors, including their disposable income. A study by Morris *et al.* (2007) established that the minimum wage would not facilitate the ability to make healthy choices or socially engage with others.

Case study 2.1

Minimum income for healthy living in later life

A study on minimum income for older people (Morris *et al.*, 2007) found that people over 65 are not spending enough money each week on food and have worryingly low levels of exercise. Pensioner poverty is leaving people at risk of falls, heart disease and is destroying their independence. Only 17% of people over 60 said they keep fit and 1 in 5 people aged 65 and over cannot walk 200 metres without discomfort or stopping. Up to 30% of 65–74-year-old men and women are obese. The study calculated the weekly cost of meeting a healthy diet is £32.20 a week and £63.70 for a couple – around 30% more than older people on a low income actually spend. The costs associated with physical exercise are modest: assessed as £2.10 for a single person and £4.10 for a couple – the main elements being the cost of group exercise sessions or solo swimming. Other components needed for healthy living include: a warm safe home, a good social life, interesting activities, an opportunity to play a valued role in the community, and access to health services.

The minimum income needed for healthy living (excluding rent, council tax and mortgage payments) was estimated as £122.70 a week for a single person and £192.60 for a couple. Pension credit guarantee provides people aged 60 and over with a minimum income of £109.45 a week for a single person and £167.05 for a couple and in addition there are entitlements to other payments such as winter fuel payments. However, the government estimates that 1 in 5 people entitled to pension credit guarantee have not claimed it.

The behavioural/cultural explanation

This explanation for health inequalities will be very familiar to most health and social care professionals and has been the one most favoured by successive governments. In this explanation for health inequalities, it is suggested that the health of the individual is determined by personal behaviour such as:

- smoking;
- drinking excessive amounts of alcohol;
- being physically inactive;
- consuming high levels of refined foods;
- not using preventative health care services such as antenatal clinics, family planning clinics, immunization/vaccination clinics or screening.

All of these behaviours are linked to subsequent morbidity and mortality and are more common among lower social classes. Smoking among adults in the UK continues to be much more prevalent among manual groups compared with middle-class people, who are more likely to be able to quit. Risky health behaviours such as drug taking or drinking excessively are also much more common among lower social groups. A simple explanation might suggest irresponsibility or a lack of information on health risks on the part of the individual. However, research has shown that such behaviours are a response to social situations such as unemployment, social upheaval and stress. People use addictive behaviours such as cigarette smoking, drug taking and drinking excessive amounts of alcohol to "*numb the pain of harsh economic and social conditions*" (WHO, 2003).

Scenario 2.1

Sandra is a single unsupported parent, living in a third floor council flat, with three children under five years and with very little disposable income. Sandra visits her GP several times in the course of three months complaining that her children have recurrent chest infections and her middle child has glue ear.

It is noted by her GP that Sandra is a heavy smoker and consequently her children are passive smokers. The GP tells Sandra that unless she stops smoking and attends the smoking cessation clinic run by the practice nurse, she will not give her any more repeat prescriptions for antibiotics for chest infections for her children. When challenged about her smoking and faced with unfilled prescriptions, Sandra becomes defensive and leaves the surgery angry and upset.

- Is the ill health of Sandra's children her fault?
- How could the GP and practice nurse support Sandra in light of her current health behaviour?
- What are the other influences on health that the GP and practice nurse need to be aware of?
- What might be the problem of adopting a behavioural explanation of health inequalities to account for your patient's poor health?

Discussion

This health behaviour on the part of Sandra may seem irresponsible and reckless, but faced with a life full of difficult decisions and a lack of choices and resources, it may be that smoking is health-enhancing to Sandra's mental health, be it at the expense of the physical health of both her and her children.

It is too simplistic to assume that smoking is entirely a result of Sandra's irresponsible or reckless behaviour. Sandra's health behaviour could be as a result of her understanding of health, education or expectations. This blaming the victim approach can be very unhelpful for the nurse and patient as it may influence the way nurses respond to or care for patients – and it may mean patients defer seeking care and attention because they are afraid of being judged.

The psychosocial explanation

This explanation focuses on the ways in which contemporary society can produce stresses that affect different groups unevenly and can contribute to ill health. The Whitehall II Study (Marmot *et al.*, 1991) examined the reasons for the social gradient in health and disease, i.e. that higher occupational groups were less likely to suffer from CHD than lower occupational groups. This study highlighted the fact that health inequalities can occur because of the way work is organized and the work climate, i.e. those with a lack of autonomy, a lot of monotony and fewer relationships with superiors are more likely to experience stress at work. These groups are also less likely to have access to material and personal resources to manage stress, and the stresses affect cardiovascular, endocrine and immune systems potentially leading to diseases such as CHD and diabetes.

Wilkinson (1997) argues that the psychosocial effects of social position account for the major part of health inequalities. It is the relationship between income, social position and health that is associated with an increased risk of CHD, stroke, hypertension, obesity and duodenal ulcers. Therefore, if an individual is relatively poor in comparison to others within their society, they are more likely to be at risk of developing any of these conditions. This may be a result of chronic stress and the physiological response to this stress, e.g. increased secretion of cortisol, elevated blood pressure, a change in the ratio of high-density and low-density lipoproteins, and a suppressed immune system.

Evidence 2.1

The spirit level: why more equal societies almost always do better

A book of evidence by Wilkinson and Pickett published in 2010 with the equivocal title, *Why More Equal Societies Almost Always Do Better*, was in a subsequent edition revised to *The Spirit Level: Why Equality Is Better for Everyone*. The book achieved huge publicity and considerable criticism by arguing that health and well-being outcomes are significantly worse in more unequal rich societies. It argued that higher levels of income inequality damage the social fabric that contributes so much to healthy societies. People with stronger social relationships were half as likely to die as those with weaker social ties. Social relations such as marital status, feeling lonely, the size of one's social network, and participation in social activities were at least as important influences on survival as that of smoking, and much more important than heavy drinking, physical activity or obesity. The book also reported that social cohesion – as measured by levels of trust – seemed to provide the causal link between income inequality and homicide rates. The most plausible explanation for income inequality's apparent effect on health and social problems is "status anxiety". This suggests that income inequality is harmful because it places people in a hierarchy that increases status competition and causes stress, which leads to poor health and other negative outcomes (Wilkinson and Pickett, 2010).

Activity 2.3

- How can the nurse ensure that their patients feel valued and included when they are admitted to the ward?
- How can this help the nurse to address health inequalities?

Discussion

In order to enhance the psychological health of patients and address the effects of stress because of their feelings of helplessness, nurses need to encourage a sense of belonging, control and inclusion. In order to make patients feel valued and included, it is important for the nurse to devise individual care plans that take into account patients' cultural, social and psychological needs as well as their physical health needs. By planning care jointly with patients, i.e. care that takes on board their expressed needs, values and beliefs, the nurse will be demonstrating a commitment to tackling health inequalities.

So far we have considered possible explanations for health inequalities and concluded that health inequalities could be due to:

- Life course explanations, which suggest that the health status of the individual is determined by the environment that the individual is exposed to in utero to adulthood. Therefore, those experiencing adverse economic conditions in early life are likely to be even more disadvantaged in adulthood.
- Materialist explanations of health inequalities, which suggest that the socio-economic background of the individual, the distribution of wealth and the impact of poverty influence the health status and well-being of the individual, thus accounting for the poorer health of lower socio-economic groups.
- Behavioural explanations of health inequalities, which suggest that it is the health behaviour of the individual such as smoking, physical inactivity, drinking in excess or eating an unhealthy diet, which will determine the health status of the individual and that these behaviours are more common in lower socio-economic groups.
- Psychosocial explanations, which suggest that stress at home or work can contribute to long term ill health.

Tackling health inequalities

In recent decades, there have been a number of government inquiries examining health inequalities and the differences in health experienced by different population groups:

- The Black Report (Black, 1980) showed that although improvements in health had been made overall, there were widespread inequalities in health outcomes, as well as in access to health services. The review highlighted differences in health related to social class.
- The Acheson Report (1998) *Independent Inquiry into Inequalities in Health* found that overall the nation's health had improved and morbidity and mortality rates from infectious diseases

had made impressive improvements. However, health inequalities had actually increased between rich and poor since the Black Report was published in 1980. The report specifically focused on the needs of mothers, children and families.

- The Wanless Report (2004) *Securing Good Health for the Whole Population*, an independent report to government, focused on prevention and the wider determinants of health in England and the cost effectiveness of action that could be taken to improve the health of the whole population and to reduce health inequalities.
- *Tackling Health Inequalities: 10 Years On* (DH, 2009) examined developments in health inequalities since the publication of the Acheson Report.
- *Equity and Excellence: Liberating the NHS* (DH, 2010a) proposed moving health improvement responsibilities to local government, which took place in 2013.
- *Healthy Lives, Healthy People: Our Strategy for Public Health in England* (DH, 2010b) follows earlier White Papers on Public Health and responds to the challenges laid out by the Marmot Review Team in *Fair Society, Healthy Lives*. Strategies to tackle health inequalities include: the creation of a Public Health England.
- The Public Health Outcomes Framework proposes several indicators that cover the wider determinants of health, requiring the combined efforts of all public services (https://www.gov.uk/government/uploads/system/uploads/attachment_data/file/216159/dh_132362.pdf).

Case study 2.2

The Marmot Review of Health Inequalities

An independent review, chaired by Professor Sir Michael Marmot, was commissioned by the UK government in response to the World Health Organization's report, *Closing the Gap in a Generation* (2008) which showed that countries with more equitable policies and more just societies were healthier.

The Marmot Review report, *Fair Society, Healthy Lives* (Marmot, 2010), emphasizes the *"causes of the causes"* of health inequalities, and the need to address these wider determinants. To tackle inequalities and reduce the steepness of the social gradient, the Marmot Review recommends actions of sufficient scale and intensity to be universal but also proportionately targeted. Strategies need to target those at the lower end of the gradient as well as throughout the whole of society, according to the level of disadvantage.

The report specifically proposed action on six policy objectives:

1. Give every child the best start in life.
2. Enable all children, young people and adults to maximise their capabilities and have control over their lives.
3. Create fair employment and good work for all.
4. Ensure a healthy standard of living for all.
5. Create and develop healthy and sustainable places and communities.
6. Strengthen the role and impact of ill health prevention.

As well as being a matter of fairness and social justice, achieving health equality would bring clear economic and social benefits nationally, such as improved productivity, lower welfare payments and health care costs, and increases in revenue.

Global perspective on tackling health inequalities

So far we have focused on public health and health promotion policies and initiatives in the UK that were developed to tackle health inequalities. However, it is important to note that these policies and initiatives were developed as part of a global perspective aimed at tackling the health inequalities of disadvantaged groups across the world. The leading organization charged with developing health care policy globally is the World Health Organization (WHO). As part of their public health policy development role in 2004, the WHO commissioned global research to investigate the issues behind health inequalities.

The WHO found that there is evidence of health inequalities from across nations in relation to infant mortality rates and across the life span (WHO, 2004). For example, the infant mortality rate for American-Indians and Alaskan natives is almost double that of White Americans. Mortality rates from cancer are 30% higher for African-Americans than for White Americans (Smedley *et al.*, 2003). In Northern Ireland, women from social class V were more than 60% more likely to experience some form of neurotic disorder than women from higher social classes (Age Concern/London School of Hygiene and Tropical Medicine, 2005).

The world is becoming smaller and the effects of globalization are being felt worldwide, for example:

- the impact of enterprises such as food chains and restaurants on the diet and health of communities (Beaglehole and Yach, 2003);
- the effects of the tobacco industry specifically targeting previously untapped markets and younger smokers (ASH, 2002);
- the arms trade and sports industries are increasingly using workforces composed of children to manufacture their goods (Kawachi and Wamala, 2007).

Nurses have an important and influential role as public health advocates to speak out against health-damaging and irresponsible behaviour on the part of industry. Brundtland (1999), cited by the RCN (1999), argues in relation to tobacco control that:

> *Nurses have many opportunities to play a leadership role in combating the tobacco epidemic. Nurses throughout the world have access to the population at all levels of the health care system, and enjoy a high degree of public trust. Indeed, there are several examples of nurses successfully initiating and implementing tobacco prevention and treatment programmes with specific target populations, such as school children, pregnant women and people recovering from cardiac diseases and cancer. The International Council of Nurses has urged nurses to get involved at all levels of tobacco control: prevention, cessation, and policy, encouraging them to be at the forefront of tobacco control at the local, national and international level, building partnerships with other professional and advocacy groups, governmental and non-governmental organisations.*

The International Council of Nurses' position statements (http://www.icn.ch/publications/position-statements/) reflect the range of issues with which nurses are involved and regarding which they may need to challenge to change global policy, e.g. female genital mutilation, the use of breast milk substitutes, the arms trade and conflict, and climate change.

The role of the nurse in tackling health inequalities

It is widely concluded that interventions at the structural levels that include changes in policies or regulations (such as food supplementation or bans on smoking in public places) are more likely to reduce inequalities than simply offering advice and information where more advantaged groups find it easier to adopt health promotion advice. However, what role does this leave for the nurse? The nurse may try to influence policy both nationally or locally to tackle health inequalities. This may include writing to policy-makers to highlight issues which promote health inequalities. Evidence suggests that lobbying as a tool for change can be effective – some researchers, for example, believe that lobbying from the public health field brought about an acknowledgement by the Conservative Government regarding variations in health, as the government had previously refused to acknowledge that health inequalities existed (Baggott, 2010). There is currently an active campaign to keep the National Health Service (NHS) public (www.keepournhspublic.com) and nurses and international organizations such as UNICEF have successfully lobbied international formula milk companies in relation to the companies' promotion of bottle feeding in developing countries.

Improving access and availability to health care involves the nurse first of all acknowledging that disadvantaged groups may not have the same access to good quality health care provision as more affluent groups. The nurse should aim to ensure equal access by:

- developing explicit guideline referrals;
- employing positive discrimination principles such as prioritising disadvantaged groups;
- making sure services are more accessible through such measures as out-of-hours clinics;
- screening high risk groups;
- ensuring that health information is accessible to high risk and disadvantaged groups.

Nurses should involve their patients as much as possible in planning their care to ensure that the care plan meets the patient's needs. Other considerations for the nurses include ensuring that in their everyday dealing with their patients that they adopt anti-discriminatory practice principles which include, being flexible, including the views of marginalized and excluded groups, challenging existing stereotypes and practices and reflecting on organizational structures and the way that structure may reinforce health inequalities.

Partnership working involves the nurse working collaboratively with other agencies to form local strategies to tackle health inequalities. Nurses may join forces with social workers, community workers, charities and leisure services to devise projects that tackle health inequalities, e.g. community nurses have successfully collaborated with organizations such as the Child Accident Prevention Trust to produce a training programme and resources for health visitors and other community nurses to use to tackle children's accidents at home.

On placement: checklist

- ❑ Are you aware that the nurses understood the health needs of their local population?
- ❑ Are patients seen as part of defined populations who might benefit from upstream approaches? Which populations?
- ❑ Did nurses work in partnership with other members of health and social care organizations to tackle the wider determinants of health, e.g. housing?
- ❑ Do nurses use public health evidence in everyday practice, and not just evidence for treating illness?
- ❑ Did other health care professionals get involved in local community action, non-governmental organizations (NGOs) or research projects?

Key learning points

1. Patients do not have equal opportunities to address their health problems.
2. Ill health is concentrated in disadvantaged groups: those on low income, those living in remote parts of the country, Black and ethnic minority groups, and older people.
3. The early years, e.g. breastfeeding and good parenting, can reduce the likelihood of ill health later.
4. Where there are apparently unfair differences in wealth and advantage, people experience stress which can lead to ill health.

Chapter summary

This chapter has considered some of the evidence that demonstrates that ill health is concentrated in the poorer sections of society. It has outlined some policy initiatives that aim to improve the health of those living in disadvantaged communities. Nurses need to have an understanding of the ways in which the context and environment in which patients live and work can influence their life chances, their behaviours and their health status. While community nurses are ideally placed to promote health in these communities as they have good access to families, all nurses need to be aware of the impact of social factors on the health of their patients.

Further reading and resources

CSDH (Commission on Social Determinants of Health) (2008) *Closing the Gap in a Generation: Health Equity Through Action on the Social Determinants of Health. Final Report of the Commission on Social Determinants of Health.* World Health Organization, Geneva. Available at: http://whqlibdoc.who.int/publications/2008/9789241563703_eng.

London is one of nine regional Public Health Observatories set up in England in 2001 by the Department of Health. The London Health Observatory takes the national lead role in monitoring health inequalities, ethnicity and tobacco use. See http://www.lho.org.uk. Since April 2013, public health observatories have become part of Public Health England.

The Marmot Review (2010) *Fair Society, Healthy Lives* is available online at: http://www.instituteofhealthequity.org/projects/fair-society-healthy-lives-the-marmot-review.

The RCN is committed to tackling health inequalities. *Going Upstream: Nursing's Contribution to Public Health* (RCN, 2012) sets out the value of nursing in preventing poor health and minimising the impact when illness occurs. Available at: http://www.rcn.org.uk/_data/assets/pdf_file/0007/433699/004203.pdf.

References

Acheson, D. (1998) *Independent Inquiry into Inequalities in Health*. The Stationery Office, London.

Age Concern/LSHTM (2005) *Minimum Income for Health Living for Older People.* Available at: http://www.ageuk.org.uk/documents/en-gb/for-professionals/money-and-benefits/1005_minimum_income_for_healthy_living_older_people_2005_pro.pdf?dtrk=true.

ASH (2002) *World Health Organization Briefing: Tobacco Industry Youth Smoking Prevention Programmes – A Critique*. Available at: http://www.ash.org.uk/files/documents/ASH_646.pdf.

Baggott, R. (2010) *Public Health: Policy and Politics*, 2nd edn. Palgrave Macmillan, Basingstoke.

Beaglehole R. and Yach, D. (2003) Globalisation and the prevention and control of non-communicable disease: the neglected chronic diseases of adults. *The Lancet*, **362**, 903–908.

Black, D. (1980) *Inequalities in Health: Report of a Research Working Group*. DHSS, London.

Cancer Research UK (2006) *Cancer and Health Inequalities: An Introduction to Current Evidence.* Cancer Research UK, London. Available at: http://www.cancerresearchuk.org/prod_consump/groups/cr_common/@nre/@pol/documents/generalcontent/crukmig_1000ast-3344.pdf.

Dahlgren, G. and Whitehead, M. (1991) *Policies and Strategies to Promote Social Equity in Health.* Institute for Futures Studies, Stockholm.

DH (Department of Health) (2008) *Working for a Healthier Tomorrow: Dame Carol Black's Review of the Health of Britain's Working Age Population.* TSO, London. Available at: https://www.gov.uk/government/uploads/system/uploads/attachment_data/file/209782/hwwb-working-for-a-healthier-tomorrow.pdf.

DH (Department of Health) (2009) *Tacking Health Inequalities Ten Years On.* DH, London. Available at: http://ec.europa.eu/health/archive/ph_determinants/socio_economics/documents/uk_rd01_en.pdf.

DH (Department of Health) (2010a) *Equity and Excellence: Liberating the NHS*. DH, London. Available at: https://www.gov.uk/government/uploads/system/uploads/attachment_data/file/213823/dh_117794.pdf.

DH (Department of Health) (2010b) *Healthy Lives, Healthy People: Our Strategy for Public Health in England*. CM7985. TSO, London. Available at: https://www.gov.uk/government/uploads/system/uploads/attachment_data/file/216096/dh_127424.pdf.

Graham, H. and Power, C. (2004) *Childhood Disadvantage and Adult Health: A Lifecourse Framework*. Health Development Agency, London.

Greater London Authority (2005) *Health in London: Review of the London Health Strategy High Level Indicators*. Health Commission, London.

Kawachi, I., Subramanian, S.V. and Almeida-Filho, N. (2000) A glossary for health inequalities, *Journal of Epidemiology and Community Health*, **56**, 647–652.

Kawachi, I. and Wamala, S. (2007) *Globalisation and Health*. Oxford University Press, New York.

Marmot M.G. (2010) *Fair Society, Healthy Lives*. Department of Health, London.

Marmot, M.G., Davey Smith, G., Stansfield, S.A. *et al.* (1991) Health inequalities among British civil servants: the Whitehall II Study, *Lancet*, **331**, 1387–1393.

Morris, J.N., Donkin, A.J.M., Wonderling, D.P., *et al.* (2000) A minimum income for healthy living, *Journal of Epidemiology and Community Health*, **54**, 885–889.

Morris, J.N., Wilkinson, P., Dangour, A.D., *et al.* (2007) Defining a Minimum Income for Healthy Living (MIHL) in older age, England. *International Journal of Epidemiology*, **36**, 1300–1307.

NHS Health and Social Care Information Centre (2005) *Health Survey for England 2004: The Health of Minority Ethnic Groups: Headline Tables*. NHS Health and Social Care Information Centre, Public Health Statistics, London.

RCN (Royal College of Nursing) (1999) *Clearing the Air*. RCN, London.

RCN (Royal College of Nursing) (2012) *Going Upstream: Nursing's Contribution to Public Health*. RCN, London.

Shelter (2006) *Chance of a Lifetime: The Impact of Bad Housing on Children's Lives*. Shelter, London.

Smedley, B.D., Smith, A.Y. and Nelson, A.R. (2003) *Unequal Treatment: Confronting Racial and Ethnic Disparities in Health Care*. National Academic Press, New York.

Wanless, D. (2004) *Securing Good Health for the Whole Population*. HM Treasury, London.

WHO (World Health Organization) (2003) *The Social Determinants of Health: The Solid Facts*. WHO, Copenhagen.

WHO (World Health Organization) (2004) *Closing the Health Inequalities Gap: An International Perspective*. WHO, Venice.

WHO (World Health Organization) (2008) *Closing the Gap in a Generation: Commission on the Social Determinants of Health*. WHO, Geneva.

Wilkinson, R. (1997) *Unhealthy Societies: The Afflictions of Inequality*. Routledge, London.

Wilkinson, R. and Pickett, K. (2010) *The Spirit Level: Why Equality Is Better for Everyone*. Penguin, London.

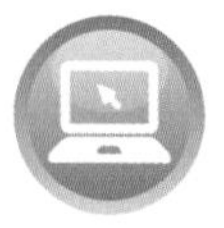

Don't forget to visit the companion website for this book: www.wileyfundamentalseries.com/healthpromotion where you can find self-assessment tests to check your progress.

3

Approaches to promoting health

Susie Sykes

Senior Lecturer, Public Health and Health Promotion, London South Bank University, London, UK

Learning outcomes

By the end of this chapter you will be able to:

1. Describe the difference between biomedical, behavioural and social approaches to health promotion
2. Describe different aspects of health promotion in relation to theoretical models available
3. Use an understanding of different health promotion models and theories in order to design and plan health promotion interventions that can be used in the role of a nurse

Introduction

This chapter will consider in more detail the different perspectives that practitioners have towards health and the ways in which these may influence how nurses interpret the conditions that patients present with. There are a number of different approaches to health promotion that may be adopted according to the perspective of health that is held, the objectives that

Fundamentals of Health Promotion for Nurses, Second Edition. Edited by Jane Wills.

Companion website: www.wileyfundamentalseries.com/healthpromotion

need to be met, or political persuasion. This chapter will look at medical approaches to health promotion that focus on: preventing disease and treating illness; behavioural approaches which concentrate on strategies for changing people's behaviour in favour of healthier lifestyles; and socio-environmental approaches that aim to effect change on the wider social and cultural environment within which health is constructed. Students will be encouraged to consider how different theoretical approaches to health promotion can be applied through their roles as nurses.

Perspectives of health

There are a number of ways of conceptualizing and understanding health. These different perspectives consider health and prioritize determinants of health in various ways. They foster different approaches to responding to health issues. This chapter will focus on three of these perspectives:

- preventative medical;
- behavioural;
- socio-environmental.

As we saw in Chapter 1, health is often viewed as the absence of disease and disability which is achieved largely through clinical measures. For those operating within this framework, health is seen as being determined primarily by physiological risk factors. A behavioural perspective, on the other hand, acknowledges the importance of this medical model of health but sees health as being influenced by the way in which people live their lives. This perspective sees lifestyle as key in determining health alongside physiological risks. Others, however, take biomedical and behavioural perspectives further and include within their definition of health the social quality of life. This socio-environmental perspective sees health as being primarily influenced by the social and economic environment within which people live and the constraints and opportunities such structural factors create. People's economic situation, housing conditions, education and employment, for example, all impact on people's health and contribute to how easily they are able to take on board health messages and adopt healthier lifestyles. Many of these structural issues may be beyond a patient's immediate control.

Consider, for example, a patient who is suffering from coronary heart disease (CHD). The condition can be interpreted differently according to the three perspectives of health that are outlined in Table 3.1.

Most professionals do not operate solely within the confines of just one of these perspectives but are likely to be influenced by one perspective more than the others. It is important to reflect upon and understand one's own perspective in order to consider why we respond to issues and prioritize actions in the way that we do.

Table 3.1 Perspectives on coronary heart disease.

Perspective	Cause of CHD	Interventions
Preventative medical	Hypertension	Screening
	Arterial plaque	Treatment with statins and/or surgery
Behavioural	Smoking	Smoking cessation
	Sedentary lifestyle	Physical activity programme, e.g. "Let's Get Moving"
	High fat diet	Lower cholesterol diet
Socio-environmental	Stress caused by employment/ unemployment, poverty, housing, conflict	Welfare benefits Environmental improvements

Activity 3.1

Health perspectives

- Reflect on which of the three perspectives of health (preventative medical, behavioural or socio-environmental) influences your thinking most when you are considering a patient's condition.
- Why does this perspective influence your thinking more than others?
- Are there times when more than one perspective influences your thinking?
- What difference would viewing a patient's condition from a different health perspective make?

Discussion

For those working in a hospital environment with an emphasis on clinical targets and outcomes, the preventative medical perspective of health can often dominate a nurse's thinking. Taking time to reflect upon how behavioural and socio-environmental factors may also have played a part in a patient's condition, enables the nurse to identify appropriate and sustainable health promotion responses.

Approaches to health promotion

The particular perspective of health that is held directly influences the approaches that are taken in health promotion interventions and will affect the way strategies are planned and implemented. Table 3.2 shows a range of approaches that may be adopted and these differ according to what is perceived to be the determinants of health and the aim of the intervention.

Table 3.2 Summary of perspectives of health and approaches to health promotion.

Perspective of health	Determinants of health viewed in terms of	Aim	Examples of health promotion interventions
Preventative medical	Physiological risk factors Family history/genetic risk factors Exposure to pathogens	To reduce morbidity and premature mortality	Clinical interventions Immunization and screening programmes Drug treatments
Behavioural	Lifestyle and behavior such as: • Smoking • Diet • Activity levels • Sexual activity • Stress levels	To encourage individuals to adopt healthy behaviours	Health education programmes Campaigns One-to-one advice Small group work/self-help groups
Socio-environmental	Social and economic environment e.g.: • Economic deprivation • Housing • Employment conditions • Low educational levels • Social exclusion and isolation	To bring about changes in the environment that enables people to enjoy better health	Policy and legislation change Advocacy Lobbying and petitioning

Adapted from Ontario Health Promotion Resource System.

Preventative medical approaches to health promotion

A preventative medical approach to health promotion has as its primary focus the prevention of ill health and disease rather than prioritizing the promotion of positive health and well-being. In working to achieve this, a preventative medical approach does the following:

- addresses physiological risk factors;
- uses clinical interventions to prevent disease;
- tends to be expert-led, i.e. initiated and led by professionals rather than by the patient.

Typical interventions are those that target whole populations or which are focused on high-risk target groups, e.g. immunisation and screening programmes. As such, interventions tend to be based on and driven by epidemiological evidence and are usually target-driven. For example, the annual influenza immunization campaigns are based on epidemiological data and target certain groups such as those over 65 years, and those in particular clinical risk groups. The campaign has epidemiologically driven targets including the immunisation of over 70% of people over 65 years (DH, 2005).

Case study 3.1

The use of statins in the prevention of coronary heart disease

Tackling vascular disease is seen as key to reducing health inequalities relating to life expectancy. Reducing smoking levels and increasing the use of statins are regarded as the two key interventions that can rapidly reduce the number of early deaths in disadvantaged groups.

Statins are the main types of medicine for lowering cholesterol in the prevention and treatment of CVD. They help to reduce harmful low-density lipoprotein (LDL) levels in the body and increase the levels of "good" high-density lipoprotein cholesterol.

The amount spent on statins and other lipid-regulating drugs that are used in the prevention of CVD has soared and is now 15 times higher than 10 years ago. In 2007, the NHS spent £500 million on statins, representing the single biggest drug cost.

Preventative medical interventions are the most acceptable approach to public health priorities as their impact is able to be assessed in terms of levels of morbidity and mortality and other clinical indicators. The clinical nature of this approach to health promotion means that it fits comfortably within a hospital setting and as a result can dominate how clinicians plan and implement health promotion initiatives.

Activity 3.2

What might be the criticism of this approach to public health?

Discussion

Critics argue that an emphasis on this approach results in an over-medicalization of issues without considering the context of how people live their lives or taking into account the wider social, cultural and economic factors that contribute to and determine health.

Behavioural approaches to health promotion

Behavioural approaches to health promotion are based on a recognition of the impact that people's lifestyle and behaviour have on their health. Health promotion interventions based on this perspective do the following:

- seek to change people's behaviour and encourage the adoption of healthier lifestyles and therefore prevent ill health;
- promote positive health and well-being;

- may target whole populations through health education messages such as quit smoking or at risk groups.

The focus of behavioural approaches to health promotion may be:

- *educational* – giving people accurate information about the impact of their behaviour on their health so that they are able to make informed choices about their lifestyle, e.g. nutritional information about what is required to ensure a healthy diet.
- *to develop the skills and strategies* that people require to implement and sustain changes in their lifestyle, e.g., cooking skills and strategies to develop menu options that appeal to all family members.

The agenda and process of this approach tend to be expert-led though this is not always the case and client-led approaches to health education with patients can occur. For example, Chapter 12 describes motivational interviewing which is widely used in primary care and in relation to rehabilitation.

Hospital settings are often seen as appropriate settings within which to undertake a behavioural approach to health promotion, in part because the high prestige and credibility of hospital staff give an authority to behavioural and lifestyle messages and because patients can be targeted at a time when their health is at the forefront of their minds.

Activity 3.3

Making Every Contact Count (MECC)

"Making Every Contact Count" (MECC) is an NHS initiative to encourage frontline workers to initiate conversations based on behavioural change methodologies (ranging from brief advice, to more advanced behavioural change techniques), empowering healthier lifestyle choices.

- ❑ Do you think nurses may be viewed as less "credible" by recipients of advice if they have clearly not chosen to engage with healthy behaviours themselves?

Discussion

Nurses and patients alike have suggested that patients are more likely to listen to, respect and follow the advice of a health adviser who models the same health habits and behaviours that they are recommending, and, conversely, will "tune out" to those who do not. In addition, healthcare professionals who are overweight or obese have reported feeling less willing, or even less able, to promote healthy diet and exercise in their patients (Zhu et al., 2011).

The effectiveness of this approach is, however, dependent on individuals being at a point at which they are ready and able to make changes in their behaviour. Critics claim that such interventions tend to focus on an individual's behaviour without looking more widely at the structural circumstances that influence those behaviours. For example, interventions that encourage people to adopt a healthier diet and eat five portions of fruit and vegetables a day as recommended by the Department of Health's 5-A-Day programme may not necessarily explore structural barriers to doing so. These may include: the cost of fresh food; public transport to out-of-town supermarkets where food might be cheaper and media messages to children which promote fast food. Chapter 12 discusses the ways in which practitioners can promote healthy lifestyles without victim blaming and seeing the individual as solely responsible for their situation.

Activity 3.4

Initiating breastfeeding

Current UK policy is to promote exclusive breastfeeding (feeding only breast milk) for the first six months, continuing for as long as the mother and baby wish while gradually introducing a more varied diet. Some 81% of mothers start breastfeeding but only 50% are breastfeeding at six weeks and by six months it has reduced to 26%. A rapid fall in breastfeeding occurs soon after birth – 12% in 4 days, with 22% stopping by two weeks and 37% by six weeks.

- What would be the objectives of an intervention to support new young mothers to breastfeed?

Discussion

The first stage for a health care professional in planning how to address an issue is to identify the contributing factors (which may be any aspect of behaviour, society or the environment) that explain why women may not initiate or sustain breastfeeding and then identify intervention points. Research studies and the National Infant Feeding Survey have identified many reasons that include:

- *perceived insufficient milk so new mother may need reassurance about the stimulating effect of suckling;*
- *difficulties in feeding, e.g. cracked nipples;*
- *a return to work;*
- *restricted freedom;*
- *embarrassment.*

Socio-environmental approaches to health promotion

Advocates of a socio-environmental approach to health promotion emphasize the view that medical and behavioural interventions should take place alongside interventions that address the wider structural social and economic factors that impact on the health of individuals, communities and populations. This approach is based on an argument that the determinants of health are highly complex and include individual, social, economic, cultural and environmental influences and, as such, require complex responses. The focus of this approach is to bring about change at a policy or structural level in order to create an environment in which it becomes both possible and realistic for individuals to make and sustain healthy choices and lifestyles, e.g. baby-friendly hospitals.

Interventions that operate within this approach and which seek to address a number of the wider determinants of health may be:

- complex
- long-term
- requiring support at a strategic level
- dependent on intersectoral commitment.

For this reason, many nurses may see it as being beyond their ability or remit to adopt this approach. It has been argued that nurses have, in the past, tended to adopt a limited, traditional health education-based approach that focuses on the giving of information (Whitehead, 2005). While it is indeed difficult for a nurse to directly bring about large-scale structural change through ward-based hospital work, there are opportunities at every level to influence or lobby for change.

Case study 3.2

A specialist asthma nurse

A specialist asthma nurse describes how she played a part in addressing the wider structural determinants of health.

In my capacity as a paediatric asthma nurse I was asked to go and review a 3-year-old boy in the children's ward who had been admitted with an asthma attack. I did all my usual education – what asthma is, looked at what things may have precipitated that attack, necessary treatments, inhaler techniques, management plan, etc. This also included looking at the home environment. During that time, the child's mother became very upset and told me about the damp and mould in their flat. The child's mother invited me to their home to see the damp for myself. The flat was covered in damp and mould from an ongoing leak from the balcony above. She felt that she was getting nowhere with the council regarding being re-housed. This was wearing her down mentally and emotionally and she was finding it harder to cope with her son's illness. She reported feeling suicidal and unable to go on. I wrote a letter to the Housing Department stating the child's medical needs, enclosing a medical paper about the effects of damp housing, and also the psychological state of the mother and the possible impact that would be having on her ability to cope with her son's needs.

The family did get re-housed within quite a short space of time. The child's mother's mood changed after this and the child's asthma is much better controlled – I don't see him now. It is always difficult to determine direct cause and effect but we cannot look at any of these things in isolation and need to treat them as a whole within their family and environment.

While the intervention described in Case study 3.2 did not bring about policy change, it did impact on the implementation of a policy that influences the wider determinations of health. Ongoing involvement in this way has the potential to influence longer-term policy review or development.

There is an overlap between these three different approaches and planned health promotion interventions may not sit solely within one of these perspectives. The type of intervention chosen will vary according to the circumstances and the objectives that need to be met. However, this provides a useful framework within which to consider the direction from which work is currently undertaken and the potential for it to be undertaken differently.

Models of health promotion

The perspectives discussed represent broad approaches to health promotion but it is useful to go beyond this and look at more detailed models of health-promoting activity. Models provide a theoretical framework through which to view health promotion as a whole and help us consider, not only how different perspectives of health can be actioned but also how our political philosophy, values and beliefs influence the way we develop and implement strategies for health promotion. They provide a tool for questioning practice and the assumptions that form the basis of practice. Through such models, a framework can be provided for developing new strategies. Theoretical models should, however, also be viewed critically. They are intended to support thinking but an over-reliance on one particular model may close minds to alternative visions. It should also be remembered that they are not, unlike nursing models, a guide to what to do.

Activity 3.5

Consider health promotion interventions with the objectives of tackling obesity

- What advantages and disadvantages exist in targeting health promotion interventions at:
  - individual levels, e.g. weight loss programmes or nutritional counselling? population levels, e.g. local food cooperative schemes or campaigns to improve school meals?

What advantages and disadvantages exist in health promotion interventions that are:

- "top-down", decided upon and led by professionals and experts (such as healthy eating campaigns)?
- negotiated with patients and based on principles of involvement and participation (such as weight loss programmes)?

Discussion

Interventions targeted at individuals can be tailor-made and can be targeted at those most in need in a way that ensures they meet the specific needs of the individual. An individual focus assumes, however, that behaviour is voluntarily chosen or inherent in cultural or social norms. Population-based interventions mean that large numbers of people can be targeted but require rather general objectives that may not meet the specific needs of minority or vulnerable groups within that population.

Top-down approaches to health promotion mean that work is usually based on epidemiological evidence of what most needs to be addressed and what has been found to work. This approach does not, however, allow patients the same degree of ownership and commitment that may come from a more negotiated and user-led approach.

Tannahill's model of health promotion

Tannahill's model (Figure 3.1) was developed to illustrate the scope of health promotion (Downie *et al.*, 1996).According to this model, health promotion is made up of three overlapping areas: health education, health protection and prevention.

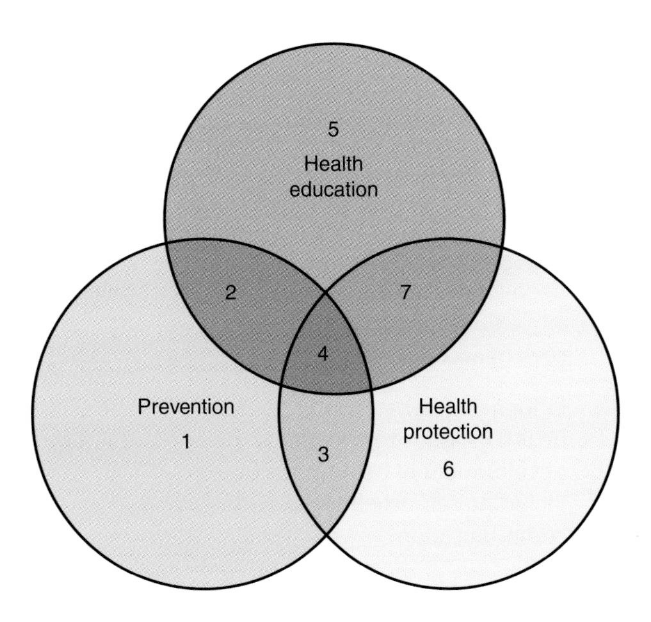

Figure 3.1 Tannahill's model of health promotion. Source: *Health Promotion, Models and Values*, 2nd edn, by Downie, Tannahill and Tannahill (1996), Figure 4.1, p. 59. Reproduced with permission of Oxford University Press.

- *Health education* is defined as work to promote positive health and well-being and to prevent or reduce ill health through the influencing of beliefs, attitudes and behaviours.
- *Health protection* includes regulatory work through legislative and policy-based interventions to protect the health and well-being of individuals, communities and populations.
- *Prevention* broadly refers to work through services to reduce the likelihood of poor health.

A feature of this model is that it distinguishes throughout between enhancing positive health and preventing ill health and sees health promotion as aiming to undertake both these objectives. Within the three overlapping circles there are seven different domains, each of which refers to a different type of activity and all of which form a part of what defines health promotion. Each of the domains is described in Table 3.3.

Table 3.3 Domains of health promotion activity in the Tannahill model.

Domain	Characteristics	Examples of typical interventions
1. Prevention services	Programmes and services designed to prevent disease and ill-health	Immunization screening programmes Nicotine replacement therapy
2. Preventive health education	Education to influence lifestyles to prevent ill-health combined with encouragement to use prevention services	Smoking cessation advice in conjunction with the provision of nicotine replacement therapy
3. Preventive health protection	Policies and regulation to prevent disease and ill-health	Fluoridation of water supplies to prevent dental health problems
4. Health education for preventive health protection	Educating policy-makers for the need for preventive regulations while educating a community to seek or accept changes	Lobbying for policies on seat belts
5. Health education	Influencing behaviour on positive health grounds to encourage the development of healthy attributes including self-esteem and communication	Life skills and relationship training
6. Positive health protection	Regulations and policies that promote positive health and well-being	Workplace smoking policy
7. Health education for positive health protection	Educating policy-makers on the need for positive health regulations while educating a community to accept or seek change	Lobbying for a smoking ban in public places

The Tannahill model is designed to present the different domains of health promotion without judgement of one being of more value than another. It provides an explicit acknowledgement that there is an overlap between the different activities that define health promotion. It does not represent within it different political philosophies that may underpin different approaches.

Beattie's model of health promotion

Beattie's model (Beattie, 1991) presents four quadrants of activity derived from two axes on a grid (see Figure 3.2). The vertical axis represents modes of interventions that range from authoritarian, top-down, expert-led interventions to bottom-up, negotiated, participatory approaches to health promotion. It could be suggested that nurses have traditionally been associated with fairly authoritarian, top-down interventions, but they also have the potential to play an important role in more participatory forms of health promotion as the following examples will demonstrate.

MODE OF INTERVENTION
Authoritative
MODE OF THOUGHT
Objective knowledge

HEALTH PERSUASION

- To *persuade* or encourage people to adopt healthier lifestyles
- Practitioner is in the role of expert or 'prescriber'
- Conservative political ideology
- Activities include advice and information

LEGISLATIVE ACTION

- To *protect* the population by making healthier choices more available
- Practitioner is in the role of 'custodian' knowing what will improve the nation's health
- Reformist political ideology
- Activities include policy work, lobbying

FOCUS OF INTERVENTION

Individual ← → Collective

PERSONAL COUNSELLING

- To *empower* individuals to have the skills and confidence to take more control over their health
- Practitioner is in the role of 'counseller' working with people's self-defined needs
- Libertarian or humanist political ideology
- Activities include counselling and education

COMMUNITY DEVELOPMENT

- To *enfranchise or emancipate* groups and communities so they recognise what they have in common and how social factors influence their lives
- Practitioner is in the role of 'advocate'
- Radical political ideology
- Activities include community development and action

MODE OF INTERVENTION
Negotiated
MODE OF THOUGHT
Participatory, subjective knowledge

Figure 3.2 Beattie's model of health promotion. Source: Naidoo and Wills, 2009. Reproduced with permission of Elsevier.

The horizontal axis represents the focus of activities ranging from interventions targeting individuals, to those focused on tackling the social determinants of health. Again, the nurse's role is often seen to fit more comfortably with a focus on individuals despite a shifting emphasis to collective approaches within the field of health promotion. Within Beattie's model there are four domains of health promotion activity:

- health persuasion
- legislative action
- community development
- personal counselling.

Health persuasion

Health persuasion activities can be seen as sitting within the behavioural perspective and have as the primary objective convincing an individual to change their behaviour and adopt a healthier lifestyle. This approach is based on the premise that the expert knows best and epidemiological evidence is likely to be used to target high-risk patients and health issues (for more discussion on this, see Chapter 12). A health persuasion intervention is often based on the giving of information about behaviour, for example, trying to persuade a patient to undertake more exercise by outlining to them what the benefits to their health might be. This is a popular technique as it is possible for it to be relatively quick, delivered as part of a consultation and it appears to address high risk factors and individuals while offering a relatively cheap form of intervention. It also does not rely on any shift in organizational commitment to become a health promotion setting (see Chapter 4). Health promotion strategies in hospitals tend to rely heavily on this technique to the exclusion of other methods.

Critics argue that if used in isolation, attempts to persuade patients to change behaviours that are expert-driven and medically approved, are likely to be limited in their effectiveness (Whitehead, 2005) and point to the fact that this technique is less likely to explore whether the patient is ready or skilled enough to make changes in their lifestyle. In addition, it has been argued that the focus on the responsibility of the individual to change their behaviour does not recognise the relative powerlessness of some people and the lack of choice that their situation in society may give them (Lavarack, 2005). This is because of a failure to explore the issues within the context of the patient's life and circumstances and a failure to address the wider social and economic determinants of health that we outlined in the previous chapter.

Legislative action

Legislative action is also concerned with changing behaviour but through the benevolent actions of the state or an organization. This approach includes actions to bring about changes to national legislation, the development of national, local or organizational policies and supportive environments for health (see Chapter 4) and the provision of adequate resources to support national programmes. Such actions aim to make healthier choices easier, such as food labelling.

Activity 3.6

Think of legislative or regulatory action to promote healthy eating. Do you think people's behaviour should be controlled?

Discussion

While interventions at this level can encourage change, universal measures are often unable to meet the specific needs of all minority groups or individuals within a population. When enforcement underpins this approach, such interventions may be met with resistance from sections of the population. A danger is that prohibitive legislation may have the effect of driving certain behaviours underground and so making it harder to access vulnerable groups and potentially increasing inequalities in health. You may have thought of examples such as bans on the advertising of "junk food" during children's television viewing time or bans on vending machines in school. While some may argue that what we eat should be a matter of choice, others argue that health problems such as the rising obesity epidemic demand intervention by the state.

Community development

Community development is committed to bottom-up, community-led, participatory approaches (Laverack, 2005). Such interventions are based on the empowerment of communities to identify and prioritise their own needs, to work together to seek solutions to those needs and implement change as part of an ongoing process. The community involved may be a geographical community but may also be a community defined by culture, interest or social identity. Advocates argue that interventions are therefore more relevant, create a sense of ownership and are more likely therefore to be effective and sustainable. Chapter 17 discusses ways in which the nurse may work with communities.

The community development process is based on principles of social justice and equity, and requires professionals to be led by the communities they work with. This therefore becomes a potentially radical approach to health promotion which may present certain challenges for some, particularly if the priorities of the community do not match those of the professional or current health policy agenda. Community development can be a complex process that requires long-term commitment and specific resources and skills. It is also often an intersectoral approach that involves partnerships with other health agencies as well as other statutory and voluntary bodies. A nurse involved in such an approach is likely to be one among a number of key professionals undertaking work as part of a planned project and as such, involvement often requires an organizational and policy commitment.

Personal counselling

Interventions within this sphere are also led by, or negotiated with, the patient and are based on one-to-one work. The role of the nurse in this situation is to listen to the patient and work to empower that individual to make the changes they feel they need to make. This might involve problem-solving strategies, skills development tools as well as confidence and self-esteem building. Such approaches can be used either to promote positive health and well-being or to prevent ill health through disease management. Developing partnerships with patients and their family in the management of long-term conditions may be an example of such a technique (see Chapter 9). Motivational interviewing, described in Chapter 12, has also been described as a client-led change strategy. Limitations of such an approach are the ability of individuals to sustain such changes when faced with structural social or economic issues that are beyond an individual's control but which create barriers to change.

Each of the quadrants of the Beattie model gives rise to a different approach. Each of these four approaches can be seen to be based on a distinct set of values, objectives and political persuasions. In reality, none are likely to be effective in promoting health and reducing inequalities in health if they are adopted as the only approach. Rather, a combination of interventions is necessary. Beattie's model provides a useful framework for considering the options available when planning a project.

Activity 3.7

The role of the nurse in health promotion

- Which of the following do you regard as health promotion activity?
- What are your reasons for saying yes or no?
- Can you identify the criteria you are using for deciding whether an activity is health promotion?

1. a leaflet to encourage people to be more physically active following a myocardial infarction;
2. campaigning for a minimum price for alcohol;
3. explaining to patients how to take their medication;
4. providing toothbrushes to early years centres;
5. supporting the local cycle-to-work initiative and raising awareness of the impact of carbon emissions;
6. establishing a patient garden and setting up a patient gardening club;
7. educating school children about the risks of smoking;
8. immunising children against infectious diseases such as measles;
9. running a Tai Chi class for older people in residential care;
10. campaigning to ban vending machines in the hospital.

Discussion

This chapter has shown that health promotion encompasses a range of activities and may work at different levels. It may be directed towards action on the determinants of health such as carbon emissions or making healthy choices easier by making the environment more health promoting, e.g. by banning vending machines. It may also be directed towards encouraging patients to adopt healthier lifestyles, whether being more physically active or promoting oral health. Building social networks may also be part of the role of the nurse.

The Tannahill and Beattie models, as well as other models available in the literature (Naidoo and Wills, 2009; Ewles and Simnett, 2010) show that health promotion incorporates a broad range of activities that go beyond simple health education and lifestyle messages. The potential for nurses to be involved in all aspects of this has not been seized upon in the past and there have been calls for nurses to develop their role to include health promotion. This may involve nurses contributing to the structural development of environments that are supportive of health, encouraging participation of communities and individuals in health issues and contributing to the development of healthy public policies. While some of these activities allow the nurse to act independently and opportunistically and to become an intrinsic part of ongoing hospital work, others require the nurse to be one part of a larger, ongoing process. The latter does make it much harder for the individual nurse to see clearly how their input affects a final outcome, but is no less important.

The nurse's contribution to promoting health, whether at a direct patient level or a more strategic level, should be based on clear aims and objectives with identified goals and desired outcomes. Achieving this requires a nurse to reflect upon and be clear about the values and perspectives that underpin practice.

On placement: checklist

- ❑ What approach to health promotion did you observe to be most common while on placement?
- ❑ Are interventions to promote health more likely to be top-down or bottom-up?
- ❑ To what extent and how are socio-environmental factors that influence health addressed?
- ❑ Are there any examples from practice of nurses lobbying for health changes?

Key learning points

1. Health promotion activities may be preventative primarily through medical interventions such as screening, educational and encouraging behaviour change, or attempt to influence the environment.
2. Models of health promotion are tools that help to describe its range of activities and what they aim to achieve.

Chapter summary

Health can be understood from a number of different perspectives, each of which has a different focus and results in a different approach being taken to promote health. A biomedical perspective sees health as being determined primarily by physiological risk factors and thus leads to health promotion approaches that focus on preventing disease using clinically based interventions such as immunisation programmes. A behavioural perspective focuses on the ways in which people live as being key to determining their health. Promoting health is then seen as encouraging healthier lifestyles. A socio-environmental perspective, on the other hand, places emphasis on the social and economic context in which people live their lives and while recognizing the importance of biomedical and behavioural interventions, would argue for the need for change at a more structural level. Models of health promotion are useful in scoping the field of activity and analytic models such as that of Beattie (1991) can help practitioners to interrogate their practice and be more able to justify the actions they take to promote health.

Further reading and resources

Naidoo, J. and Wills, J. (2009) *Health Promotion: Foundations for Practice*, 3rd edn. Ballière Tindall, London.
This is a clear and accessible textbook which is easy to read and provides lots of examples of the application of theory to practice.

Scriven, A. (2005) *Health Promoting Practice: The Contribution of Nurses and Allied Health Professionals*. Palgrave Macmillan, Basingstoke.
A text that explores the health promotion role of numerous health care professionals with some case studies of practice.

References

Beattie, A. (1991) Knowledge and control in health promotion: a test case for social policy and social theory, in *The Sociology of the Health Service* (eds J. Gabe, M. Calnan and M. Bury), Routledge, London.

DH (Department of Health) (2004) *Choosing Health: Making Healthy Choices Easier.* The Stationery Office, London.

DH (Department of Health) (2005) The Influenza Immunisation Programme: letter from Chief Medical Officer. Available at: www.dh.gov.uk.

Downie, R.S., Tannahill, C. and Tannahill, A. (1996) *Health Promotion, Models and Values.* Oxford University Press, Oxford.

Ewles, L. and Simnett, I. (2010) *Promoting Health: A Practical Guide,* 6th edn. Ballière Tindall, London.

Lavarack, G. (2005) *Public Health, Power, Empowerment and Professional Practice.* Palgrave Macmillan, Basingstoke.

Naidoo, J. and Wills, J. (2009) *Health Promotion: Foundations for Practice,* 3rd edn. Ballière Tindall, London,

Ontario Health Promotion Resource System (n.d.) *Health Promotion 101 Online Course.* Available at: www.ohprs.ca/.

Scriven, A. (2005) *Health Promoting Practice: The Contribution of Nurses and Allied Health Professionals.* Palgrave Macmillan, Basingstoke.

Whitehead, D. (2005) The culture, context and progress of health promotion in nursing, in *Health Promoting Practice: The Contribution of Nurses and Allied Health Professionals* (ed. A. Scriven), Palgrave Macmillan, Basingstoke.

Zhu, D.Q., Norman, I.J., and While, A.E. (2011) The relationship between doctors' and nurses' own weight status and their weight management practices: a systematic review. *Obesity Reviews,* **12** (6), 459–469.

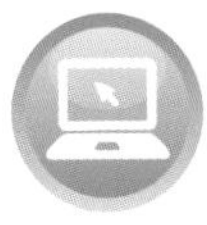

Don't forget to visit the companion website for this book: www.wileyfundamentalseries.com/healthpromotion where you can find self-assessment tests to check your progress.

4

Creating supportive environments for health

Amanda Hesman

Senior Lecturer, Adult Nursing, London South Bank University, London, UK

Learning outcomes

By the end of this chapter you will be able to:

1. Describe environments that are conducive to health
2. Discuss how the nurse and wider inter-professional team can contribute to creating supportive environments for health that make it easier for people to make healthier choices
3. Discuss how national policy has a local impact in creating supportive environments for health
4. Describe the limitations of the settings concept and barriers to its implementation

Introduction

Health promotion takes place in settings – environments where people learn, work, play and love. Understanding the nature of these settings helps us to understand how to best reach populations and how the setting itself can influence health messages, health approaches and health philosophy. This chapter will explain the origins of the World Health Organization's

Fundamentals of Health Promotion for Nurses, Second Edition. Edited by Jane Wills.

Companion website: www.wileyfundamentalseries.com/healthpromotion

(WHO) healthy settings approach and illustrate the concept with examples from schools, prisons, the health service and the workplace. Within each chosen setting, examples of good public health practice will be identified together with the organizational systems needed to create an environment supportive of health, within and between settings.

Creating supportive environments

The Ottawa Charter (WHO, 1986) describes creating supportive environments as a key action for health promotion, recognizing that an individualistic philosophy to promoting health and well-being focuses on the individual, their lifestyle, their risk behaviour, and runs the risk of blaming the individual for any ill health. The environmental, socio-economic and social context in which people live creates and maintains individual health behaviours such as smoking as a response to social expectations or drug use as a response to unemployment. The following statement from the Ottawa Charter recognizes this interplay between health, context and setting: "*Health is created and lived by people within the settings of their everyday life: where they learn, work, play and love.*"

As we saw in Chapter 2, health is determined by the interplay of environmental, organizational and personal factors. The WHO use the term "*settings*" to describe environments that can enable health and well-being. We all live in such settings whether it is the place we work, the place we live or the place we play. At a national level, the following environments have been identified as appropriate health-promoting "settings":

- schools
- prisons
- universities
- hospitals
- workplaces
- local neighbourhoods.

These settings are not merely opportunities for the delivery of health education. A health-promoting setting is one that embraces a "systems" approach towards health. A systems approach towards health is one that addresses:

- the creation of a healthy working and living environment;
- the integration of health promotion and health development into the daily activities of the setting;
- the development of links with other settings and with the wider community.

Figure 4.1 is adapted from the National Health Service (NHS) in Scotland (www.healthscotland.com). It shows how health (the tree) has its roots in biological, social and environmental factors. The trunk of the tree is supported by key health promotion principles – participation, equity, empowerment, partnerships and sustainability. The branches of the tree illustrate some of the key activities necessary to promote health in settings, such as policy development, improving the environment, building relationships and communication, involving patients and the public, monitoring and auditing services.

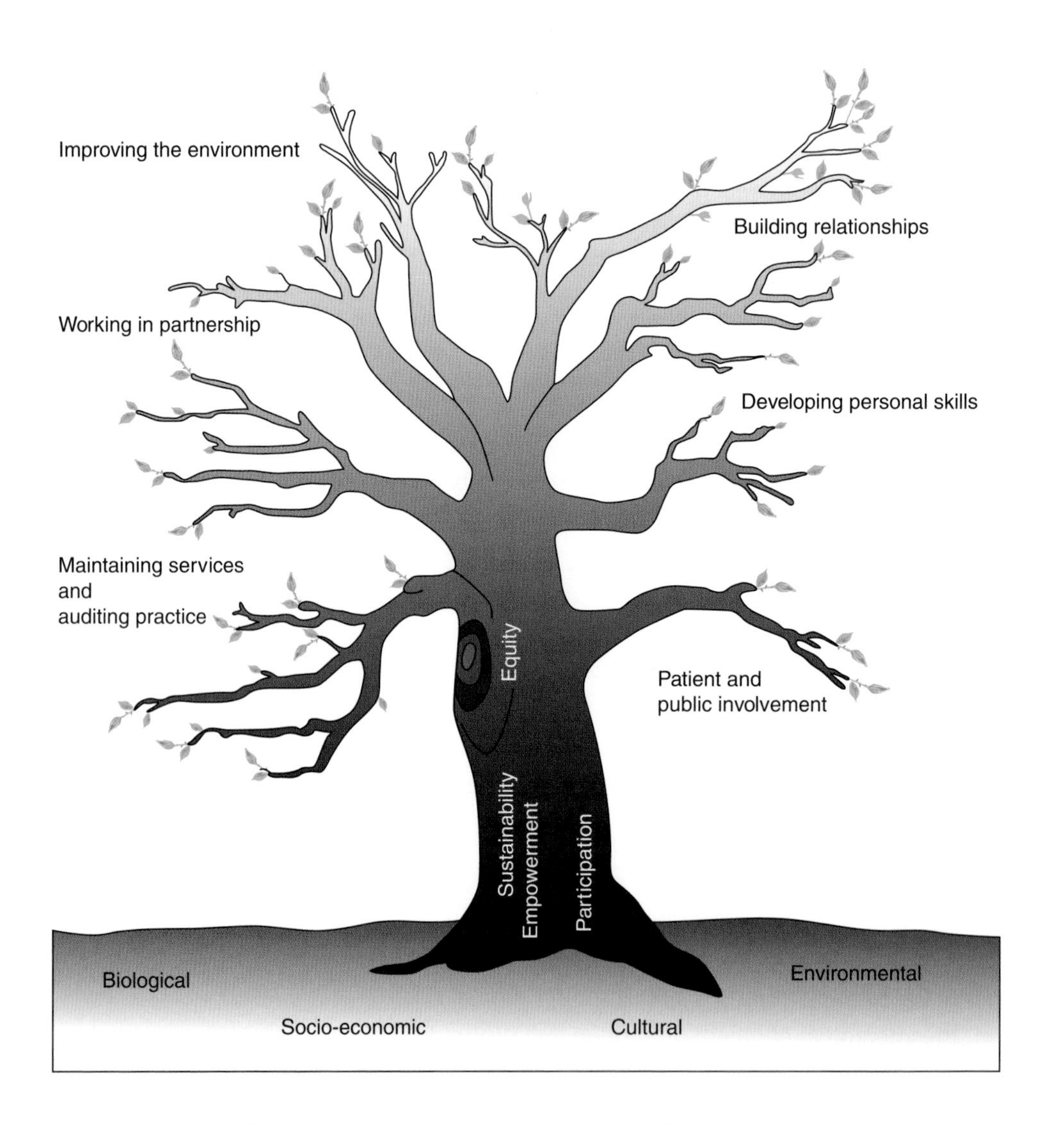

Figure 4.1 The Tree of Health Promotion. Source: adapted from NHS Scotland, 2005.

Activity 4.1

Consider your work environment, how does it facilitate the health and well-being of staff and patients?

Discussion

You might like to think about:

- *how policies and structures can enable health promoting actions, e.g. a no-smoking policy;*
- *how the physical environment impacts on those in the setting, e.g. the ward layout, lighting;*
- *how the setting can make partnerships with other agencies and the community to enable it to become more health promoting, e.g. a prison may link with the NHS to promote health;*
- *ways in which individuals can be empowered to take control over their health in the setting, e.g. flexible working arrangements;*
- *ways in which individuals can participate and be involved in determining the shape of the setting, e.g. Patient Advice and Liaison Services (PALS);*
- *ways in which the setting can contribute to sustainable development and be made more environmentally health promoting, e.g. waste management policies;*
- *ways in which healthy behaviours are encouraged, e.g. healthy food in the canteen, walking routes round the hospital.*

Creating supportive environments for health means adopting a wider and more holistic approach that sees health as "*not merely the absence of disease*" (WHO, 1948). An environment can be identified as being supportive to health if it enables healthier choices to be made and therefore sustains healthier living. Case study 4.1 has used the example of cycling as the healthier choice. Cycling has many health benefits not only for the individual but also for the environment. Individual health benefits from cycling include increased cardiovascular output, reduced coronary heart disease (CHD) risk factors and maintenance of body weight. At a collective level, benefits for the environment include fewer carbon emissions, less traffic pollution, less noise and less congestion).

Case study 4.1

Promoting the health of staff through an integrated transport policy

- *Policy*: cycle helmets are currently VAT exempt. A travel expenses policy may reimburse work-related travel by bike such as that adopted by Kings College NHS Trust, London. A health and safety policy will provide additional staff insurance for those cycling to and from work.
- *Environment*: the work environment supports cycling to work with sufficient and secure bike sheds, showers and changing room facilities. Also by the provision of bikes at work that can be used by staff for meetings between sites.
- *Partnership building*: working with local authorities in order to provide training for employees and their families on how to cycle safely. Working with local transport planners to ensure that the hospital and surrounding roads facilitate safer cycling.
- *Empowerment*: a consultation exercise that actively seeks the views of its employees on barriers to cycling to work and then consults on an action plan to overcome these barriers.
- *Participation*: having a cyclists user group that informs management of the needs of those cycling to work, for example, Newham Trust London has such a group. In conjunction with the police and transport planners, organize a "critical mass demonstration" for your local area.
- *Sustainable change*: in order to bring about sustainable change, cycling to work needs to be the easier choice for the majority of employees, and this means prioritizing the needs of the cyclist above those of the car driver.

Consider the approaches to health promotion outlined in Chapter 3. The spectrum of health promotion responsibility can be seen as if on a continuum – at one end, the health problem and solution so that the health problem lies with the individual and their behaviour. At the other end of the "Solution Spectrum", the health problem and solution lie within the setting. Figure 4.2 is a diagrammatic representation showing how public health/health care promotion can be framed. For example, traditional approaches to tackling workplace stress tend to see the individual as unable to manage the stresses and demands of the job and thus the answer is to offer counselling and stress management programmes. A "settings" approach locates the problem clearly in the organization itself in workplace cultures that inhibit decision-making or control and the solutions might be improving communication strategies or task work groups. The health promoting activity that is used will depend on how the problem is framed.

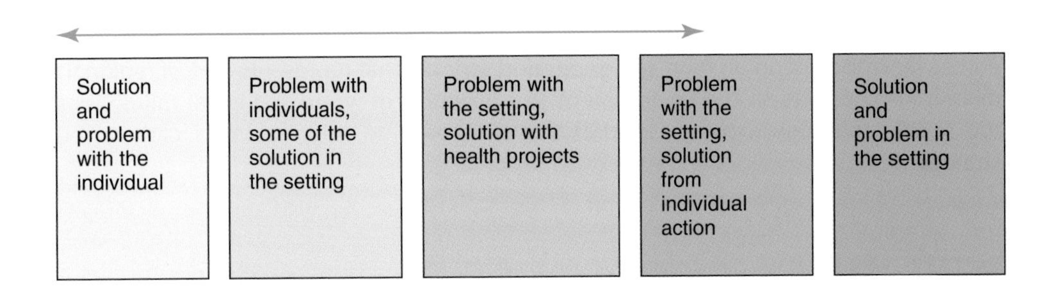

Figure 4.2 The solution spectrum. Source: based on Whitelaw *et al.*, 2001.

A health promoting health service

There is a clear role for the NHS as a health promotion service that makes the most of the 74.4 million outpatients appointments, attended from April 2012 to March 2013 (HSCIS, 2013). During the same period, 18.3 million A&E attendances were recorded. Of these, 3.8 million resulted in admission to hospital for inpatient treatment, 3.7 million resulted in a GP follow-up, and 7.1 million were discharged with no follow-up. (HSCIS, 2013) The NHS is the biggest employer in Europe and as such, has an enormous health promotion potential for its 3.1 million workforce.

For the NHS, a typical day includes:

- over 835000 people visiting their GP practice or practice nurse;
- almost 50000 people visiting accident and emergency departments;
- 49000 outpatient consultations;
- 94000 people admitted to hospital as an emergency admission;
- 36000 people in hospital for planned treatment.

Current levels of sickness absence among NHS staff mean that 10.3 million working days are lost in the NHS in England each year. The annual direct cost of absence is estimated to be £1.7 billion a year. Reducing this sickness and absence by one-third would make direct cost savings of £555 million (DH, 2011).

The Boorman Report (2009) emphasizes achieving physical, mental and social "contentment" for all NHS employees and recognizes that employment needs to be good for mental and physical health. Indeed, good employment is protective of good health and poor employment is detrimental to health and well-being. This report makes clear the links between the workforce well-being and key outcome measures such as patient satisfaction and Trust performance. The report highlights case studies of interventions for NHS staff ranging from the provision of complementary therapies, mindfulness training, on-site access to physiotherapy, and even to a fruit van.

The NHS is also enormous. It has a huge impact on local economies as an employer and purchaser with a spend on food and goods and services that represents 10% of regional economies. It also impacts on the environment as a producer of waste and in car miles –issues that the Sustainable Development Unit of the NHS aims to address in its carbon reduction strategy.

Activity 4.2

Debate the following: "health services are designed to deal with health" or "health services are designed to deal with illness". Which statement do you agree with and why?

The hospital setting

Traditionally hospitals have adopted a "downstream approach" to health and have only been curative environments for patients. This has meant that hospitals have lacked an emphasis on sustaining and improving health and well-being for staff, patients and the wider community.

The WHO Health Promoting Hospital (HPH) Network was launched in recognition of the impact that the hospital can have on the health and well-being of its staff, patients and the wider population (see WHO, 2007). In appreciation of the wider public health role that hospitals can have in tackling the broader determinants of health, the European Network of Health Promoting Hospitals was launched in 1990 and subsequently the English Network of Health Promoting Hospitals and Trusts was established.

Apart from improving the quality of care delivered, hospitals can also contribute to the health of the population as follows. First, hospitals exist within a community and an HPH should be establishing alliances and partnerships with their community to promote "concepts of cure, care and prevention". For example, the HPH should:

- actively seek user representation from minority and disadvantaged groups such as the intellectually impaired, and provide meaningful involvement from the community when new services are planned;
- provide free first aid training for child minders or provide free falls prevention training for elderly groups;
- create a calm and pleasing environment using nature and the arts.

Second, as a major source of employment for local populations, the NHS is ideally placed to improve their health through health and safety measures at work and via sustainable terms and conditions of employment. For example, the HPH should:

- implement healthy working initiatives such as promoting a healthier workplace by providing exercise facilities or offering subsidized membership to local sports facilities;
- implement health and safety policies such as control of substances hazardous to health regulations (COSHH) and have no lifting policies;

- support individuals back to work after periods of sustained illness;
- provide a comprehensive occupational health service;
- support staff in career development;
- provide on-site child care.

Third, an HPH has the potential to work with the local community to lobby and influence local and regional policy on issues such as:

- transport planning;
- smoke-free environments;
- the provision of healthy catering in private and public care homes;
- access to affordable, high quality fruit and vegetables.

The reality of the hospital setting is one where there are many barriers to improving the health and well-being of staff, patients, visitors and the local population. These include financial, physical, organizational and motivational barriers.

- *Staff*: lack of readily available lifting equipment, poor standard of induction programmes for new members of staff, poor communication and consultation procedures, poor supervision of learners, shift work.
- *Patients*: high rates of hospital-acquired infection that delay recovery, long periods of unnecessary immobility, insufficient information on their condition, prognosis and progress, insufficient hydration, insufficient pain relief.
- *Visitors*: unduly restrictive visiting times, insufficient signposts on hospital grounds, poor access by public transport, which can be expensive or due to a lack of a car.

Activity 4.3

What might a health-promoting hospital look like?

Discussion

You might consider some of the following:

- *A staff restaurant that offers a range of healthier choices prominently positioned and competitively priced.*
- *Free breakfasts offered to cyclists during "Bike to Work Week" when bike maintenance classes are held.*
- *A waste policy on pharmaceutical waste, incineration, water use.*
- *A partnership with a local fitness and leisure club scheme.*
- *A Green Hospital Transport policy would include secure bike stands, interest-free loans for a bike, a car sharing scheme and pedometers to encourage staff to walk to work.*
- *Staff groups on working conditions.*

The pharmacy setting

The Pharmacy White Paper (DH, 2008) clearly sets out the direction that the pharmacy service should take, which includes a shift from dispensing to the provision of clinical services that make more use of the clinical skills of pharmacy staff. To achieve this, pharmacies will promote health, well- being and self-care, will be the first port of call for minor ailments and will support patients with long-term conditions. Community pharmacists are well placed to do this:

- An estimated 1.2 million people visit a pharmacy each day for health-related reasons.
- Pharmacists may have established relationships and rapport with many of their regular customers. Regular customers will include those people with long-term conditions such as CHD and those that have physical and intellectual disabilities that require pharmacological support and advice on health management.
- Pharmacists are considered experts on medicines by health workers and the public alike, which puts them in an influential position to promote health and prevent ill health.

Activity 4.4

How might a pharmacy contribute to health promotion?

Discussion

An individual with diabetes may benefit from secondary or tertiary health interventions, a discussion of lifestyle changes, management of poly pharmacy and referral to a long-term condition management programme such as the Expert Patient Programme (EPP). Reasons for non-concordance with medication are varied and may include:

- *lack of understanding;*
- *forgetfulness;*
- *lack of information;*
- *fear of side effects;*
- *"feeling better";*
- *denial of need;*
- *an attempt at regaining some autonomy.*

Evidence indicates that participation in self-management programmes does increase a sense of empowerment and symptom control (see Chapter 9). There are two national structured educational programmes for diabetics: Diabetes Education and Self Management for ongoing and Newly Diagnosed Diabetics (DESMOND) aimed at type 2 diabetics and Dose Adjustment For Normal Eating (DAFNE) aimed at type 1 diabetics (DH, 2007).

Table 4.1 Pharmacy services and health promotion.

Primary prevention	Health education	Health protection
Advice on immunizations and vaccinations Chlamydia screening Access to emergency contraception Identification of individuals who would benefit from "over the counter" statins	Medication concordance, adherence and the management of poly pharmacy Advice on the management of long-term conditions such as asthma Participation in media campaigns such as Medicines Awareness Week, how to deal with the flu and the taking of folic acid in pregnancy Skills training, e.g. inhaler technique for people with asthma Advice on methadone programmes and benzodiazepine reduction Symptom management Local knowledge of statutory and non-statutory health services	Cessation programmes that use nicotine replacement therapy and behaviour modification intervention Ensuring antibiotics are prescribed appropriately and by actively participating in the monitoring of antibiotic prescriptions Ensuring that the pharmacy is accessible in location, has appropriate opening times and has an atmosphere that facilitates open communication Pregnancy testing

Although a pharmacy has the potential to promote health (Table 4.1), there are barriers to its development as a health-promoting setting: often a pharmacy may lack a confidential area for discussion; pharmacists do not routinely receive training in health promotion specifically on models of behaviour change; and despite new contractual arrangements to broaden the health improvement role of pharmacies, they are nevertheless set up as commercial businesses.

Case study 4.2

The Healthy Living Pharmacy (HLP) initiative

The Healthy Living Pharmacy (HLP) initiative started in Portsmouth in 2010. To qualify to become a healthy living pharmacy, the pharmacy needs staff trained as health champions and it must have suitable facilities such as a consultation area where people can speak to a member of the pharmacy team in private. Pharmacies should provide high quality NHS services such as weight management, stopping smoking programmes, emergency contraception and NHS health checks, in addition to the medicine supply service and advice on self-care that are provided as core.

Early evaluation results have been promising; a person walking into a HLP in Portsmouth is twice as likely to set a quit date and stop smoking than in a traditional pharmacy. In just one month, pharmacies in Portsmouth made more than 3600 alcohol interventions and directly referred 29 individuals to a specialist alcohol service (http://www.hantslpc.org.uk/uploads/Portsmouth%20HLP%20interim%20outcomes.pdf).

The school setting

The school setting has clearly been identified and supported in national policy as an environment that should be supportive to health. The Healthy Child Programme 5–19 (DH and DfCSF, 2009) is such a policy in which school nursing has been identified as crucial to the effective delivery of the key public health issues for children:

- bullying;
- emotional health and well-being;
- dental decay;
- obesity and weight management;
- teenage pregnancy;
- sexually transmitted infections;
- smoking;
- drug and alcohol misuse.

School nurses are specialist public health nurses responsible for delivering public health programmes or interventions that improve health outcomes for school-aged children. This includes assessing the school-aged population health and well-being needs and championing health promotion activities both in and out of school settings (see Chapter 17).

Health promoting schools (HPS) aim to link the day-to-day living of the child in the school to the home and to make education a route to healthy values and beliefs becoming established. HPS can support health by:

- incorporating health issues into classroom teaching, e.g. sexual health and smoking;
- offering school health services, e.g. vaccination and screening programmes;
- providing the physical space and building, e.g. sufficient areas for recreation;
- identifying vulnerable pupils, e.g. those at risk from malnourishment;
- establishing a network of partnerships within the school, e.g. with catering staff and with the local community and with environmental health officers;
- ensuring that policies that impact on staff, pupils and parents have a health framework; involving parents and carers in policy formulation, such as the provision of nutritious meals may also impact on their own health promoting behaviour.

The healthy schools initiative is a global one and widely supported in some countries. In England, it started in 1999 and schools were expected to meet the National Healthy Schools Standard (NHSS) and to demonstrate a whole school approach showing how the school tackles:

- personal, social and health education, including sex and relationship education and drug education (including alcohol, tobacco and volatile substance abuse);
- healthy eating promotion;
- physical activity promotion;
- emotional health and well-being (including bullying).

Although aspects of this are still included in the inspections by OFSTED that schools undergo, it is no longer a quality standard and schools are simply encouraged by the Department for Education under their support for pastoral care.

The prison setting

Prisons may not be immediately identified as a setting to promote health but the significant health problems experienced by prisoners both on remand and in prison demand a health improvement role. The majority of prisoners have experienced major problems prior to incarceration to a far greater extent than the general population:

- 20–30% of all offenders have learning disabilities or difficulties that interfere with their ability to cope with the criminal justice system.
- 49% of women and 23% of male prisoners in a Ministry of Justice study were assessed as suffering from anxiety and depression. This can be compared with 16% of the general UK population (12% of men and 19% of women).
- In the 12 months ending September 2012, there were a total of 23134 incidents of self-harm in prisons. Women accounted for 30% of all incidents of self-harm despite representing just 5% of the total prison population.
- A Prisons and Probation Ombudsman study found that in the 92 cases of prisoners dying from natural causes, restraints were used during final inpatient stays in outside hospitals on 29 out of 52 occasions (Prison Reform Trust, 2013).

In addition, the majority of prisoners are far more likely than the general population to experience major problems including debt, violence, sexual abuse, unemployment, homelessness, or relationship breakdown. These problems do not resolve during imprisonment and their psychological effects may become exacerbated during incarceration or upon release. The situation is compounded by being in prison, adding to the sense of isolation and hopelessness. Socio-economic deprivation is also over-represented in the prison population and dispersal to different prison settings can add to the feeling of loneliness particularly in those people who do not have the right to remain in the UK and who do not speak English. The prison has been identified internationally (WHO, 2007) as an environment that needs to be supportive for health. The Prison Service Order for Health Promotion (DH, 2003) gives advice on how to put into practice this guidance and the DH (2009) plan, "Improving Health, Supporting Justice" is a strategic framework for national coherence. It recommends a cross-cutting approach across the judicial system in order to do the following:

- reduce health inequalities;
- reduce risk behaviour;
- reduce mortality in prison and the community from suicide, accidental drugs overdose, blood-borne viruses, chronic liver disease and coronary artery disease;
- increase participation, empowerment and self-esteem for offenders and their families.

The health promoting prison has the potential to address the health needs of those who are hardest to reach in the community but a degree of tension exists between a desire for the appropriate level of security and the need for a positive health promoting environment.

Activity 4.5

How could the prison nurse be involved to improve the mental health and well-being of clients and staff?

Discussion

Prison mental health is a priority and there are numerous initiatives to promote health, including Walking the Way to Prison Health, gardening clubs, music education and Storybook Dads, an initiative to enable fathers to maintain the vital emotional bond between parent and child by enabling parents to make bedtime story CDs, DVDs and other educational gifts for their children (http://www.storybookdads.org.uk/).

Chapter summary

This chapter has discussed settings-based health promotion. This has a particular philosophy that focuses on "whole systems" with particular emphasis on participation, partnerships internally and externally, the physical environment and structures. Yet often the root causes of ill health that arise from the setting are not addressed and the setting is simply a delivery site targeting interventions at the individual rather than the setting itself. The settings approach provides a practical way to think about health promotion within specific settings such as hospitals, prisons, pharmacies, neighbourhoods, workplaces and schools. The complexities of such large organizations provide challenges that can limit the potential for improving health and wellbeing. The nurse can contribute to the health-promoting environment in three ways:

- as a nurse giving direct patient care, which includes promoting and sustaining behaviour change;
- as a responsible employee;
- as an active citizen.

It is necessary for the nurse to recognize their contribution to health and well-being as a member of an interdisciplinary team and to be conscious of their role and responsibilities in respect to the setting's core values. A nurse is, of course, responsible to individual patients and clients but needs to remain mindful and be critically aware of the "bigger picture" and reflect upon how they can contribute to the health setting's philosophy. Aspects of the "bigger picture" that the nurse needs to actively reflect upon and contribute to include the following:

- policy, e.g. implementing health and safety legislation;
- the environment, e.g. identifying physical barriers to care for people with sensory impairment;
- partnership building, e.g. understanding and respecting the different roles within the interdisciplinary team;
- empowerment, e.g. ensuring that patients and their relatives know about the PALS;
- participation, e.g. seeking out service user views;
- sustainable change, e.g. making sure changes are to systems and thus sustainable.

The nurse is able to contribute both directly and indirectly towards an environment supportive of health. Health and well-being can be sustained and improved upon while participating in direct individual care and indirectly by contributing to the setting's philosophy.

On placement: checklist

- To what extent is your placement a 'setting' in which health could be promoted?
- How health promoting were: (a) the physical environment; (b) relationships; (c) opportunities to participate?
- Was there evidence of an approach to sustainability, e.g. waste management, carbon reduction?
- How did the placement setting promote your well-being?

Key learning points

1. Health promotion takes place in settings: socially and culturally defined geographic and physical areas of social interaction such as a school. Instead of just working to change the problems of those individuals in the setting, the nurse can seek to change these social systems which can support health.
2. Each setting can promote health through its policies, ethos, environment and the ways in which it encourages staff and patients to be involved.
3. Healthy settings include hospitals, health services, workplaces, schools, universities, prisons, cities, neighbourhoods, villages and markets.

Further reading and resources

Health in Prisons Project (HIPP, 2004) *Promoting Health in Prisons: A Good Practice Guide*. Available at: http://www.hipp-europ.org.

Scriven, A. and Hodgins, M. (2012) *Health Promotion Settings: Principles and Practice*. Sage, London.

A book that considers health promotion work in a variety of settings from neighbourhoods and cities to prisons to workplaces. The book will provide many leads to further reading and examples of innovative projects.

Ubido, J., Winters, L., Ashton, M. *et al.* (2006) *Top Tips for Healthier Hospitals*. Liverpool Public Health Observatory/Cheshire and Merseyside Public Health Network, Liverpool. Available at: http://www.nwph.net/champs/Publications/Top%20tip2%20for%20healthier%20hospitals%20-%20FULL%20report.doc.

The University of Central Lancashire has a research centre devoted to the study of health promotion in different settings. Available at: http://www.uclan.ac.uk/research/environment/groups/healthy_settings_unit.php.

References

Boorman S. (2009) *NHS Health and Wellbeing*. DH, London. Available at: http://www.nhshealthandwellbeing.org/pdfs/Staff%20H&WB%20Case%20Studies%20VFinal%2023-11-09.pdf.

Department of Health (2003) *The Prison Service Order for Health Promotion (PSO 3200)*. HMS Prison Service, London.

Department of Health (2007) *Improving Diabetes Services: The NSF Four Years on London*. DH, London. Available at: http://www.bipsolutions.com/docstore/pdf/16198.pdf.

Department of Health (2008) *Pharmacy in England: Building on Strengths, Delivering the Future*. CM 7341. TSO, London. Available at: http://www.official-documents.gov.uk/document/cm73/7341/7341.pdf.

Department of Health (2009) *Improving Health, Supporting Justice: The National Delivery Plan of the Health and Criminal Justice Programme Board*. DH, London. Available at: http://www.nmhdu.org.uk/silo/files/improving-health-supporting-justice.pdf.

Department of Health (2011) *NHS Health and Well-being Improvement Framework*. DH, London. Available at: https://www.gov.uk/government/uploads/system/uploads/attachment_data/file/216380/dh_128813.pdf.

Department of Health and Department for Children, Schools and Families (2009) *Healthy Child Programme (From 5–19 Years Old)*. DH, London. Available at: http://webarchive.nationalarchives.gov.uk/20130107105354/http://www.dh.gov.uk/prod_consum_dh/groups/dh_digitalassets/documents/digitalasset/dh_108866.pdf.

HSCIS (2013) *Provisional Monthly Hospital Episode Statistics for Admitted Patient Care, Outpatients and Accident and Emergency Data, April 2012 to March 2013*. Information Centre, London.

Prison Reform Trust (2013) Bromley Briefings Prison Fact File. Available at: http://www.prisonreformtrust.org.uk/Publications/Factfile.

Whitelaw, S., Baxendale, A., Bryce, C. *et al.* (2001) "Settings" based health promotion: a review. *Health Promotion International*, **16** (4), 339–352.

World Health Organization (1948) *Constitution.* WHO, Geneva.
World Health Organization (1986) Ottawa Charter for Health Promotion. *Health Promotion*, **1** (4), i–v.
World Health Organization (2007a) *Health in Prisons.* WHO, Copenhagen.
World Health Organization (2007b) *Integrating Health Promotion into Hospitals and Health Services: Concept, Framework and Organization*. WHO, Copenhagen. Available at: http://www.euro.who.int/_data/assets/pdf_file/0009/99801/E90777.pdf.

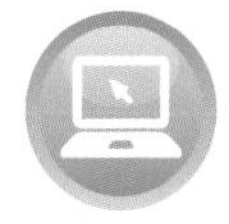

Don't forget to visit the companion website for this book: www.wileyfundamentalseries.com/healthpromotion where you can find self-assessment tests to check your progress.

Part Two

Public Health Priorities

Introduction

Health priorities in the UK are largely determined by morbidity and mortality data. As we have seen in Chapter 2, a range of factors such as socio-economic status, age and ethnicity as well as lifestyles and health behaviour can influence these rates of illness and death.

Public health priorities are those issues that are the greatest cause of disease and death. They may become a public health concern because of:

- their impact on the health of the population as a whole;
- their impact on the health budget;
- public or professional concern about the issue.

Obviously, public health priorities change over time and some may become obsolete if, for example, a disease is eradicated such as diphtheria, smallpox or cholera due to improved sanitation and vaccination programmes. Conversely, some health problems become much greater public health concerns and as a result, have become priorities such as obesity, which has reached epidemic proportions and trebled in the last two decades.

Deaths from cancers, coronary heart disease (CHD) and stroke have risen in the last couple of decades also. They now account for around two-thirds of all deaths. Cancer, stroke and heart disease not only kill, but also are also major causes of ill health, preventing people from living their lives to the full and causing avoidable disability, pain and anxiety. These diseases are largely preventable as their greatest risk factors arise from individual behaviours and the way that people lead their lives.

We know the most significant factors as shown in Figure 0.1 that lead to poor health: smoking; high blood pressure; obesity; poor diet; lack of exercise; and excessive alcohol consumption.

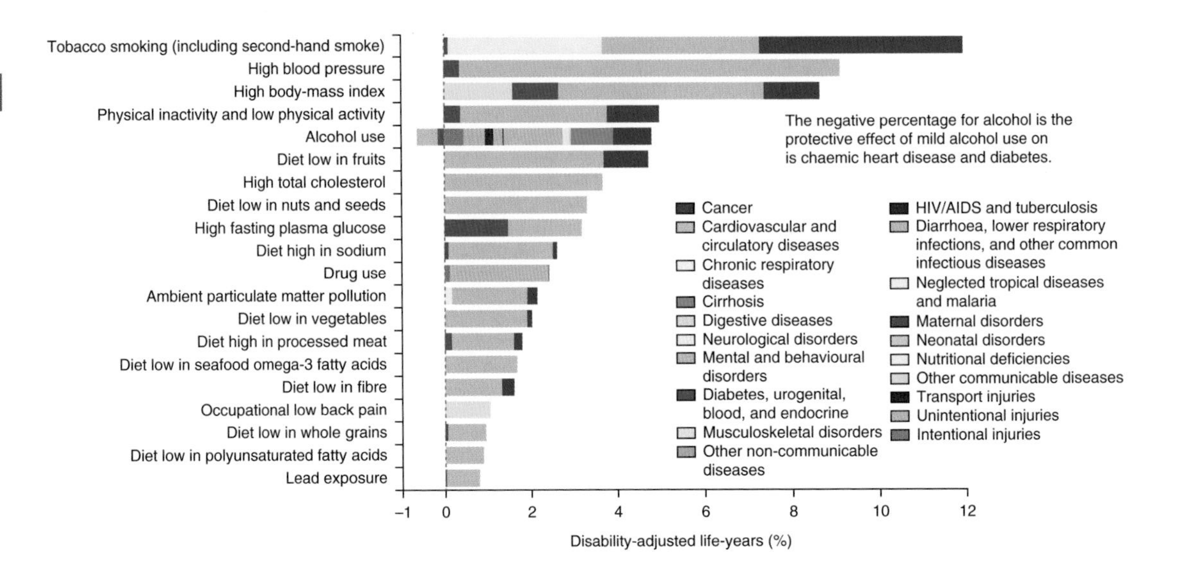

Figure 0.1 The burden of disease attributable to 20 leading risk factors. Source: Murray *et al.*, 2013, Figure 7, p. 19. Reproduced with permission of Elsevier.

Smoking remains the single biggest preventable cause of ill health and there are approximately 114000 premature deaths from smoking in the UK every year. Most deaths from smoking are related to lung cancer, CHD and chronic obstructive pulmonary disease. Alcohol is a factor in 20–30% of accidents and thus places a particular strain on accident and emergency departments. Alcohol-related deaths cause between 20000–40000 deaths in England and Wales from stroke, cancer and liver disease. Beyond these the wider determinants of health (poor early childhood experience, poor education, lack of work and poor environments) have been described in the Marmot Review, *Fair Society, Healthy Lives* (Marmot, 2010)(see Chapter 2) and it is these that lie behind the marked health inequalities between the richest and the poorest.

There are numerous ways in which these issues are addressed from medical assessments such as NHS Health Checks that are offered to men and women aged 40–74. Everyone receiving an NHS Health Check receives individually tailored advice and support to help manage their risk of heart disease, stroke and diabetes. There are also interventions that seek to regulate the environment such as a ban on cigarette vending machines in order to make healthier choices easier.

The traditional focus of health promotion has been on modifying those behaviours such as smoking and diet that are known to have an impact on people's health. The English national public health strategy *Healthy Lives, Healthy People* (DH, 2010) emphasizes the role that individuals play in determining their health choices. Even when we know what would be healthy choices, we do not necessarily choose them. All sorts of factors influence the choices we make. People respond to the social context in which they live and may participate in health-damaging behaviours in order to cope with the pressures of their everyday lives. Graham (1993), for example, found in her studies about women and smoking, that women from lower socio-economic groups reported that it was the only thing they had for themselves in a world of insurmountable difficulties. Marsh and McKay (1994) found that 70% of lone parents smoke compared to 28% of the rest of the population. Many nurses feel that smoking is their only pleasure in an otherwise stressful day and allows them to acquire their much-needed breaks (McKenna *et al.*, 2003). Protective health behaviours are also less common among people living in disadvantaged circumstances. It is not simply that people do not know that their health behaviour is damaging to their health, but access to and availability of healthy opportunities such as exercise facilities or fresh fruit and vegetables may be less obtainable. The Whitehall Study of civil servants found that lower grades report more stress and have less social support and personal resources to deal with the sources of stress (Cabinet Office, 1997).

The NHS and every health care professional are being urged to "make every contact count": use every contact with an individual to maintain or improve their mental and physical health and well-being where possible, whatever the nurse's specialty or the purpose of the contact with the patient. This will mean that the nurse needs to reassess how they use their time with the public and with every contact, aim to offer advice and support to maintain or improve a person's mental and physical health and well-being, which might mean looking outside their initial symptom or concern. Nurses are trained in their own field and develop clinical skills but may not feel confident in other health areas, such as nutrition and obesity, or the signs of unhealthy stress or anxiety. Nurses now receive universal training in child safeguarding or patient safety and, increasingly, there will be an expectation that the nurse is confident in public health and health promotion.

Health promotion is an inherently political activity, reflecting current ideologies about the organization of society and the extent to which people are connected to each other, society's health and social care provision, the extent of personal responsibility, legitimate means to encourage choice and the role of government legislation (Naidoo and Wills, 2009). An understanding of the national and local policy agenda will help the nurse identify how they can make an explicit contribution to meeting targets and priorities for health improvement (e.g. childhood obesity, sexual health, smoking). Part Two discusses current public health priorities and some of the many targets set by the government aimed at improving the health of the population contained in a number of policy documents such as the public health White Paper, *Healthy Lives, Healthy People* (DH, 2010). Chapters 6–9 discuss why certain health issues become national priorities, why the nurse should be involved and some examples of actions they can take as advocates for public health and health promotion initiatives.

References

Cabinet Office (1997) *Work Stress and Health: The Whitehall II Study*. London Public and Commercial Services Union, London.

Department of Health (2010) *Healthy Lives, Healthy People: Our Strategy for Public Health in England.* TSO, London.

Graham, H. (1993) *Hardship and Health in Women's Lives*. London, Wheatsheaf.

Marsh A. and McKay S. (1994) *Poor Smokers*. London Policy Studies Institute, London.

Marmot, M. (2010) *Fair Society, Healthy Lives*. DH, London. Available at: http://www.instituteofhealthequity.org/projects/fair-society-healthy-lives-the-marmot-review.

McKenna, H., Slater, P.. McCance, T. *et al.* (2003) The role of stress, peer influence and education levels on the smoking behaviour of nurses, *International Journal of Nursing Studies*, **40**, 359–366.

Naidoo, J. and Wills, J. (2009) *Foundations for Health Promotion*. Elsevier, London.

5

Smoking

Jenny Husbands

Senior Lecturer, Health Adult Nursing, London South Bank University, London, UK

Jane Wills

Professor, Health Promotion, London South Bank University, London, UK

Learning outcomes

By the end of this chapter you will be able to:

1. Understand the reasons why people smoke
2. Have an overview of the policies designed to address smoking and tobacco control
3. Have an overview of the strategies designed to help patients stop smoking
4. Consider the role of the nurse in health promotion

Introduction

Smoking is the most important risk factor for coronary vascular disease (CVD), cancer, respiratory diseases and low birth weight. Although the health risks of smoking are the focus of numerous health education campaigns and successive governments have attached high importance to reducing smoking rates, some people are unable or unwilling to stop smoking.

Internationally cigarette smoking is increasing in some countries and for some communities which has led to the international community led by the WHO drafting policies aimed at helping people to stop smoking and to challenge the role of the tobacco industry. This chapter will

Fundamentals of Health Promotion for Nurses, Second Edition. Edited by Jane Wills.

Companion website: www.wileyfundamentalseries.com/healthpromotion

discuss the prevalence of smoking and the approaches used to address smoking through attempts to help people quit and tobacco control policies.

Factors influencing smoking

Activity 5.1

Why do people smoke? List as many reasons as you can think of.

Discussion

- *Addiction: Nicotine in cigarettes is a stimulant that affects the brain quickly, releasing dopamine, giving a feeling of pleasure. This means that smokers start to make a link between the act of smoking and its effects and even the taste of cigarettes, the holding of a cigarette or the feeling of smoking. Because it is addictive, smokers may dislike the symptoms that come from giving up nicotine including cravings, irritability, anxiety, difficulty concentrating, restlessness and disturbed sleep.*
- *Stress: Many people claim that smoking helps them to cope with stress. People smoke at times of anxiety or distress or when they need a break which partly explains why nurses and lone parents smoke. Because nicotine is a stimulant, cigarettes will not actually help a person relax.*
- *Peer group: Young people start to smoke in the teenage years if those around them smoke, including their parents, or if they believe that smoking will raise their self-esteem and make them appear mature. Smoking is more common among those with low educational achievement (Kobus, 2003). Some young women start smoking as a means of suppressing their appetite and controlling their weight (PHRC, 2009) in societies where being thin is socially desirable and where being overweight is stigmatized.*
- *Tobacco marketing: Despite attempts to control the promotion of tobacco, cigarettes still seem glamorous, appealing, fashionable and attractive and designed to appeal to the young.*

Tobacco use in the United Kingdom dates back to the sixteenth century when it was imported from Asia and commonly consumed by pipe smoking, as snuff or was chewed, all of the above predominately by men. By the nineteenth century, tobacco consumption changed with the advent of the Industrial Revolution and the mass production of cigarettes. Cigarette smoking was also moving away from a male-dominated and predominantly middle-class domain to a cross-cultural behaviour taken up by both males and females and across the social strata (WHO, 2011). Smoking was seen as socially desirable and acceptable and was actively encouraged in the media as both fashionable and stylish and a means of coping with life's stresses.

Case study 5.1

Shisha and chewing tobacco

Other products are sometimes thought to be safer than cigarettes. Shisha pipes use tobacco sweetened with fruit or molasses sugar, which makes the smoke more aromatic than cigarette smoke. Smoking shisha means that the person and anyone near them are inhaling smoke that contains nicotine, tar, carbon monoxide and heavy metals, such as arsenic and lead. Because people smoke shisha for much longer periods of time, in one hour they may inhale the same amount of smoke as 100 cigarettes.

"Smokeless tobacco" is typically used by people of South Asian origin where a wad of tobacco is placed in the mouth or nose and chewed. Betel quid, paan or gutkha is a mixture of ingredients including betel nut (also called areca nut), herbs, spices and often tobacco, wrapped in a betel leaf. Smokeless tobacco raises the risk of mouth cancer and oesophageal cancer (NICE, 2012).

Prevalence of smoking

Currently, in the United Kingdom, approximately 20% of the adult population smoke:

- In England, 22% of men and 18% of women smoke.
- In Wales, 25% of men and 22% of women smoke.
- In Scotland, 22% of men and 23% of women smoke.
- In Northern Ireland, 24% of men and 25% of women smoke (ONS, 2013).

Current smokers smoked an average of 12.7 cigarettes per day. Among pupils aged 11–15, in England, in 2011, 5% were regular smokers (smoking at least one cigarette a week).

In the UK there is a direct correlation between smoking rates and social class; data from the General Lifestyle Survey shows that in 2010 28% of smokers were from manual occupations, whereas 13% were from managerial and professional backgrounds. Smokers from manual backgrounds started smoking early in their lives; 48% of men and 40% of women were smoking by the age of 16, compared to 33% of men and 28% of women from managerial and professional backgrounds (ONS, 2013). Figure 5.1 illustrates the clear step-wise

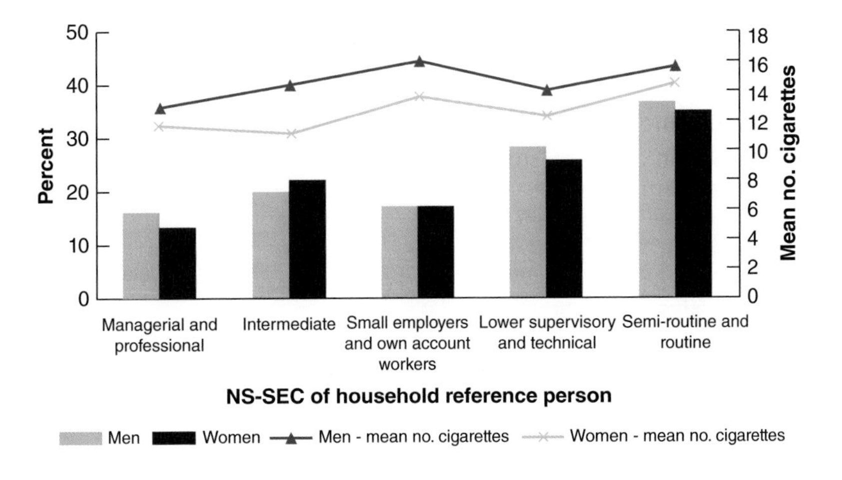

Figure 5.1 Cigarette smoking by social class and gender in Scotland 2011. Source: Dowling, 2012; Figure 4A, p. 108. Reproduced under the Open Government Licence.

gradient in smoking prevalence with social class in Scotland in 2011. Smoking rates are greatest among those in greatest hardship. Smoking accounts for nearly half of the health inequalities experienced by lower socio-economic groups (Jha *et al.*, 2006). Almost 80% of the world's smokers live in low- or middle-income countries and if current trends persist by 2030, it is estimated that eight million people will die as a result of tobacco inhalation both actively and passively; and 80% of those people will be from low- or middle-income families (Cancer Research UK, 2013).

Activity 5.2

What do you think accounts for the greater prevalence of smoking among lower socio-economic groups?

Discussion

This has very little to do with education or motivation – knowledge of smoking risks and motivation to quit are similar across all social groups. People from lower socio-economic groups are far less likely to quit smoking, possibly because hardship makes it less likely for them to attend cessation groups; a higher proportion of smokers in their social network and/or their spouse or partner may be more likely to smoke; and disadvantaged smokers are often more highly addicted, for example, they may smoke more cigarettes a day.

Activity 5.3

Figure 5.2 shows a decline in smoking over the last few decades. What do you think are the reasons for the decline in cigarette smoking?

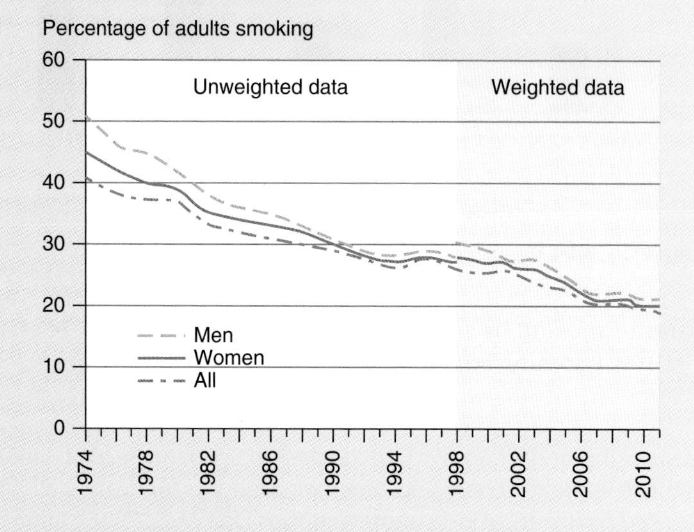

Figure 5.2 The decline in smoking in UK, 1974–2010. Source: Office for National Statistics, 2013, Figure 1.1, p. 4. Reproduced under the Open Government Licence.

Discussion

The decline in cigarette smoking since the 1970s can be attributed to:

- *improved public awareness of the health risks and better health promotion and public health campaigns;*
- *improved access to smoking cessation services, including nicotine replacement therapy;*
- *the rise in tobacco taxation and the price of cigarettes;*
- *the control of smoking in public places.*

There are other differences in smoking prevalence (Cancer Research UK, 2013):

- *Ethnicity differences*: 20% of Indian men smoke; 40% of Bangladeshi men smoke, whereas only 2% of Bangladeshi women smoke.
- *Geographic differences*: UK smoking rates are higher in Scotland and Wales, and higher in the North West and Yorkshire and Humberside.

This indicates that smoking is deemed socially acceptable for some ethnic groups and that there are gender differentials in the social acceptability of smoking. In some cultures, smoking is both acceptable and desirable and may be viewed as a status symbol, indicating wealth or position;

it could be argued that some minority ethnic groups smoke because of the inequalities and discrimination they face and use smoking as a coping mechanism. These figures demonstrate the strong association between tobacco consumption, income and the strategies individuals adopt to cope with their overwhelmingly difficult lives.

Case study 5.2

Smoking in pregnancy

In the UK, approximately 25–30% of pregnant women smoke; the effects of smoking in pregnancy include pre-term labour; a low birth weight baby; foetal inter-uterine growth retardation and maternal hypertension. Interventions to support pregnant women to stop smoking include smoking cessation groups which could be either based in hospital or primary care; telephone counselling; demonstrating empathy, unconditional positive regard and support and nicotine replacement therapy.

A systematic review of how to stop smoking in pregnancy and following childbirth (Baxter *et al.*, 2009) found that a high proportion (but not all) staff routinely ask about smoking status. There is the suggestion that concerns about damage to the relationship between professional and pregnant woman may be important and prevent staff from raising the issue. There is also evidence of differences in approach between professionals, such as cutting down versus quitting and the importance attached to quitting. Differences between women regarding preferences for information and follow-up discussion suggest the importance of individual tailored advice and the challenge of providing content appropriate to each woman's needs/ wishes.

Smoking as a public health priority

Smoking accounts for:

- 80% of deaths from lung cancer;
- 80% of deaths from bronchitis and emphysema;
- 17% of deaths from heart disease;
- 25% of all cancer deaths. These include cancer of the lung, mouth, lip, throat, bladder, kidney, pancreas, stomach, liver and cervix.

Other effects of smoking include:

- Women smokers go through the menopause up to two years earlier than non-smokers and are at a greater risk of developing osteoporosis;
- Smoking has been associated with increased sperm abnormalities and is a cause of impotence.
- Smokers are more likely to develop facial wrinkles at a younger age and have dental hygiene problems (London Health Observatory, 2012).

Passive smoking in children costs at least £9.7 million each year in UK primary care visits and asthma treatment costs, and £13.6 million in UK hospital admissions. The cost of providing asthma drugs for children who develop asthma each year as a result of passive smoking up until the age 16 in the UK is approximately £4 million annually. Two million children in the UK under 16 still live in a household where they are exposed to SecondHand Smoke(SHS) (ASH, 2011). In children, second-hand smoke (SHS) can cause:

- asthma
- sudden infant death syndrome (SIDS)
- middle ear disease
- bronchitis
- pneumonia
- coughing and wheezing.

Activity 5.4

How would you explain the impact of smoking to a patient?

Discussion

The oxygen in the body is transported around by the haemoglobin within the red blood cells. Every time a person breathes in smoke, they absorb the carbon monoxide (CO) through their lungs. CO sticks to red blood cells 200 times more easily than oxygen. So when a person smokes, the CO passes across into the red blood cells and takes some of the oxygen's space. When blood cells are carrying CO, they cannot carry as much oxygen, therefore, meaning that smokers are often managing on lower levels of oxygen.

Figure 5.3 shows what happens to the human body when smoking and the possible associated diseases. There are numerous benefits of stopping smoking in the short and longer term:

1. Return to normal pulse and blood pressure rates after 20 minutes.
2. Nicotine and carbon monoxide reduced by 50% after eight hours.
3. Oxygen levels returned to normal after eight hours.
4. Carbon monoxide rates eliminated from the body after 24 hours.
5. Lungs start to clear mucus and other debris after 24 hours.
6. No nicotine left in the body after 48 hours.
7. Taste and smell sensations greatly improved after 48 hours.
8. Circulation improvement and increased oxygen levels after 2–12 weeks.
9. Coughs, wheezing and breathing problems improve and lung function increases by 5–10% by 3–9 months.
10. The risk of lung cancer decreases by 50% and the risk of myocardial infarction is on a par with that of a non-smoker after ten years.

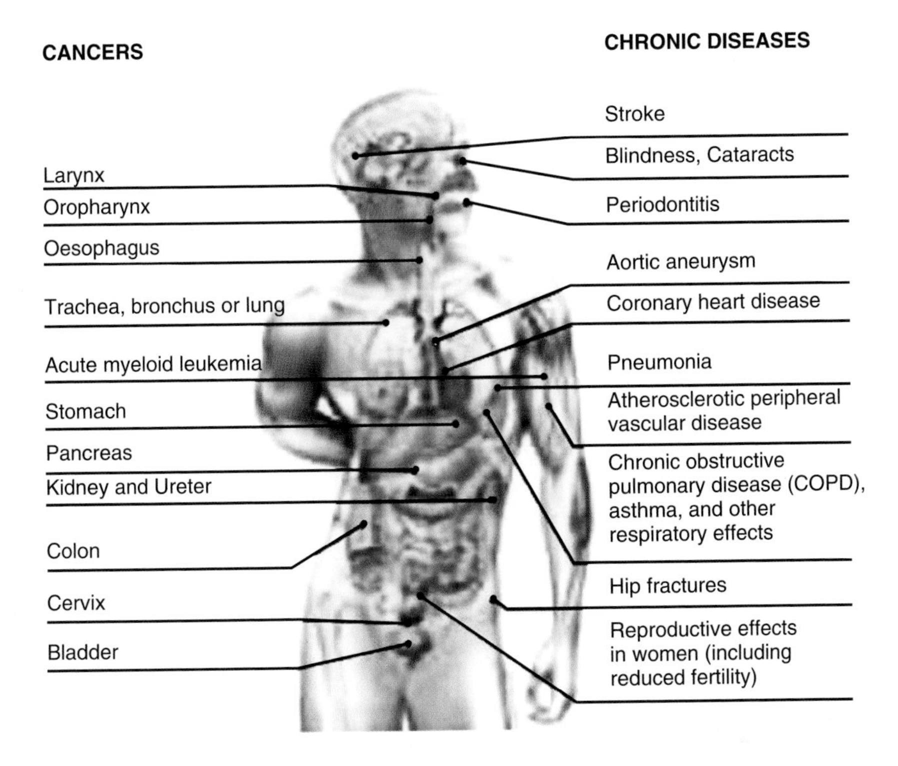

Figure 5.3 The impact of smoking on the body.

Many patients who smoke may be reluctant to quit because of their anxiety about some of the side effects of withdrawal which may include tearfulness, cough, light-headedness, mouth ulcers, sleep disturbance and increased appetite or weight gain. The main reasons people can put on weight are because:

- Nicotine suppresses the natural appetite and increases the body's metabolism.
- When people stop smoking, their appetite often increases.
- People often find that food is tastier and so eat more after they stop smoking.
- Some people replace cigarettes with snacks and sweets.

Addressing smoking: tobacco control

Tobacco control is a worldwide initiative and the WHO Tobacco Free Initiative (TFI) aims to develop smoking cessation initiatives, treat tobacco dependence, and address the issue of tobacco control. In the European Union, health policy is set by the member states but in the UK, overall tobacco control and smoking cessation policy fall under the remit of the following government departments:

- the Department of Health
- the Treasury
- Her Majesty's Revenue and Customs
- the UK Border Agency
- the Department of Education and Industry.

The Health and Social Care Act (2012) changed the structure of the NHS in England and will inevitably have an impact on the delivery and management of tobacco control strategies, for example, stop smoking services which are managed and primarily delivered by public health departments have moved into the local authority domain. With the demise of the primary care trusts and the transfer of the roles and responsibilities of the primary care trusts to clinical commissioning groups, smoking cessation work will be transferred to the commissioning groups. This may have an impact on which services are available and how services are delivered (ASH, 2013a).

Joossens and Raw's (2011) study of 30 European countries found that the United Kingdom scored the highest in the range of tobacco control measures. These measures are different within government departments and each department will inevitably have different agendas and approaches to tobacco control and smoking cessation. For example, the Department of Health will have a health remit and will place their emphasis on:

- health improvement;
- education to enable people to make informed choices;
- the prevention and treatment of smoking-related disease;
- managing long-term conditions related to smoking;
- supporting people to stop smoking.

Because smoking is so embedded in society, a comprehensive approach is needed to reduce public acceptability. In recent years this has entailed a three-pronged approach that includes reducing access to cigarettes and tobacco products for young people; using taxation to raise the price; and ending all tobacco advertising and promotion. In addition, smoking is no longer allowed in public places. The dates of some of the actions taken to control tobacco in the UK are outlined in Table 5.1.

Current UK stop smoking policy includes the following aims:

- to reduce rates of smoking in adults to 18.5% by 2015;
- to reduce smoking rates in 15-year-old or younger age groups to 12% by 2015;
- to reduce smoking rates in pregnant women to 11% or less by 2015;
- to hold public consultations on the plain packaging of cigarettes;
- to ban cigarette vending machines;
- to ban cigarette displays at the point of sale, in large shops, e.g. supermarkets from 2012 and in small shops from 2015 (DH, 2011; ASH, 2012).

Table 5.1 Tobacco control in England, 2000–2013.

Year	Policy
2002	Ban on tobacco advertising
2004	Tackling tobacco smuggling
2007	Ban on smoking in public places
2007	Rise in the legal age for tobacco purchase to 18
2009	Ban on cigarettes in vending machines
2012	Tax on tobacco raised to 5% above inflation
2013	Phased introduction of ban on display of cigarettes in supermarkets and shops
2013	Postponement of the introduction of plain packaging for cigarettes

Activity 5.5

Would you support an extension of legislation to include the following bans?:

- No smoking in cars where there are children.
- No smoking in the vicinity of hospital grounds.
- No smoking in parks.
- Electronic cigarettes.

Discussion

Although widely supported and producing some health benefits, particularly for those working in the hospitality industry, legislation to prohibit smoking in indoor public places and workplaces has not reduced the proportion of children exposed to damaging levels of second-hand smoke (Sims et al., 2012). There is, therefore, a lobby to extend protection for children from SHS.

NICE is currently investigating new guidance on how to help people stop smoking when using hospital services, which may include the recommendation to ban smoking in all hospital grounds.

Electronic cigarettes will be licensed as a medicine in the UK from 2016 and available as an aid to quitting. They will not be able to be used in public spaces and will be controlled by advertising restrictions. Many health care professional organizations are concerned that they may make smoking appear acceptable.

Addressing smoking: creating supportive environments

In order to help people to quit smoking, the environment has to be conducive and supportive. This is particularly true of hospitals which can encourage patients to quit by being completely non-smoking areas, by treating nicotine withdrawal and by offering referral services to patients prior to surgery, and to those attending out-patient clinics such as respiratory and cardiac rehabilitation.

NICE guidelines (2008) recommend that:

- All patients who smoke should be given information about smoking cessation.
- All patients should routinely have their smoking status recorded and offered brief opportunistic interventions to help them to make an informed choice.
- All patients should be offered a referral to a specialist service.
- Nicotine withdrawal should be recognized and patients offered appropriate treatment, e.g. nicotine replacement therapy.
- Staff should be made aware that nicotine affects the metabolism and therefore drug interactions may be compromised.
- The discharge plan for patients leaving hospital should include advice and offer continuity, liaison with community services, and of course on-going support.
- Follow-up for patients should include recording the patient's smoking status.

It is important to remember patients may not be aware of the services available or all the health problems associated with smoking, so nurses must ensure patients are given information so that they can make an informed choice.

Case study 5.3

Stop smoking in secondary care

In 2009, Blackpool Teaching Hospitals NHS Foundation Trust implemented an organizational public health strategy. A key element of this strategy has been the delivery of the stop smoking in secondary care service. The service aimed to embed the assessment of smoking status and offer support to smokers in every clinical contact; to improve uptake to effective forms of support either via referral or medication; and to offer clinical support to smokers who are in hospital and experiencing forced abstinence. It was recognized that patients who smoked spent an average of two days longer in hospital and it was further acknowledged that the hospital setting provided an excellent opportunity to influence the health behaviour of patients as they may be more receptive to health advice and support while in hospital. The scheme included training for all clinical and non-clinical staff across the Trust on the "stop smoking care pathway"; the establishment of a stop smoking specialist adviser post; a publicity campaign under the brand name "a better tomorrow" with a strapline for stopping smoking,

"Stop smoking, start living a better tomorrow". Over a 12-month period, the service trained 385 staff in brief intervention, encouraged 500 clients to set a quit date and saw 232 proceed to stop smoking. The ward-based support received by clients saw an average quit rate of 64%, one of the highest quit rates in the area.

(RCN, 2012)

Addressing smoking: developing personal skills and stopping people from starting to smoke

It is estimated that every year more than 205000 children in the UK start smoking (ASH, 2013b). Among adult smokers, about two-thirds report that they took up smoking before the age of 18 and over 80% before the age of 20. The latest survey of adult smokers shows that almost two-fifths (40%) had started smoking regularly before the age of 16 (ONS, 2013). Smoking rates among young people are also not declining and the Department of Health has set a target to reduce the number of young people who smoke to 12% by 2015 (compared to 15% in 2009). Smoking rates for this age group may be underestimated and under-reported: found saliva tests on 15-year-old boys that 21% were smokers and 19% of girls were smokers.

Evidence suggests that girls have higher smoking rates than boys, and the reasons for this are linked to a desire to control their weight and body image (NHS Information Centre for Health and Social Care, 2012; PHRC, 2009). Other contributory factors that may influence young people to smoke are having parents, siblings and/or friends who smoke and it is closely associated with school truancy and social deprivation.

Activity 5.6

Given the information on smoking prevalence and young people, what might be effective interventions to stop people starting to smoke?

Discussion

- *Knowledge: Knowledge about smoking is a necessary component of anti- smoking campaigns and it may deter young people from starting to smoke but smoking is not a rational behaviour where information about risks will act as a deterrent as explained in Chapter 12 (NICE, 2010).*
- *Role modelling: Many school-based programmes are based on the principles of social learning theory which predicts that young people adopt smoking as part of the socialization process into adolescence. Many school-based programmes attempt to influence behaviour*

(Continued)

by presenting positive role models who reject smoking in typical situations where smoking is encouraged, in the hope that the rejecting behaviour will be modelled by the target audience. Whether or not the target audience pays attention to the model depends upon the characteristics of both the model and the individual observer.

- *Building self-esteem: Another approach focuses on building self-esteem and decreasing feelings of alienation that might prompt a young person to start smoking to fit in with a peer group or feel more mature.*
- *Reducing availability: High prices can deter children from continuing smoking or the amount they smoke, since young people do not possess a large disposable income.*
- *Mass media: Using the mass media (TV, radio, newspapers, billboards) to influence the image of non-smoking though the evidence of effectiveness is limited (Brinn et al., 2011).*

Addressing smoking: developing personal skills and enabling people to quit

Of all smokers, 46% try to quit: of these, 8% use NHS support, 15% use medication over the counter and 23% quit without the use of a stop smoking medication. For this reason, considerable emphasis is placed on using brief advice that will encourage smokers to think about giving up, and if they find it difficult, to refer them to available help to address their addiction and psychological dependence.

The development of personal skills for smoking cessation could include skills such as:

- developing coping strategies, e.g. relaxation and stress management;
- developing new ways of dealing with or managing problems;
- self-monitoring, i.e. record keeping to become aware of triggers or cues to smoking;
- having or developing an awareness of environmental influences on smoking, e.g. where people are most likely to smoke;
- anticipating barriers and challenges to smoking cessation, e.g. unsupportive family or friends.

Case study 5.4

Brief interventions

The Department of Health recommends that all nurses use a 30-second approach of very brief advice used opportunistically with smokers. There are three elements known as the 3 As:

1. **A**sking about smoking status.
2. **A**dvising about how to stop.
3. **A**ct or offering help.

There is almost always an opportunity to ask a patient about their smoking: whether it relates to a presenting problem, when taking a history, or an alert from the computer. Asking someone if they want to stop can put them on the defensive and may also entail a long story. Very brief advice is recommending to the patient that they can have support and medication. There is no-need for in-depth knowledge – very brief advice just means that you are helping to point someone in the right direction.

The NHS recommends groups and a nicotine replacement therapy as the treatment for smoking (NICE, 2008). Groups provide a smoker with intensive support generally in the form of one hour over a period of 6–7 weeks. Smokers attending this type of group are not expected to quit smoking until week 3. A couple of weeks are spent preparing for a quit attempt by helping smokers to plan and prepare for life without cigarettes. The group is encouraged to quit together at week 3 and then support continues for a further 3 or 4 weeks. Pharmacological therapy in the form of NRT and bupropion (Zyban) is discussed in the group. Group facilitators equip clients with sufficient information about all the products to assist their decision about which, if any, is most appropriate to aid their quit attempt. Carbon monoxide monitors are a common feature of groups and are useful for demonstrating the early benefits of quitting. Some services offer relapse prevention meetings, for example, a once a month session, or a regular drop-in session.

Scenario 5.1

Jo, age 35, visits her GP complaining of breathlessness. She is bringing up three young children alone and she is living on income support in a third floor flat in local authority housing.

Jo admits to smoking 30 cigarettes a day and she has a history of high blood pressure. One of Jo's children is asthmatic.

Jo's GP advises her to give up smoking and suggests that she joins a smoking cessation group run by the practice nurse. She appears to listen to the GP's advice and agrees that she must think seriously about her lifestyle. After the first group session, the practice nurse informs the GP that Jo did not attend.

Two weeks later, Jo takes her youngest child to the GP surgery because he has a chest infection. The GP asks if Jo has managed to cut down on her smoking. Jo laughs and says:

"Well, it's all very well from where you're sitting. Look, if I come up on the lottery, perhaps I'll take myself off to a health farm and get myself sorted. But in the meantime, I reckon I'll just have to take my chances!"

- Why might Jo be reluctant to attend a smoking cessation group?
- What support could the practice nurse offer?
- How would you feel about Jo continuing to smoke?

The role of the nurse in addressing smoking

Activity 5.7

Should nurses who smoke be encouraged to quit? Consider the following arguments – which do you agree with?

- Patients see nurses as "normal people" and have no expectation of them as role models.
- Nurses are more likely to smoke because they have stressful jobs and are poorly paid – two of the high-risk factors for nicotine addiction – and so should not be unfairly stigmatized.
- Nurses should be public health champions.

Discussion

Smoking among nurses is as high as in the general population and several studies have revealed clear links between nurses' smoking status and their knowledge and attitudes to issues relating to smoking cessation. Nurses who smoke rate the health risks of smoking lower than non-smokers and ex-smokers. They are more likely to have negative attitudes to smoking-related issues and rate the benefits of cessation much lower. However, most nurses who smoke do want to quit and have tried to do so several times.

The NMC (2012) requirements state that nurses:

- Must give advice based on the best available evidence.
- Must deliver care based on the best available evidence or best practice.
- Must recognize and work within the limits of their competence.
- Must not discriminate in any way against those in their care.

Nurses need to take opportunities to offer health education advice and referral both opportunistically and during planned health education sessions. Such advice needs to be realistic and non-judgmental, taking into consideration the very real difficulties that people have in quitting smoking and the role that it plays in their lives and the limited choices some patients have. While quitting smoking is the most important action people can take for their health, nurses need to work with the patient and recognize those who are not ready or able to change their health behaviour (see Chapter 12). As with all issues, the nurse needs to be evidence-informed and ensure they follow current guidelines and ideally take up smoking cessation training. The NHS workforce potentially has considerable power and influence over smoking services and policies and the nurse can get involved in tobacco lobbying.

On placement: checklist

- Did you observe any nurse giving advice both opportunistically and during planned health education sessions?
- What support was available for smoking patients?
- Did you observe any patients leaving the ward to smoke? What happened?
- Was smoking status part of assessment? Was this followed up?

Key learning points

1. Smoking may be a response to social conditions and demanding personal lives.
2. High risk groups such as pregnant women, young people and people with potentially life-threatening conditions such as obesity, diabetes mellitus and CVD should be targeted for smoking interventions.
3. Opportunities should be taken to discuss smoking status which should be recorded for all patients.
4. Understanding rather than judgement should be the guiding principle of health promotion encounters.

Chapter summary

This chapter suggests that there needs to be a supportive environment to enable people to quit smoking that takes into account the socio-economic determinants of health and health behaviour and the impact these determinants have on the patient's ability to make health choices. Patients need education and support to enable them to make informed health choices and viable and acceptable alternatives to smoking. The alternatives need to be realistic and sustainable so that patients see them as credible and meaningful. In order to successfully challenge smoking, nursing interventions need to be targeted at high risk groups such as pregnant women and children and people with other potentially life-threatening conditions such as obesity, diabetes mellitus and CVD. This is in addition to the support for tobacco control policies that seek to make the healthier choice easier.

Further reading and resources

Action on Smoking and Health (www.ash.org.uk), the British Heart Foundation (www. Bhf.org.uk) and Cancer Research UK (www.cancerresearchuk.org) all provide briefings and research reports.

The Department of Health (2011) *Healthy Lives, Healthy People: A Tobacco Control Plan for England* is available at:

https://www.gov.uk/government/uploads/system/uploads/attachment_data/file/213757/dh_124960.pdf.

The National Centre for Smoking Cessation and Training includes training at http://www.ncsct.co.uk and there are also e-learning modules at http://www.nhshealth.org.uk/StopSmoking/.

RCN (2011) *Clearing the Air: Smoking and Tobacco Control* is available at:
http://www.rcn.org.uk/__data/assets/pdf_file/0011/78554/001945.pdf.
This has lots of information about smoking prevalence and prevention methods.

Up-to-date statistics on the prevalence of smoking and many other conditions are available from www.statistics.gov.uk.

References

ASH (2011) *Secondhand Smoke: The Impact on Children.* Available at: http://www.ash.org.uk/files/documents/ASH_596.pdf.

ASH (2012) *Public Support for Putting Tobacco Products in Plain Packaging*. Available online at http://www.ash.org.uk/files/documents/ASH_765.pdf.

ASH (2013a) *ASH Briefing: UK Tobacco Control Policy and Expenditure*. Available at: http://www.ash.org.uk/files/documents/ASH_667.pdf.

ASH (2013b) *Young People and Smoking*. Available at: http://www.ash.org.uk/files/documents/ASH_108.pdf.

Baxter, S., Blank, L., Guillaume, L., *et al.* (2009) *Systematic Review of How to Stop Smoking in Pregnancy and Following Childbirth*. ScHARR Public Health Evidence Report 4.1. Available at: http://www.shef.ac.uk/polopoly_fs/1.43298!/file/Smoking-4_1.pdf.

Brinn, M.P., Carson, K.V., Esterman, A.J. *et al.* (2011) Mass media interventions for preventing smoking in young people. *Cochrane Database of Systematic Reviews*, **11**. (Art. No.: CD001006). DOI: 10.1002/14651858.CD001006.pub2.

Dowling, S. (2012) Smoking, in *The Scottish Health Survey 2011*, vol. 1 *Adults* (eds L. Rutherford, C. Sharp and C. Bromley), Edinburgh: Scottish Government, pp. 101–133.

HSCIC (Health and Social Care Information Centre) (2012) *Statistics on Smoking, England, 2012*. Available at: https://catalogue.ic.nhs.uk/publications/public-health/smoking/smok-eng-2012/smok-eng-2012-rep.pdf.

Jha, P., Peto, R., Zatonski, W., *et al.* (2006) Social inequalities in male mortality, and in male mortality from smoking: indirect estimation from national death rates in England and Wales, Poland, and North America. *Lancet*, **368** (9533), 367–370.

Joossens, L. and Raw, M. (2011) *The Tobacco Control Scale 2010 in Europe*. Association of European Cancer Leagues, Brussels. Available at: http://www.krebshilfe.de/fileadmin/Inhalte/Downloads/PDFs/Kampagnen/TCS_2010_Europe.pdf.

Kobus, K. (2003) Peers and adolescent smoking. *Addiction,* **98** (Suppl. 1), s37–55.

London Health Observatory (2012) *Smoking in England*. Available at: http://www.lho.org.uk/LHO_Topics/National_Lead_Areas/NationalSmoking.aspx.

NHS Information Centre for Health and Social Care (2012) *Smoking, Drinking and Drug Use Among Young People in England in 2011*. Available at: http://www.natcen.ac.uk/media/975589/sddfull.pdf.

NICE (2008) *Smoking Cessation PH 10*. NICE, London. Available at: http://www.nice.org.uk/nicemedia/live/11925/39596/39596.pdf.

NICE (2010) *School-Based Interventions to Prevent the Uptake of Smoking Among Children.* PH 23. NICE, London. Available at: http://www.nice.org.uk/PH23.

NICE (2012) *Smokeless Tobacco Cessation: South Asian Communities.* PH 39. NICE, London. Available at: http://publications.nice.org.uk/smokeless-tobacco-cessation-south-asian-communities-ph39.

NMC (Nursing and Midwifery Council) (2012) *The Code: Standards of Conduct, Performance and Ethics for Nurses and Midwives*. NMC, London.

ONS (Office for National Statistics) (2013) *General Lifestyle Survey Overview: A Report on the 2011 General Lifestyle Survey* Available at: http://www.ons.gov.uk/ons/rel/ghs/general-lifestyle-survey/2011/rpt-chapter-1.html.

PHRC (Public Health Research Consortium) (2009) *A Review of Young People and Smoking in England*, DH, London. Available at: http://phrc.lshtm.ac.uk/papers/PHRC_A7-08_Final_Report.pdf.

RCN (Royal College of Nursing) (2012) *Going Upstream: Nursing's Contribution to Public Health*, RCN, London. Available at: http://www.rcn.org.uk/__data/assets/pdf_file/0007/433699/004203.pdf.

Sims, M., Bauld, L. and Gilmore, A. (2012) England's legislation on smoking in indoor public places and work-places: impact on the most exposed children. *Addiction,* **107** (11), 2009–2016.

WHO (World Health Organization) (2002) *Tobacco Free Initiative*, WHO, Geneva. Available at: http://www.who.int/tobacco/en/.

WHO (World Health Organization) (2011) *Gender, Health, Tobacco and Equity*. Available at: http://www.who.int/tobacco/publications/gender/gender_tobacco_2010.pdf.

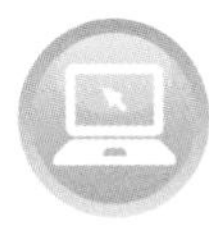

Don't forget to visit the companion website for this book: www.wileyfundamentalseries.com/healthpromotion where you can find self-assessment tests to check your progress.

6

Alcohol

Jane Wills

Professor, Health Promotion, London South Bank University, London, UK

Learning outcomes

By the end of this chapter you will be able to:

1. Understand the reasons for alcohol being a public health priority
2. Have an overview of the measures used to tackle alcohol-related harm and drinking behaviours
3. Consider the role of the nurse in health promotion on alcohol

Introduction

The consumption of alcohol is an established part of many people's lives. Alcohol misuse is, however, a major cause of disease, injury and harm. For the individual, harmful drinking may lead to cancer, liver cirrhosis and heart disease. It can cause break down in relationships and in families and contribute to domestic violence. For communities, alcohol can fuel crime and disorder and it can also have an effect in the workplace on productivity. This chapter will discuss the prevalence of alcohol-related harm and the public health policies and initiatives that address this. The role of the nurse in initiating brief interventions about alcohol and in providing information will be discussed.

Fundamentals of Health Promotion for Nurses, Second Edition. Edited by Jane Wills.

Companion website: www.wileyfundamentalseries.com/healthpromotion

The impact of alcohol on health

Alcohol or ethanol is a depressant drug that diffuses from the stomach and small intestine to parts of the body containing water. It peaks in the blood within an hour of consumption and will interact with nerve cell membranes and neurotransmitter pathways, resulting in sedation, impaired judgement and reduced muscular control. Most alcohol is metabolized in the liver at

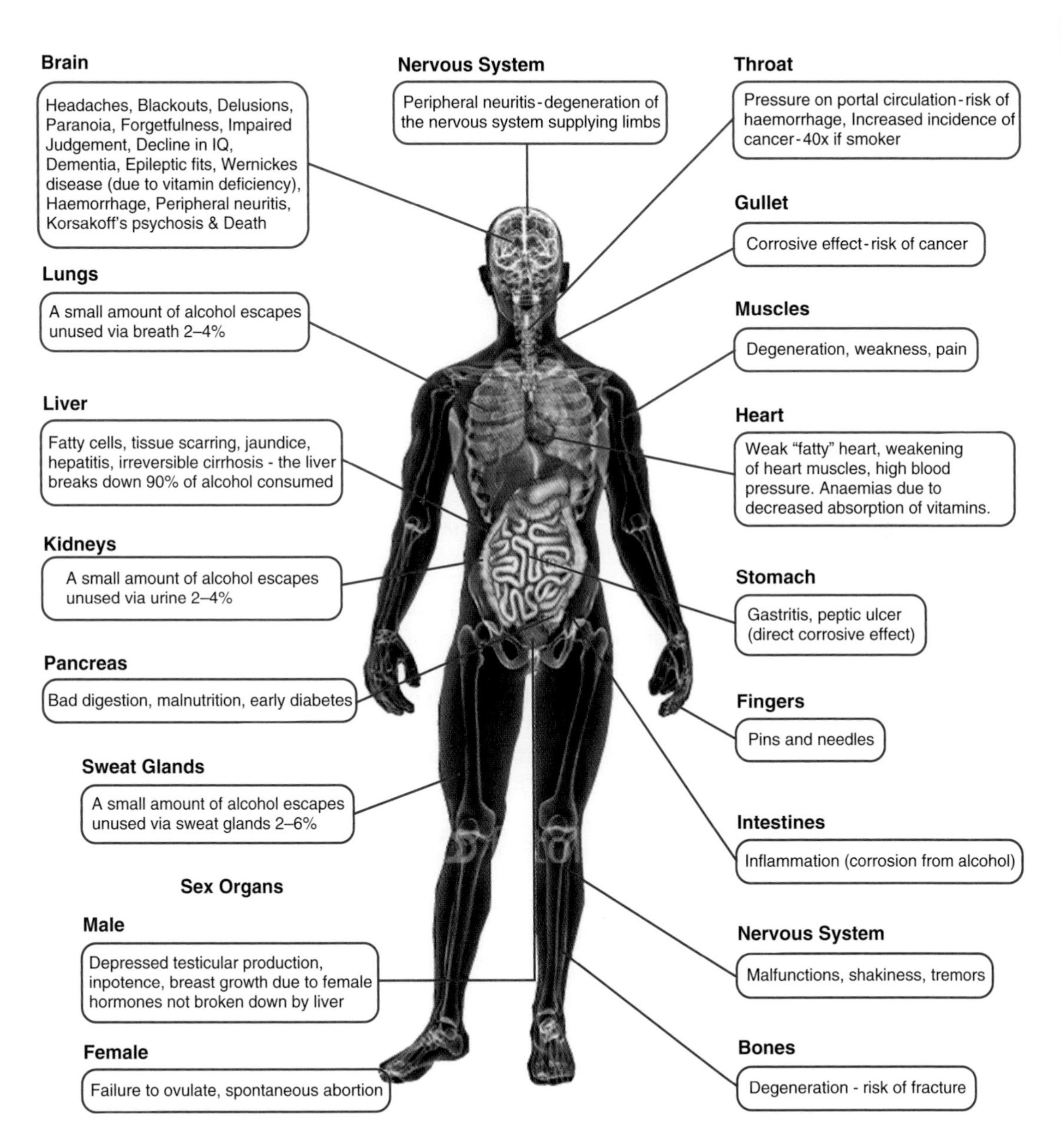

Figure 6.1 The impact of alcohol on the body.

roughly one unit per hour but prolonged excessive use will have an impact on body cells and organs throughout the body. Alcohol intoxication can affect many parts of the body, including:

- motor function
- emotion
- balance
- problem-solving skill
- memory
- judgement
- social control
- sexual control
- vision
- language.

Prolonged use can have an impact on many organs and body functions as shown in Figure 6.1

Defining alcohol-related harm

The World Health Organization uses the following terms to describe drinking:

- hazardous
- harmful
- dependent.

Table 6.1 shows the definitions of these categories and trends in their prevalence.

Alcohol in the UK is measured in units. One alcohol unit is measured as 10 ml or 8 grams of ethyl alcohol. This equates to about a single measure of spirits or about half a pint of beer or less than a small glass of wine. Current guidance states that men should not exceed 3–4 units per day on a regular basis and women should not exceed 2–3 units per day on a regular basis. It is recommended that a person has at least 48 hours per week with no alcohol. The limits are given as daily figures for regular consumption in order to discourage the idea that a week's units can be saved up and drunk all at once. Harmful drinking means regularly drinking above these limits and hazardous drinking means drinking more than 6 units per day for women and 8 units per day for men. Figure 6.2 shows the guidelines for "sensible" drinking levels or low risk.

Knowing how much alcohol people actually drink is essential in evaluating the harm it may cause. Yet population surveys consistently find that drinkers' own estimates of the total amount consumed account for only 40–60% of the alcohol actually sold (Bloomfield *et al*., 2003). People who drink a lot of alcohol may say they drink less when asked, because excessive drinking is disapproved of in most societies.

Table 6.1 Definitions of different categories of drinkers and trends in their prevalence.

Type of drinker	Definition	Trend
Hazardous	Those who drink over the sensible drinking limits, either regularly or through less frequent sessions of heavy binge drinking, but have so far avoided significant alcohol-related problems	For women, the binge drinking rate (twice over the recommended limit once a week) increased from 7% in 1998 to 16% in 2006, similarly, in men, the proportion rose from 20% to 24% over the same period
Harmful	Harmful drinkers drink at higher levels than most hazardous drinkers and exhibit signs of alcohol-related harm	Heavy drinking rose among men from 19% in 2005 to 24% in 2007 and from 8% to 15% for women over the same period
Dependent	Those who are likely to have increased tolerance of alcohol, suffer withdrawal symptoms, and have lost some degree of control over their drinking. In severe cases, they may have withdrawal fits and may drink to escape from or avoid these symptoms	There was a 24% increase in moderate to severe drinkers between 2000 and 2007

Women	Should not regularly drink more than **2 to 3** units of alcohol a day. That's no more than a standard **175 ml** glass of wine (ABV 13%).
Men	Should not regularly drink more than **3 to 4** units of alcohol a day. That's not much more than **a pint** of strong lager, beer or cider (ABV 5.2%).

Regularly means drinking this amount most days or every day. ABV is the percentage of alcohol in the drink.

PREGNANT WOMEN If you are pregnant or trying to conceive, it is recommended that you avoid drinking alcohol. But if you do drink, it should be no more than 1-2 units once or twice a week.

Figure 6.2 Low risk guidelines for drinking.

Activity 6.1

Estimating alcohol consumption accurately is very difficult. Why might this be so?

Discussion

- *The concentration (strength) of alcohol varies between types of drink and few people know the difference.*
- *The standard volume of a "drink" varies between types of drink and between countries.*
- *Different ways of referring to the amount of alcohol in a drink make comparison difficult. For example, wine, beer and spirit labels usually give the alcohol content as a percentage of the liquid in the bottle. Drinking safely advice generally refers to units of alcohol often quoted in terms of "a glass of wine" or "a half-pint of beer" or "a measure of spirits".*
- *When drinks are poured at home, the "measure" is often uncontrolled and estimates tend to be even more inaccurate.*

As important as knowing about the volume a person drinks is knowing about the pattern of their consumption. Drinking large amounts in one go – particularly of spirits –has a much higher health risk than drinking the same quantity of alcohol in a more dilute form (e.g. beer or wine) in smaller amounts spread over several days. Binge drinkers may consume very little alcohol on most days of the week, but get extremely drunk at weekends or on festive occasions. The rapid rise to a high level of alcohol in the bloodstream is particularly dangerous.

Case study 6.1

Pregnant women and drinking

Excessive alcohol consumption during pregnancy can damage the developing foetus as alcohol passes freely across the placenta. Possible outcomes of excessive alcohol consumption may include miscarriage, still birth, low birth weight, learning disabilities and hyperactivity as well as foetal alcohol spectrum disorder (FASD). According to an evidence review for Public Health Wales (Jones, 2013), there is no evidence of a "dose-response"– that the more a woman drinks, the more likely she is to have a problem with pregnancy or the child. Any serious consequences of alcohol during pregnancy are complicated by the fact that women who misuse substances heavily are known to have poorer obstetric and neonatal outcomes, along with late booking and poor attendance for antenatal care.

- NICE recommendations (2008) state that pregnant women and women planning to get pregnant should avoid drinking alcohol in the first 3 months of pregnancy.
- If women choose to drink while pregnant, they should drink no more than 1–2 units once or twice a week.
- They should be advised not to get drunk or binge drink while pregnant.

Alcohol as a public health priority

Alcohol is one of the leading causes of disease, injury and death and is a major public health priority. The numbers of people who drink at levels likely to present a risk to their health have risen steadily over the last couple of decades and liver disease is the only major cause of death and illness which is increasing in England while decreasing in Europe (Davies, 2012). Alcohol accounts for the following statistics:

- 5792 men's deaths and 2956 women's deaths could be attributed to alcohol in 2011, double the number of alcohol-related deaths in 1992 (ONS, 2013);
- 27% of men's deaths and 15% of women's deaths in the age group 16–24 were from alcohol-attributable causes (NHS Information Centre, 2012);
- 1.2 million hospital admissions in 2011/2012 were related to alcohol consumption, double that of 2002/2003;
- 15% of the people killed in road traffic accidents are as a result of drink driving;
- 44% of all violent incidents are committed by people who have been drinking (Chaplin *et al.*, 2011).

It is clear that alcohol has a major impact on the health and well-being of individuals, and the estimated cost is around £2.7 billion in hospital admissions, attendance at A&E, primary care and treatment of related conditions such as hypertension (DH, 2008). Beyond the individual, alcohol is linked to domestic violence and over a third of those reporting domestic violene perceive their attacker to be under the influence of alcohol (Cabinet Office, 2004) and over a quarter of children ringing Childline are worried about a parent's drinking.

Groups that are more disadvantaged are far more likely to suffer from alcohol-related harm: there are nearly four times as many alcohol-related deaths among men in routine occupations than among men in higher managerial roles. There is considerable geographic difference in the UK with far higher numbers of dependent and hazardous drinkers in the North of England and Scotland.

The prevalence of drinking

Drinking levels have doubled since the 1950s and though consumption is levelling off, the impact of drinking on health is beginning to show in an alarming rise in hospital admissions. Figure 6.3 shows the steady increase in related conditions.

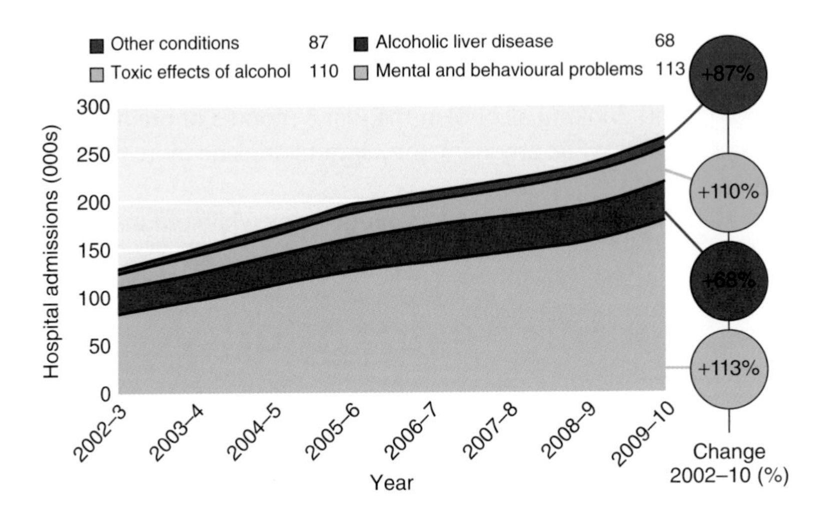

Figure 6.3 Hospital admissions wholly attributable to alcohol in England, 2002/03–2009/10. Source: Appleby, 2012, Figure 4. Reproduced with permission of BMJ Publishing Group Ltd. (Source data: NHS Information Centre).

Excessive alcohol consumption and drunkenness are characteristic of what is thought of as British drinking behaviour. Although not unique to the UK, the UK is one of the heaviest alcohol-consuming countries in Europe. The majority of the population (60%), however, drink in line with recommended lower levels and about 14% do not drink at all. One of the most significant trends in recent years is the rise in the number of women who drink and the amount they drink.

Scenario 6.1

When Lucy went out with her friends as a 16-year-old following her GCSE exams, she drank three bottles of "alcopops" (fruit-flavoured drinks containing a spirit such as vodka, 1.5 UK units each) at home, followed by a "large glass" of white wine (250 ml, around 3 units) – and a tequila 'slammer' (2 units). She was picked up by the police slumped on a verge, unconscious, and taken to A&E where she spent the night on a drip.

- What risks are there in Lucy's behaviour?
- What might account for this behaviour?

Discussion

There are risks for Lucy in becoming unconscious as she may choke on vomit, have a respiratory arrest if her brain slows down, she may be vulnerable to sexual assault and, should she regain consciousness, she may be unsteady and at risk of injury.

There are many psychosocial factors that may account for why this young woman celebrates her exams in this way:

- *Temperament and personality traits including the "sensation-seeking trait".*
- *Emotional and behavioural problems such as depression which cause her to use alcohol.*
- *Familial factors – Family attitudes that favour the use of alcohol, particularly if her parents abuse it; or poor or inconsistent parenting.*
- *Peer-group members using alcohol is a strong predictor of alcohol misuse in young people.*
- *Price – the low price of alcohol means it is possible for a young person on limited income to drink excessively.*
- *Availability – alcohol regulation is lax and though sales are illegal to those under 18 years old, most alcohol is consumed in the home.*

The policy context

A national alcohol strategy in 2007 entitled "Safe, Sensible, Social" (DH, 2007) attempted to tackle the harms of alcohol by addressing price and availability, point of sale and through public health education. The government's 2012 strategy (Home Office, 2012) more strongly focuses on binge drinking and the impact of alcohol on town centres and communities and the demands placed on A&E departments by violent incidents, road traffic accidents, self-harm and psychiatric disturbances fuelled by alcohol. It includes a raft of recommendations on the licensing of premises that sell alcohol.

Addressing alcohol-related harm: control

Alcohol taxation is an effective public health measure as it raises prices and suppresses demand. Demand for alcohol is inversely related to price and consequently to alcohol-related harm. But when there are high taxes on alcohol, this effect is lost if retailers do not pass on the additional cost. Very cheap alcohol enables the heaviest drinkers to maintain their consumption and it also means that young people with limited money have access to cheap, strong drink.

Evidence 6.1

Minimum price for alcohol

A systematic review investigated the relationship between tax/price and alcohol consumption. Booth *et al.* (2008) concluded that *"there is evidence to suggest that price increases (including through taxation) have a significant effect in reducing demand for alcohol"* (p. 33). It found that problem drinkers seek out the cheapest ways to get drunk as they tend to be either young or those who drink a lot, and therefore would change their behaviour in response to price increases more than moderate drinkers would.

A commitment to a price of at least 50p per unit was part of the government's alcohol strategy but was shelved in 2013 despite reports from Canada where it is claimed that a 10% increase in the minimum price resulted in a 32% fall in wholly alcohol-related deaths. It was claimed that the UK government came under pressure from the drinks industry to shelve the policy. Concern over the government's identification of the drinks industry as a key partner in tackling alcohol problems has aroused concern among professionals and agencies dealing with the consequences of alcohol misuse since 2004 , who doubted the industry's willingness and ability to perform this role (Baggott, 2006, p. 2).

In contrast to attempts to reduce the attractiveness of tobacco through the introduction of plain packaging, there has been little attention to the packaging of alcohol. There is a lack of information on alcohol product labels, making it very difficult for consumers to choose drinks with a lower alcohol content.

Again, in contrast to tobacco, there are few restrictions on alcohol advertising. Many studies have shown that alcohol advertising increases the likelihood that young people will start to consume alcohol and the media and popular culture are saturated with images of drinking. Norway is the only country in Europe with a comprehensive ban on alcohol advertising which also has one of the lowest rates of alcohol consumption in Europe. The campaigning charity, Alcohol Concern, have suggested the introduction of a model similar to France's Loi Evin, a law passed in 1991, which has banned alcohol brands from sponsoring cultural or sports events, alcohol advertising targeted at young people, and alcohol advertisements screened on TV or in cinemas.

Addressing alcohol-related harm: creating supporting environments

There are a few public spaces where drinking is not permitted. Controlled drinking zones have been widely used by local authorities to reduce drinking and drunkenness by giving police powers to intervene. In 2008, a ban on drinking alcohol on public transport was introduced in London and in 2012 it was also banned on Scottish trains at night. Alcohol has also been banned at most Scottish football matches to reduce the risk of violence between fans.

Addressing alcohol-related harm: developing personal skills

Activity 6.2

Consider the example of an alcohol education poster in Figure 6.4. What are the health promotion messages it is trying to convey?

Does this look familiar?
Regularly drinking more than your recommended daily limit of alcohol can cause liver disease, heart disease and cancer.
Men should not regularly drink more than 3-4 units a day.
Women should not regularly drink more than 2-3 units a day.
If you are concerned you can speak to your GP in confidence.
Not sure about the recommended daily limit or units?
Visit www.drinkaware.co.uk
NHS
North Yorkshire and York

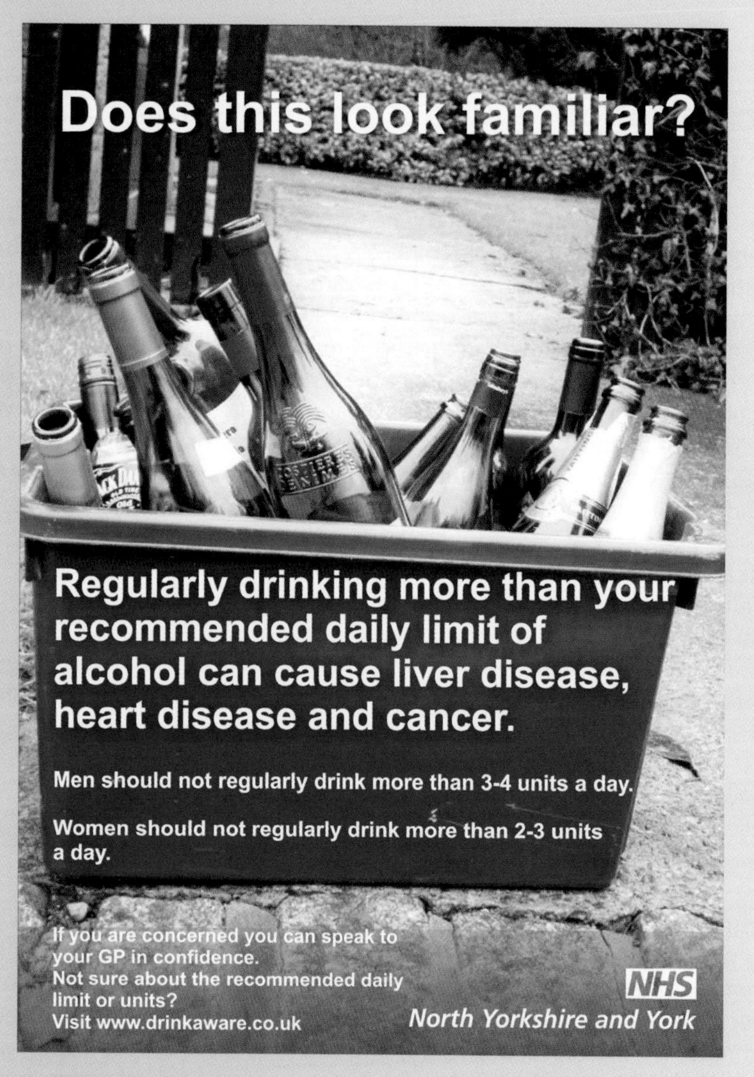

Figure 6.4 Example of an alcohol awareness poster. Source: North Yorkshire and York Primary Care Trust, 2008. Reproduced under the Open Government Licence.

(*Continued*)

Discussion

Most alcohol messages on television, posters, or billboards, are attempting to change perceptions of acceptable behaviour when drinking and the social and interpersonal consequences of excessive alcohol consumption. Rather than attempting to change people's views of the desirability of drinking, the campaigns suggest that drinking may affect a person's reputation and image through embarrassing drunken behaviour.

Addressing alcohol-related harm: early identification and brief interventions

There are many opportunities to intervene as early as possible to identify and treat alcohol dependence. Nurses have a key role to play in the prevention of alcohol misuse through early identification and offering brief advice for hazardous and harmful drinkers and, where necessary, prompt referral to specialist alcohol services.

Few people who drink more than the recommended levels of alcohol seek professional help for their drinking. They may be unaware of the long-term dangers to their health yet many will still encounter health care professionals for reasons related to their alcohol consumption. *Our Invisible Addicts* is a report by the Royal College of Psychiatrists (RCP, 2011) on the problems of substance misuse among older adults. It claims that the scale of this problem is unacknowledged and practitioners are reluctant to address the issue because of:

- ageist assumptions;
- failure to recognize symptoms;
- lack of knowledge about screening;
- discomfort with the topic;
- lack of awareness of substance misuse in older people ("If you don't think about it, you won't see it");
- misuse traditionally considered to be rare in old age;
- symptoms may mimic or be hidden by symptoms of physical illness;
- unwillingness to ask;
- absence of informants.

There is strong evidence that opportunistic early identification and brief advice are effective in reducing alcohol consumption (Kaner *et al.*, 2007). Early identification may involve a simple assessment but may also involve the administration of a short questionnaire about drinking behaviour such as AUDIT –(Alcohol Use Disorders Identification Test), followed by advice. This does not require a high level of training and can take place in A&E departments, psychiatric services, homelessness services, antenatal clinics, general hospital wards and criminal justice settings. It may be appropriate for those who present with depression, chronic conditions, digestive problems or minor injuries who may have symptoms of higher risk drinking. Because an assessment can take some time to administer, abbreviated versions are available that will reveal if an individual is likely to be a lower risk drinker, increasing risk drinker, higher risk drinker or alcohol-dependent. The questions focus on drinking patterns, feelings about drinking and the response of close others. Questions from the AUDIT assessment include:

- How often during the last year have you found that you were not able to stop drinking once you had started?
- How often during the last year have you failed to do what was normally expected from you because of your drinking?
- How often during the last year have you needed an alcoholic drink in the morning to get yourself going after a heavy drinking session?
- How often during the last year have you had a feeling of guilt or remorse after drinking?
- How often during the last year have you been unable to remember what happened the night before because you had been drinking?
- Have you or somebody else been injured as a result of your drinking?
- Has a relative or friend, doctor or other health worker been concerned about your drinking or suggested that you cut down?

A brief intervention may only be able to ascertain whether the patient is drinking above lower risk levels, give information about health risks and levels of consumption and ascertain whether they would benefit from referral to a specialist service. As discussed in Chapter 12, the approach of the nurse when discussing issues such as alcohol use is crucial to the extent to which the patient accepts a willingness to change or, alternatively, is in denial. Patients are often unaware of the risks of drinking and drinking at increasing or higher risk levels is usually not a permanent condition but a pattern into which many people occasionally fall, only for a period of time, so the practitioner should convey acceptance of the person without condoning their current drinking behaviour (http://www.alcohollearningcentre.org.uk). A practitioner may raise the issue: "Can you think of any benefits that reducing your drinking might have for you?" They may acknowledge the challenges that this change in behaviour may pose: "It can be quite hard when you're out with a crowd to keep track of your drinking, can't it?"

In a brief intervention of 5–15 minutes, a nurse should cover using motivational interviewing principles (see Figure 6.1) the potential harm caused by the person's level of drinking and their reasons for making a change and outline some practical strategies to help reduce alcohol consumption, including:

- sticking to recommended guidelines;
- having days without alcohol;
- alternating alcoholic drinks with ones containing no alcohol;
- trying not to drink on an empty stomach;
- avoid buying in rounds and drinking slowly;
- keeping a daily drinks diary to monitor consumption;
- diluting drinks;
- avoiding spirits.

The role of the nurse in health promotion

For nurses, lack of education and training and lack of confidence/experience have been cited as "barriers", ultimately resulting in low commitment to tackling alcohol misuse. Shaw *et al.* (1978) examined the lack of willingness by health care practitioners to intervene to tackle drinking problems concluding that it was influenced by practitioners' concepts of the following:

- *role adequacy* (or the extent to which practitioners feel adequately prepared and have the appropriate knowledge and skills to identify and respond in a positive and effective way);
- *role legitimacy* (the extent to which practitioners feel they have the authority to intervene in an area that is perceived to be "specialist" and outside their perceived level of professional competence);
- *role support* (perceived levels of support from specialist services and te extent of multidisciplinary working).

There has been scant provision of alcohol education in pre-registration and post-registration nursing curricula. Nurses may be taught biophysiological aspects of alcohol and alcohol-related harm in relation, for example, to liver failure or the management of delirium tremens, but the skills of brief interventions are rarely taught. The ever-increasing alcohol-related harm that is experienced by patients means this is now addressed in several online learning resources to develop skills and competences to encourage nurses to talk to patients about their use or misuse of alcohol.

On placement: checklist

- ❑ Can you identify occasions where a nurse's attitudes, beliefs, feelings and prejudices affected an opportunity to raise issues relating to alcohol misuse?
- ❑ Can you identify examples of good practice in brief interventions?
- ❑ What health education materials were used, if any, and how up to date and appropriate are these to patient's needs?
- ❑ Can you identify examples of liaison with substance misuse specialist services?
- ❑ On what occasions were substance misuse topics raised?

Key learning points

1. Many conditions that present in health care settings may be related to alcohol-related harm.
2. Drinking behaviour may be a response to social conditions and demanding personal lives.
3. No assumptions should be made about who may be drinking at high risk levels and accurate assessments should equally be made where drinking is low risk.
4. Alcohol may be a difficult issue to raise but opportunities should be taken when this seems relevant.
5. Understanding rather than judgement should be the guiding principle of health promotion encounters.

Chapter summary

This chapter has shown that alcohol may be an issue for nursing practice and that opportunities to identify and assess drinking behaviour should be more widely seized. Nurses, who have a rapport with patients, are ideally placed to use "teachable moments" to discuss behaviours, risks and willingness to change. The "FRAMES"' approach, which has much in common with motivational interviewing is being widely promoted as an easy-to-remember guide to educating about alcohol.

- **F**eedback: helping patients to make the link between their injury/condition and their alcohol misuse.
- **R**esponsibility: encouraging patients to take responsibility for their own drinking.
- **A**dvice: providing patients with individually tailored advice on issues such as keeping consumption within safe limits.
- **M**enu: providing patients with options to enable them to reduce their drinking, for example, choosing a small glass of wine instead of a large one, avoiding drinking in rounds and not relying on alcoholic drinks alone to quench thirst.
- **E**mpathy: using an empathetic approach rather than lecturing, for example, saying: "We all like a drink but being in A&E on Saturday night can't have been much fun."
- **S**elf-efficacy: emphasizing to patients that they can change their drinking habits, in the same way, for example, that patients can and often do give up smoking.

Further reading and resources

Because of the scale of the problems of alcohol misuse and the necessity for this to be addressed, there are numerous learning platforms available to the nurse:

Alcohol Learning Centre, available at: http://www.alcohollearningcentre.org.uk.
This includes a series of online modules covering the role of alcohol in society, the impact of alcohol on health, the use of screening tools and how the practitioner can address alcohol use with the patient.

http://www.healthscotland.com/topics/health/alcohol/index.aspx contains fact sheets and guides to brief interventions.

Various agencies exist that provide guides to alcohol interventions e.g. Alcohol Concern, available at: www.alcoholconcern.org.uk.

National Institute for Health and Clinical Excellence (2010) *Alcohol-Use Disorders: Preventing Harmful Drinking* (PH 24). London: NICE. Available at: www.nice.org.uk/ph24.

References

Baggott, R. (2006) *Alcohol Strategy and the Drinks Industry: A Partnership for Prevention.* Joseph Rowntree Foundation, York.

Bloomfield, K., Stockwell, T., Gmel, G. and Rehn, N. (2003) International comparisons of alcohol consumption. *Alcohol Res Health*, **27** (1), 95–109.

Booth, A., Meier, P., Stockwell, T., *et al.* (2008) *Independent Review of the Effects of Alcohol Pricing and Promotion: Systematic Reviews.* SCHARR, University of Sheffield, Sheffield.

Cabinet Office (2004) *Alcohol Harm Reduction Strategy for England.* Strategy Unit report. Cabinet Office, London.

Chaplin, R., Flatley, J. and Smith, K. (2011) *Crime in England and Wales 2010/2011*. Home Office, London.

Davies, S.C. (2012) *Annual Report of the Chief Medical Officer: On the State of the Public's Health.* Department of Health, London.

Department of Health (2007) *Safe, Sensible, Social: Next Steps in the National Alcohol Strategy*. DH, London. Available at: http://webarchive.nationalarchives.gov.uk/20130107105354/http://www.dh.gov.uk/en/Publicationsandstatistics/Publications/PublicationsPolicyAndGuidance/DH_077470.

Department of Health (2008) *Reducing Alcohol Harm: Health Services in England for Alcohol Misuse.* DH, London.

Home Office (2012) *The Government's Alcohol Strategy*. Cm 8336. TSO, London.

Jones, S.J. (2013) *Early Years Path Finder Project: Substance Misuse*. Public Health Wales, Cardiff. Available at: http://www2.nphs.wales.nhs.uk:8080/EarlyYearsDocs.nsf/85c50756737f79ac80256f2700534ea3/9ef46d6e5021cae680257b8c006ceaa5/$FILE/Early%20Years%20Programme%20-%20Substance%20misuse%20(alcohol%20and%20drugs)%20evidence%20synthesis%20v1%20June%202013.docx.

Kaner, E. (2007) Effectiveness of brief alcohol interventions in primary care populations. *Cochrane Database of Systematic Reviews.* **2**. CD004148.

NHS Information Centre (2012) *Statistics on Alcohol*. Available at: https://catalogue.ic.nhs.uk/publications/public-health/alcohol/alco-eng-2012/alco-eng-2012-rep.pdf.

NICE (2008) *Antenatal Care: Routine Care for the Healthy Pregnant Woman,* CG 62. Available at: http://www.nice.org.uk/nicemedia/pdf/CG062NICEguideline.pdf.

Office of National Statistics (2013) *Alcohol Related Deaths in the United Kingdom 2011*. Newport: ONS.

RCP (Royal College of Psychiatrists) (2011) *Our Invisible Addicts*. RCP, London.

Shaw, S., Cartwright, A., Spratley, T. and Harwin, J. (1978) *Responding to Drinking Problems.* London: Croom Helm.

Don't forget to visit the companion website for this book: www.wileyfundamentalseries.com/healthpromotion where you can find self-assessment tests to check your progress.

7

Sexual health

Jane Wills

Professor, Health Promotion, London South Bank University, London, UK

Learning outcomes

By the end of this chapter you will be able to:

1. Define the issue and its importance as a public health priority
2. Know how it is being addressed in national policy
3. Discuss evidence-based strategies for addressing the issue at individual, community and population levels

Introduction

A person's sexual health is intrinsic to their well-being yet it is rarely discussed and mostly sexual health is considered in relation to disease or access to contraception. With rapid increases in acute sexually transmitted infections (STIs), continued increases of new HIV diagnoses and the highest rate of teenage pregnancies in Western Europe, sexual health in the UK is highlighted as a major issue in public health policy. A key priority for all nurses is to identify patient risk factors in respect of STIs, blood-borne infections, pregnancy and use of contraception methods. Sexual health is a sensitive and potentially embarrassing area and the nurse needs to understand the potential issues of stigma and/or shame that patients may experience when discussing their sexual health. Obtaining informed consent is a core competence.

Fundamentals of Health Promotion for Nurses, Second Edition. Edited by Jane Wills.

Companion website: www.wileyfundamentalseries.com/healthpromotion

Defining sexual health

Sexual health should be distinguished from sex, which refers to the biological characteristics that define humans as female or male, sexual activity, sexual function or sexuality which is the expression of a person's gender and sexual orientation. The World Health Organization (2006) defined sexual health as:

> *A state of physical, emotional, mental and social well being related to sexuality; it is not merely the absence of disease, dysfunction or infirmity. Sexual health requires a positive and respectful approach to sexuality and sexual relationships, as well as the possibility of having pleasurable and safe experiences, free of coercion, discrimination and violence. For sexual health to be attained and maintained, the sexual rights of all persons must be respected, protected and fulfilled.*

In other words, sexual health is a positive and holistic concept but it may be challenged by differential power relations where individuals (both women and men who have sex with men) may have to negotiate concerns about safer sex or be threatened with violence or abuse. Sexual rights thus include the right of all persons to:

- choose their partner;
- decide to be sexually active or not;
- have consensual sexual relations;
- decide whether or not, and when, to have children.

Sexual health promotion is about encouraging positive attitudes to sexual health in order to facilitate more satisfying, fulfilling and pleasurable relationships. It aims to enable people to make informed choices about the sex they have, with an emphasis on making healthy decisions. The ability that people have to take control of their sexual decisions affects their emotional well-being.

Activity 7.1

Most people who come into a health care setting are not there because they have sexual ill health problems so why should this be a priority for nursing care?

Discussion

- *A person's illness or disability may well have an impact on their sexual health and/or sexuality.*
- *Facilitating good sexual health requires a proactive approach to issues such as screening and contraception.*
- *Some diseases such as HIV can cause multisystem problems that are often unrecognized.*

Despite the positive ways in which sexual health may be described, it is usually framed as issues relating to sexual ill health or disease. There is considerable prejudice, stigma and discrimination linked to sexual ill health and sexual health. For example, over 30000 young women under 18 become pregnant each year, including nearly 6000 girls under 16 and nearly 50% go on to have abortions (Office of National Statistics, 2011). For many of these young women, having children young is not unusual, as their mother and grandmother may have been teenage mothers yet there is a common public perception that some teenage mothers have greater/automatic access to housing and other services.

Activity 7.2

How might social data recorded about a patient be a source of discrimination?

Discussion

Relationship status options are usually recorded as only S/M/W/D (single, married, widowed, divorced) which reduces all people in long-standing or co-habiting relationships to single, which denies the validity of all other types of partnership and also misses recording the potential support from a partner. This type of form misses out on separated individuals, and on other sexual relationships that patients may be engaged in, and also assumes that an individual's marital status is equivalent to a monogamous union.

Why is sexual health a public health priority?

In 2001, the Department of Health published the first *National Strategy for Sexual Health and HIV* (DH, 2001). This set out five main aims, including reducing the transmission of STIs (with a national goal of a 25% reduction in new gonorrhoea infections by 2007), reducing the prevalence of undiagnosed STIs and reducing the stigma associated with STIs.

Following on from this, the White Paper *Choosing Health: Making Healthy Choices Easier* (DH, 2004) included sexual health as one of its six key priorities. In the other countries in the UK, there are similar action plans for improving sexual health and sexual health services.

While most local sexual health strategies include the promotion of sexual health through, for example, sex and relationships education (SRE) or peer education, sexual health as a public health priority is generally seen in relation to reducing:

- unintended pregnancies;
- numbers of abortions;
- transmissions of sexual transmitted infections (STIs);
- new HIV diagnoses.

In addition, sexual health promotion may be seen as reducing problems related to sexual function that may arise as a consequence of cancer, vascular or heart disease, neurological impairment, rheumatoid and arthritic conditions, hormonal dysfunctions, continence problems, difficulties with fertility and the consequences of early pregnancy or gynaecological conditions. Certain medications, surgery, radiation and chemotherapy can also affect sexual functioning, while surgery such as mastectomy, hysterectomy, amputation or stoma creation can also result in sexual problems. Yet 6% of men and 15% women report a sexual problem that has gone on for more than a year and may never raise the issue (Mercer *et al.*, 2003). In these situations, the nurse's role is to acknowledge that sexual function is a quality of life concern and to be aware of the resources that may be available to address the issue.

Scenario 7.1

Mrs Patel is a 52-year-old South Asian woman with cervical cancer who was treated with radiotherapy as an outpatient. English is not her first language. At her first outpatient's appointment Mrs Patel was assessed by a member of the outpatient nursing team, and the doctor responsible for her treatment. The nurse assumed her medical colleague would explain the side effects of the treatment, including information about its impact upon sexual function. But the senior registrar noticed that Mrs Patel was widowed, and, assuming she would not be in a sexual relationship, gave limited information about the effects of the treatment. Ten months later Mrs Patel returned to the radiotherapy clinic complaining of vaginal dryness and pain during intercourse. Vaginal examination proved difficult due to vaginal stenosis and fibrosis that had occurred as a result of the radiotherapy.

- What checks should be in place to avoid stereotyping patients in nursing care?
- What knowledge and skills should nurses have to meet Mrs Patel's needs?
- Should nursing staff have requested a female interpreter at the initial assessment?
- How does inadequate information affect the future sexual function of the patient?
- What further nursing and medical care may now be necessary?

Adapted from (RCN, 2000)

England experiences some of the poorest sexual health in Europe in relation to rates of STIs and teenage pregnancy. An STI is an infection that can be transmitted by unprotected sex and includes genital herpes, gonorrohea, and syphilis. It is important to remember, however, that not everyone with an STI will have signs and symptoms of the condition. If a person does present with symptoms, these may include increased discharge, pain or ulcers. Early diagnosis of sexually transmitted infections (STIs) reduces the risk of costly complications and reduces the risk of onward transmission and the likelihood of the progression of HIV I being present. Figure 7.1 shows the increasing numbers of STIs in England and Wales, 2003–2007.

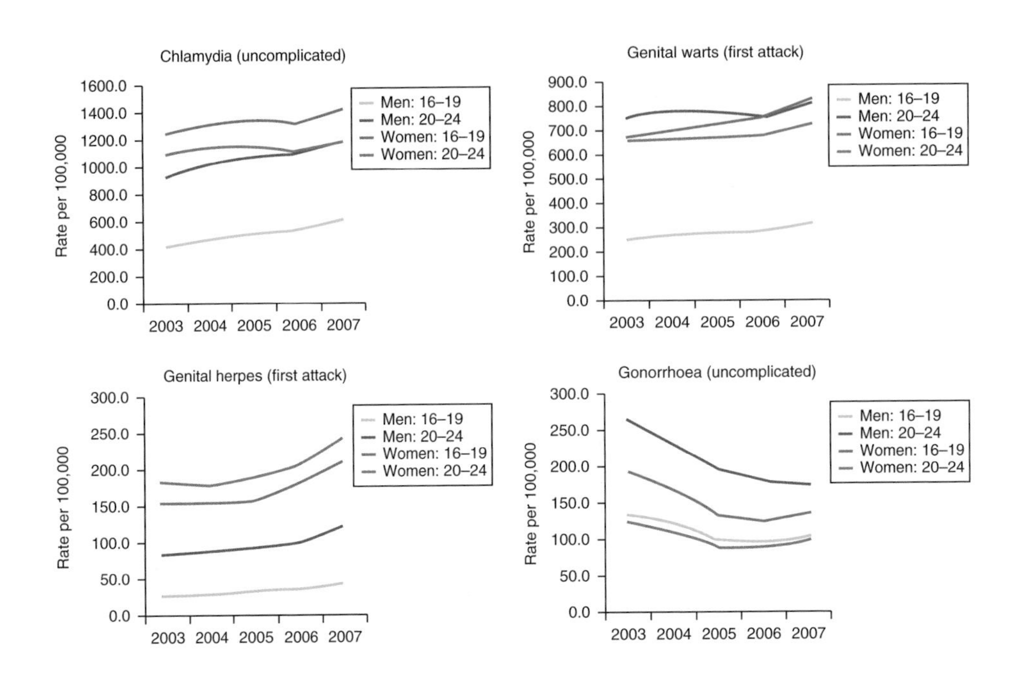

Figure 7.1 Rates of diagnoses of selected STIs in those aged under 25 years, UK, 2003–2007. Source: Health Protection Agency 2007, Figure 4. Reproduced under the Open Government Licence.

In 2011, a total of 426867 new STI diagnoses were reported to the Health Protection Agency (HPA) from sexual health clinics and chlamydia testing sites across the UK. This is just over 7000 more cases than were reported in 2010.

Activity 7.3

What general factors might account for this upward trend in STI diagnoses?

Discussion

- *increased risk taking;*
- *an increase in people seeking early diagnosis and treatment for infections;*
- *increased cases identified through screening such as the National Chlamydia Screening Programme;*
- *increased use of sensitive tests.*

Table 7.1 Total number of new HIV diagnoses in England, 2005-2011.

2005	2006	2007	2008	2009	2011
7469	7096	6927	6820	6112	6150

Source: Health Protection Agency (2012).

HIV continues to be one of the most important communicable diseases in the UK. It is an infection associated with serious morbidity, high costs of treatment and care, mortality and high number of potential years of life lost. Each year, many thousands of individuals are diagnosed with HIV for the first time. The infection is still frequently regarded as stigmatizing and has a prolonged "silent" period during which it often remains undiagnosed. Highly active antiretroviral therapies have resulted in substantial reductions in AIDS incidence and deaths in the UK. Table 7.1 shows the number of new cases of HIV, 2005–2011, which appears to be declining but it is also important to know the prevalence of HIV (the total number of people living with HIV). Some 120000 people had been diagnosed with HIV in the UK by 2012, of whom 27000 have developed AIDS and more than 20000 have died.

Activity 7.4

Which population groups do you think are most at risk of HIV?

Discussion

Half of those diagnosed in 2011 (48%, 3000) probably acquired their infection through sex between men and 47% (2890) through heterosexual contact. The overall decline in new diagnoses is largely due to fewer reported cases among heterosexuals who probably acquired their infection abroad.

While "at risk" is a commonly used term in relation to infectious diseases (see Chapter 13), focusing on at risk groups may lead to a lack of diagnosis for those who are not in these groups. Heterosexual men and women born outside of Africa are the least likely to be aware of their HIV infection or get tested. Many HIV organizations believe there should be more emphasis on partner notification to reduce undiagnosed HIV infection.

Chlamydia is the most common STI, with sexually active young people most at risk. It often has no symptoms but can lead to pelvic inflammatory disease, ectopic pregnancy or tubal damage. There has been an opportunistic national screening programme for under-25-year-olds since 2003. In 2011, 2.1 million chlamydia tests were carried out in England among young adults aged 15–24. A total of 147594 chlamydia diagnoses were made among this age group, equivalent to a diagnosis rate of 2148 per 100000 population.

Evidence 7.1

Reasons for attending chlamydia screening

Various studies have explored the factors that might prompt someone to go for chlamydia screening. Because it is mostly asymptomatic, individuals are able to deny their personal risk. Women are more likely to be informed about chlamydia than men but greater knowledge is not associated with increased likelihood to be screened. The main reason given in a study of undergraduates was not deeming it necessary because they did not consider themselves at risk. Many were unsure of their risk despite only half of the sample having used a condom in their last sexual experience.

(Greaves *et al.*, 2009)

Reducing teenage pregnancy, unintended conceptions and terminations are identified as national priorities. The figures in Table 7. 2 show that on average nearly 1 in 5 women of child-bearing age will have a termination of pregnancy. Yet there is considerable variation across age, location and ethnicity. Half of the abortions (49%) were to women with partners while 26% were to single women and 16% of abortions occurred within marriage. The vast majority of abortions take place in the very early stages of pregnancy (79% took place before 10 weeks gestation) with only 1 in 10 taking place over 13 weeks gestation. Brent in London has the highest rate – 39.4 women per 1000 had an abortion there. In 2011, 6151 women came to England for an abortion, the highest number, 4149, from Ireland where abortion is illegal.

Table 7.2 Abortion statistics, England and Wales, 2005–2009.

	2005	2006	2007	2008	2009
Total number (residents)	186416	193737	198499	195296	189100
Rate per 1000 women aged 15–44	17.8	18.3	18.6	18.2	17.5

Sexual health inequalities in England

While sexual health is a concern for most of the population, national epidemiological data and trends indicate that there are population groups who should be targeted for sexual health promotion and prevention programmes (DH, 2009):

- Young people who experience high rates of STIs, teenage conceptions and abortions.
- Older people over 50 who have increasing HIV and STI rates.
- Gay men (MSM) who experience high rates of HIV infection and STIs.
- African communities who experience high rates of HIV infection with significant numbers of late diagnoses.

- Caribbean communities who experience high rates of STIs and increasing HIV infection rates.
- People with physical and learning disabilities who experience problems accessing appropriate and relevant information and services.
- Transsexual men or women who experience problems accessing appropriate and relevant information and services.
- HIV positive people who experience high rates of STIs including repeat infections.
- Women who have repeat abortions.
- Users of sexual health services who experience repeat STI infections.

Factors contributing to sexual health

The sexual behaviour of the population is an important determinant of rates of STIs. Until the 1990s, little was known about people's sexual behaviour but prompted by the rise in HIV, the National Survey of Sexual Attitudes and Lifestyles (NATSAL) was started and the third survey is due to be published in 2013. There have been considerable changes in sexual behaviours in the past three decades: people have a greater number of lifetime partners, there is a lower median age of first intercourse, a greater proportion of the population have had concurrent partnerships in the past year (two or more partners at the same time), a greater proportion have had two or more partners in the past year and did not use condoms consistently, and a greater proportion of men report ever having had a homosexual partner.

Some of these behaviours are described as "risky". Risky sexual behaviours are defined as those which increase the chance of contracting or transmitting disease, or increase the chance of an unwanted pregnancy. Risky sexual behaviours would include:

- Having more than one sexual partner.
- Changing sexual partners frequently.
- Having oral, vaginal or anal sexual contact without a condom.
- Using unreliable methods of contraception, or contraception inconsistently.

Activity 7.5

What might account for risky sexual behaviours?

Discussion

Factors that you may have mentioned include:

- *lack of skills (for example, in using condoms);*
- *lack of negotiation skills (for example, to say "no" to sex without condoms);*
- *lack of knowledge about the risks of different sexual behaviours;*
- *alcohol or drugs leading to uninhibited behaviour;*
- *availability of resources, such as condoms or sexual health services;*
- *peer pressure to have sex or unprotected sex;*
- *attitudes (and prejudices) of society which may affect access to services.*

The factors behind England's poor sexual health have been hotly debated. Christian groups and many on the right wing complain that media culture, and increasingly sex education, promote promiscuity, which in turn makes it more likely people will have multiple partners and at a young age and will potentially transmit STIs or experience an unwanted pregnancy. Others complain that young people are not equipped to promote their own sexual good health and Sex and Relationships Education (SRE) is inadequate and "too little, too late".

As sexual health services are transferred from the NHS to local authorities in England, there is concern about access to emergency contraception and STI testing. About two and a half million people currently use NHS specialist community contraception services (family planning clinics) each year although the majority of women still choose their GP as their contraception provider.

Scenario 7.2

Janice is 16. The police who picked her up from the street where she had collapsed brought her into an A&E department. She is very intoxicated and has been placed on a drip overnight.

- Should the nurse discuss Janice's sexual health?
- If so, what should she discuss?

Janice is a vulnerable young person whose alcohol use may put her at risk of unwanted and/or unprotected sexual activity. One study by the British Youth Council found that 1 in 5 young people claimed their first sexual experience was while drunk. Raising the issue with Janice might be difficult and a sensitive approach is needed to taking a sexual history without unnecessary probing. This should be done in a private space. The nurse should be non-judgmental and supportive and avoid making any assumptions about Janice but a structured one-to-one conversation should:

- provide information about where to access emergency contraception;
- discuss risk reduction and support for decision-making;
- discuss condom use and encourage consistent use and build skills in negotiating their use.

Addressing sexual ill health and promoting sexual health

In the context of sexual health, prevention is *reducing or delaying risk of an adverse health outcome*. This can be at different levels: primary, secondary and tertiary.

Primary prevention may include:

- Supporting people to make informed decisions about sex and relationships including delay in age at first sexual activity.
- Prevention of unintended pregnancy through effective and available contraception including long-acting reversible contraception (implant or intra-uterine device).
- Preventing infection with STIs/HIV by promoting consistent condom use.
- Reducing later abortions.
- Undertaking vaccination programmes for hepatitis B.
- Working with others to protect people from sexual assault and supporting those who are harmed.

Awareness of contraception methods is quite limited and 44% women choose oral contraception and may be unaware of other methods (see Table 7.3).

The focus of most government health education campaigns on sexual health is to urge young people to use a condom. A campaign in 2006 using television and radio adverts and online messages shows couples with the name of an STI displayed on their underwear. The campaign aimed to show that infections are not so easy to spot and only a condom offers protection Figure 7.2 shows a poster reminder to carry a condom.

Table 7.3 Different types of contraceptive methods.

User dependent methods	Long-acting reversible contraception	Sterilization	Emergency contraception
Combined oral contraceptive, "the pill" Progestogen-only pill, the "mini pill" Male condoms Female condoms Diaphragm with spermicide Cap with spermicide Contraceptive patch Contraceptive vaginal ring Natural family planning	Intrauterine system Intrauterine device Contraceptive injection Sub-dermal implant	For both men and women	Emergency hormonal contraception "the morning after pill" The intrauterine device

Keys, Cash, Condom
You don't know where your night may take you, so it's best to prepare and always carry a condom with you.
It doesn't mean you're looking for sex – it just means you're looking out for yourself.
Sex
worth talking about
nhs.uk/worthtalkingabout

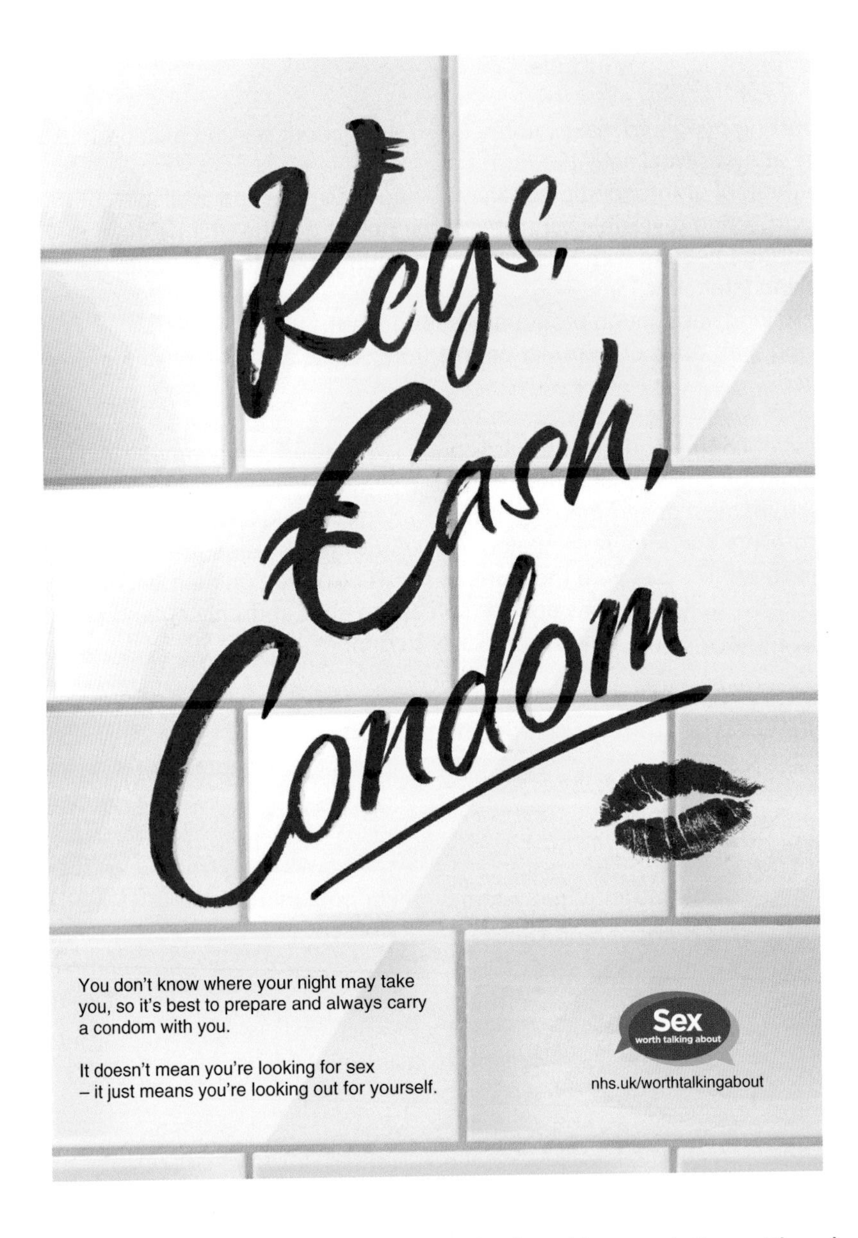

Figure 7.2 *Keys, Cash, Condom* campaign poster, displayed in association with pub chains. Source: Department of Health and Department of Education. Reproduced under the Open Government Licence.

Evidence 7.2

Reducing teenage pregnancy

Teenage pregnancy is often both the result and the cause of poverty, low achievement and low aspirations and is associated with poor long-term health outcomes for young parents and their children. A systematic review of interventions to tackle unintended teenage pregnancies (Origanje *et al.*, 2010) identified health education, skills building and improving access to contraception as the key strategies to address the issue. There is little or no good evidence that abstinence-based programmes on their own result in improved sexual health outcomes for young people. There is increased interest in the effects of interventions that target the social disadvantage associated with early pregnancy and parenthood. Teens and Toddlers (http://www.teensandtoddlers.org/about-us.html) is one such intervention where young people identified as at risk by their schools, are paired with toddlers, in a nursery setting. This builds their aspirations, to fulfil their educational attainment to achieve their potential and delay pregnancy, as well as choosing to remain in education, employment or training. A review by Harden (2009) suggests there is some limited evidence of the effectiveness of this approach.

Secondary prevention includes:

- Management and treatment of early stage STI/HIV infection through early identification by testing. The expansion of routine HIV testing outside the settings of sexual health, antenatal clinics and pregnancy termination services, and blood donors, means many nurses will be expected to offer, recommend and conduct a test (see NICE guidance). This has the potential to decrease the proportion of HIV positive individuals who are diagnosed late.
- Preventing onward transmission through partner notification programmes.
- Preventing or reducing repeat infections.
- Preventing repeat unintended pregnancies/abortions.

Case study 7.1

Point of Care HIV testing

Conventional HIV testing requires the submission of a blood sample and a follow-up return visit one or two weeks later to get the result, meaning that some people will not return for test results. Rapid HIV tests are able to test whole blood or saliva for HIV antibodies indicating HIV infection. Known as Point of Care (PoCT) or near-patient tests, results are available in minutes, allaying some patient anxiety. HIV testing is now recommended for all pregnant women, TB patients, all new GP registrants, all medical admissions in areas of high prevalence and to patients from high risk groups.

Tertiary prevention includes:

- Management of late stage and complex infections.
- Preventing onward transmission.

Treating a sexually transmitted infection as early as possible is key to reducing onward transmission. In addition, when an individual presents to sexual health services for screening or treatment, there is an ideal opportunity to discuss sexual health promotion and prevention.

The role of the nurse in health promotion

Nurses are taught to adopt a holistic approach to nursing care, and sexual health issues would be addressed as part of this. The role of the nurse is to create an environment in which the patient feels comfortable raising any concerns. This may include the disclosure of abuse or exploitation. In such circumstances, the nurse should work within professional boundaries, for example, the identification of proposed female genital mutilation (FGM) is a criminal matter and should be referred to the police.

Although there are nurses who take on specialist roles in sexual health relating to genito-urinary medicine, HIV, teenage pregnancy or family planning, many nurses may, at some point, need to take a sexual history, conduct a genital examination or undertake investigations. In this sensitive area, it is especially important that the nurse practises with due regard to codes of practice and the law. For example, the Fraser Guidelines provide for the discussion of sexual matters with a young person under 16. These state that a nurse may provide advice and care to a person under 16 without parental consent, including contraception, if they are confident that the young person is aware, competent and consents to that care (see http://www.fpa.org.uk/sites/default/files/under-16s-consent-and-confidentiality-factsheet-march-2009.pdf). The NMC code of practice sets out the need for nurses to be non-judgmental in their practice and states they have a duty of confidentiality which means being sensitive in approach and not disclosing any information without that person's consent.

On placement: checklist

- ❑ Can you identify occasions where a nurse's attitudes, beliefs, feelings and prejudices on issues of sexual health affected a specific learning encounter?
- ❑ Can you identify occasions of embarrassment in talking about sexual matters with patients?
- ❑ Can you identify examples of good practice in recognizing sexual diversity?
- ❑ On what occasions were sexual health-related topics raised and/or a patient's sexual well-being promoted?

Key learning points

1. Sexual health may be an important but embarrassing issue for a patient and so might not be raised.
2. It is important not to make assumptions about who may be at risk of sexual ill health.
3. Sexual ill health should be considered when a patient presents with another issue, e.g. alcohol-related injury.
4. Drugs/alcohol are major risk factors for sexual risk taking.
5. Many issues relating to a person's sexuality will touch upon legal issues and the nurse should abide by confidentiality and legal guidelines.
6. Many nurses will be in situations where an HIV test would be recommended.

Chapter summary

This chapter has shown that a patient's sexual health may be an issue for nursing practice in relation to sexual function or reducing risk. Where sexual health risk could be reduced, nurses will be using communication skills to take a sexual history and provide information. Nurses are increasingly involved in screening procedures, such as HIV testing, which require a discussion with patients about sexual activity. Sexual health is a complex area that can cause nurses confusion and embarrassment and may challenge personal morality and values. Support for patients' sexuality and sexual health needs is a recognized part of nursing practice and requires sensitivity and awareness of non-prejudicial practice.

Further reading and resources

The World Health Organization's definitions and goals for sexual health may be found at http://www.who.int/reproductivehealth/publications/sexual_health/defining_sexual_health.pdf.

There is a range of guidance on HIV testing:

National Institute for Health and Clinical Excellence (2011a) *Increasing the Uptake of HIV Testing among Black Africans in England*. NICE Public Health Guidance 33. Available at: www.nice.org.uk/guidance/PH33.

National Institute for Health and Clinical Excellence (2011b) *Increasing the Uptake of HIV Testing among Men Who Have Sex with Men*. NICE Public Health Guidance 34. Available at: www.nice.org.uk/guidance/PH34.

BHIVA, BASHH, BIS (2008) *UK National Guidelines for HIV Testing 2008*. Available at: http://www.bhiva.org/HIVTesting2008.aspx.

Health Protection Agency (2010) *Time to Test for HIV: Expanded Healthcare and Community HIV Testing in England*. Available at: http://www.hpa.org.uk/web/HPAweb&HPAwebStandard/HPAweb_C/1287145269283 (accessed 1 March 2011).

NICE (2007) *One to One Interventions to Reduce the Transmission of Sexually Transmitted Infections (STIs) Including HIV, and to Reduce the Rate of Under 18 Conceptions, Especially Among Vulnerable and At Risk Groups*. NICE, London.

RCN (2004) *RCN Competencies: Sexual Health Competencies: an Integrated Career and Competency Framework for Sexual and Reproductive Health Nursing*. RCN, London.

http://avert.org.uk for resources and information about HIV/AIDS.

References

Department of Health (2001) *National Strategy for Sexual Health and HIV*. DH, London.
Department of Health (2004) *Choosing Health: Making Healthy Choices Easier*. TSO, London.
Department of Health (2009) *Equality Impact Assessment for Sexual Health Strategy*. Available at: http://webarchive.nationalarchives.gov.uk/20130107105354/http://www.dh.gov.uk/en/Publicationsandstatistics/Publications/PublicationsPolicyAndGuidance/DH_111227.
Department of Health (2012) *Abortion Statistics for England and Wales*. Available at: https://www.gov.uk/government/uploads/system/uploads/attachment_data/file/211790/2012_Abortion_Statistics.pdf.
Greaves, A., Lonsdale, S., Whinney, S., *et al.* (2009) University undergraduates' knowledge of chlamydia screening services and chlamydia information following the introduction of a national chlamydia screening programme. *European Journal of Contraception and Reproductive Health Care*, **14** (1), 61–68.
Harden, A. (2009) Teenage pregnancy and social disadvantage: systematic review integrating controlled trials and qualitative studies. *BMJ*, **339**, b4254.
Health Protection Agency (2007) *Continued Increase in Sexually Transmitted Infections: An Analysis of Data from UK Genitourinary Medicine Clinics up to 2007*. Department of Health, London.
Health Protection Agency (2012) New HIV diagnoses and deaths. *Health Protection Report*, **6** (16), 20 April.
Mercer, C.H. *et al.* (2003) Sexual function problems and help seeking behaviour in Britain: national probability sample survey. *BMJ*, **327**, 426–427.
ONS (Office of National Statistics) (2011) *Conceptions in England and Wales*. Available at: http://www.ons.gov.uk/ons/rel/vsob1/conception-statistics--england-and-wales/2011/2011-conceptions-statistical-bulletin.html.
Origanje, C., Meremikwu, M., Eco, H., *et al.* (2010) Interventions for preventing unintended pregnancies among adolescents. *Cochrane Database of Systematic Reviews*, 1, 1–83.
RCN (2000) *Sexuality and Sexual Health in Nursing Practice*. RCN, London.
World Health Organization (2006) *Defining Sexual Health*. WHO, Geneva. Available at http://www.who.int/reproductivehealth/publications/sexual_health/defining_sexual_health.pdf.

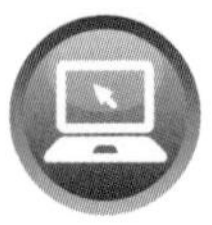

Don't forget to visit the companion website for this book: www.wileyfundamentalseries.com/healthpromotion where you can find self-assessment tests to check your progress.

8

Obesity

Jane Wills

Professor, Health Promotion, London South Bank University, London, UK

Jenny Husbands

Senior Lecturer, Adult Nursing, London South Bank University, London, UK

Muireann Kelly

Research Assistant, London South Bank University, London, UK

Learning outcomes

By the end of this chapter you will be able to:

1. Understand the causes of obesity
2. Understand the impact of obesity on health
3. Have an overview of the strategies to address diet and physical activity in the population
4. Consider the role of the nurse in addressing patients' obesity

Introduction

Being obese increases the risk of developing a number of serious and potentially life-threatening diseases, such as type 2 diabetes, heart disease, or some types of cancer such as breast cancer or colon cancer. Obese people have a much higher risk of complications following surgery such as a heart attack, wound infection, nerve injury, and urinary tract infections. Many

Fundamentals of Health Promotion for Nurses, Second Edition. Edited by Jane Wills.

Companion website: www.wileyfundamentalseries.com/healthpromotion

joint replacements are caused by obesity as more weight going through a joint leads to increased wear and tear and obesity tends to lead to a more sedentary life with less exercise and less movement, which also affects the joints. Obesity in pregnancy also carries risks, including gestational diabetes and pre-eclampsia. It is therefore a major public health priority.

Addressing obesity is about a patient gradually losing weight through a combination of a calorie-controlled diet and regular exercise. There are simple messages to achieve this including eating more fruit and vegetables and cutting down on saturated fat and doing moderate intensity exercise of 30 minutes on at least five days per week. However, as we have seen elsewhere in this book simply exhorting people to follow such messages is unlikely to be successful. This chapter will discuss behaviour change interventions alongside some of the population-level interventions that are used to encourage healthy eating and physical activity.

Defining obesity

Overweight and obesity are terms describing an excess of body fat, usually related to increased weight-for-height. The Body Mass Index (BMI) is the most commonly used method for determining obesity status, as it is a cheap, simple and non-invasive measure. BMI is the ratio of a person's weight in kilogrammes to their height in metres squared (kg/m^2). BMI is often classified as healthy, overweight, or classes of obesity.

However, the problem with this measurement as a means of determining health risk and specifically diseases that are attributed to being obese and overweight, such as coronary heart disease (CHD) and cancer, is that it depends on where the body fat is stored on the body that increases the risk of developing these diseases.

Body fat distribution can be attributed to body type and, significantly, fat distribution is a far more accurate determinant of health and health risk than body weight. For example, if a body builder's weight was measured and the body builder happened to be of short statue, their body mass index would be high, but it would not necessarily represent a significant health risk. Women generally are more likely to have a pear body type due to the influence of the female hormone oestrogen. However, post menopause when the levels of oestrogen decline, fat distribution on the body may become more central and therefore post-menopausal women have an increased risk of CHD and cancer.

Table 8.1 BMI and classification of obesity as per NICE guidance (NICE, 2006).

Classification	BMI (kg/m^2)
Healthy weight	18.5–24.9
Overweight (or pre-obese)	25.0–29.9
Obese Class I	30.0–34.9
Obese Class II	35.0–39.9
Obese Class III	40.0 or more

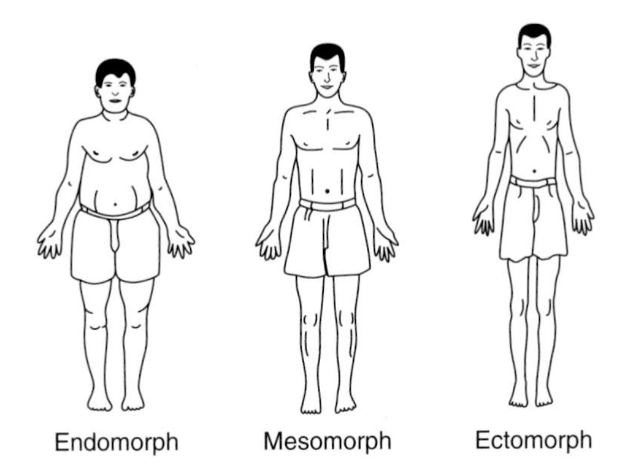

Figure 8.1 Body types and obesity.

A more useful way of understanding the significance of body type and fat distribution is taking into consideration the patient's somatotype or body type. There are three basic somatotype or body types (see Figure 8.1):

- An Endomorph is someone who has wider hips and is smaller from the waist up and has a tendency to gain weight easily. If this person gains weight, they tend to store fat on their hips and lower body and have a pear shape; this pear shape is not generally associated with any significant risk of CHD; diabetes type 2 or cancer.
- An Ectomorph is someone who has a long lean body shape and generally a lower level of body fat, but if this person becomes overweight, they have a tendency to store body fat centrally. Central body fat storage is typically referred to as apple-shaped and in terms of the health risks, people who are apple-shaped have a higher incidence of coronary heart disease, diabetes mellitus, and certain types of cancer namely breast cancer and colon cancer
- A Mesomorph is someone who has a more muscular build and generally has a lower level of body fat, but if this person does become overweight, they have a tendency to store their body fat centrally; this is referred to as apple-shaped and again in terms of the health risks is associated with a higher incidence of coronary heart disease (CHD), diabetes mellitus, breast and colon cancer.

NICE guidance on prevention, identification, assessment and management of overweight and obesity recommend combining BMI status with waist circumference measurement for judgement of obesity in individuals with a BMI of 35 kg/m^2 or less (NICE, 2006, p. 35). A raised weight circumference is defined as 102 cm in men and 88 cm in women. The hip–waist ratio refers to the circumference of the waist divided by the hip circumference and proposes that hips should be at least 0.85 cm larger than the waist in women and the hips should be greater than 0.9 cm than the waist in men . If the hip–waist ratio is less than the figures quoted, there is an increased risk of CHD, diabetes mellitus breast and colon cancer (WHO, 2008).

Activity 8.1

- Do you think defining obesity according to the waist circumference is an accurate assessment of health?
- Do you think there any potential problems with this measurement?

Discussion

The problem with this measurement as a means of determining health risks is that it is open to interpretation and also relies on the accuracy of how and where on the body the measurements are taken. For example, if the patient is immobile, it may pose a problem because it may prove difficult to take accurate waist and hip measurements.

The WHO (2008) recommends taking the hip measurement over the widest point of the buttocks and the waist measurement at a specified height from the floor with the patient standing upright. Waist circumference is perhaps a more effective and reliable measurement and assessment of health risks. This measurement solely measures the waist circumference and proposes that a waist measurement of greater than 35 inches or 85 cms in women; and a waist circumference of 40 inches or 102 cms in men is associated with an increased risk of CHD, breast and colon cancer. The problem with this measurement is the accuracy of the measurements and effective interpretation of the information. In addition, other factors may affect the waist measurement, such as fluid retention, flatulence and food. Ideally, the patient should be standing which poses a problem in patients who are less mobile or have spinal disabilities.

Prevalence of obesity

Some 26.1% of English adults are obese, and 42% of men and 32% of women are overweight (NHSIC, 2012). Based on Health Survey for England data from 2010:

- More men than women are overweight (41.6% males versus 31.7% females), but more women than men are morbidly obese (3.8% females versus 1.6% males).
- Prevalence of overweight and obesity are lowest in the 16–24 age groups, and generally higher in the older age groups among both men and women. There is a decline in prevalence in the oldest age group which is especially clear in men.
- Adults in social class V (unskilled manual) have a higher prevalence of obesity than those in social class I (professional).
- Obesity prevalence varies between ethnic groups. Obesity prevalence is highest in Black Caribbean, Black African and Pakistani populations, whereas Chinese and Bangladeshi groups have the lowest prevalence of obesity. Figure 8.2 shows the high prevalence amongst Black African women.

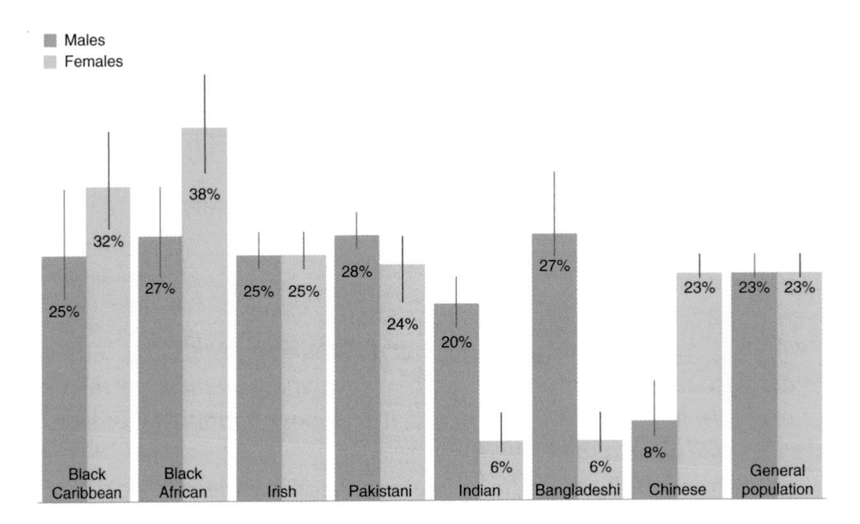

Figure 8.2 Prevalence of obesity in adults by ethnic group. Source: Public Health England, Obesity Knowledge and Intelligence, 2013. Reproduced under the Open Government Licence.

Income and social deprivation, e.g. unemployment are associated with high rates of obesity. The National Obesity Observatory report that:

- For women in particular, lower socio-economic status is associated with an increased risk of obesity.
- Obesity in women increases steadily with decreased family income.
- There is a strong correlation between obesity and educational attainment in both genders.
- The National Child Measurement Programme finds that there is a clear correlation between the geographical area's level of deprivation and levels of obesity in children.

Activity 8.2

Who do you think is most at risk of becoming obese?

Discussion

Approximately half of all pregnant women are overweight or obese at the start of their pregnancy and 15% of all pregnant women are obese (NICE, 2010), which poses risks of pregnancy-induced hypertension, gestational diabetes, premature labour, lower birth weight baby, foetal and maternal death.

People who have learning disabilities have higher rates of obesity than the general population, with rates running at 35% compared to 25% for the general population (see Chapter 14).

There is a strong correlation between obesity and overweight in women who have mental health problems, though the causal relationship between actual body weight, self perception of body weight and being stigmatized because of the body weight is complex and varies across cultures, age groups and ethnicity (National Obesity Observatory, 2011).

Causes of obesity

Obesity occurs when calorie intake through food and drink consumption exceeds calorie expenditure over a prolonged period, resulting in the accumulation of excess body fat.

Activity 8.3

What accounts for the rise in obesity over the last 20 years?

Discussion

There are various factors that combine to contribute to this process. The Foresight report referred to a "complex web of societal and biological factors that have, in recent decades, exposed our inherent human vulnerability to weight gain" (Butland et al., 2007, p. 3). The sudden increase in population obesity prevalence is now predominantly recognized as a result of social, environmental and technological changes in the past 30–40 years such as sedentary lifestyles, heavy marketing of energy-dense foods, and availability of fast food outlets.

The Department of Health (2011) recommend that the negative energy balance can be addressed by a combination of a reduction in calories and increased energy expenditure: a reduction of 100 calories per person per day and a minimum of 30 minutes five times a week of moderate intensity activity such as brisk walking, dancing, cycling, mowing the lawn or energetic housework.

Activity 8.4

Why do you think people find it hard to maintain a healthy body weight?

Discussion

Numerous studies of different population groups cite the following barriers:

- *intrapersonal (e.g. temptation, lack of discipline, low self-worth, boredom, body image, lack of confidence, illness);*
- *interpersonal (e.g. social situations, caring responsibilities);*
- *environmental (e.g. unemployment, low income, time constraints, ready access to unhealthy food).*

And enablers as:

- *intrapersonal (e.g. regulating food intake, being physically active);*
- *interpersonal (e.g. social support, time, relationships)*
- *environmental (e.g. available healthy food such as markets, green space for exercise, subsidized leisure).*

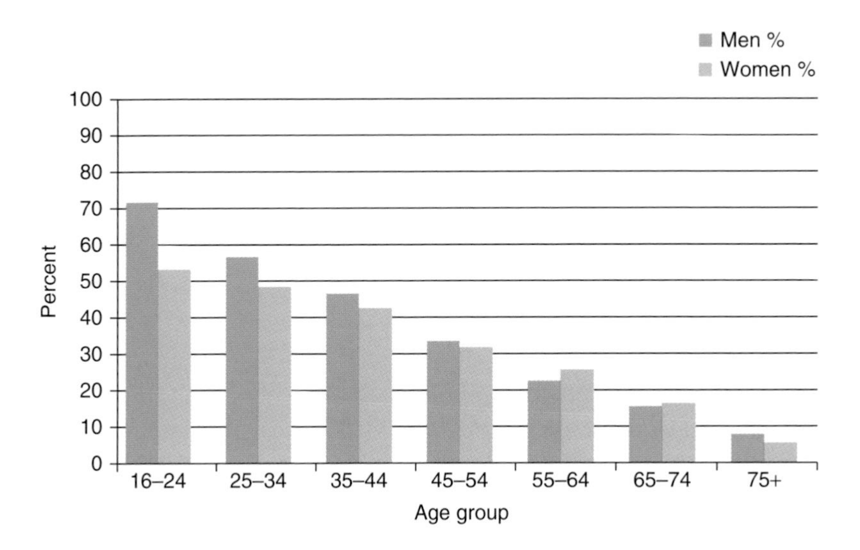

Figure 8.3 Physical inactivity in England. Source data: Joint Health Surveys Unit, 2004.

The most recent Active People Survey (Sport England, 2013) found that 39% of men and 29% of women aged over 16 met the recommended guidelines for physical activity but in the most disadvantaged boroughs only about 15% of adults were classed as active. Figure 8.3 shows how even these low levels of activity decline with age.

The majority of the public believe their own diet to be "quite" healthy yet only 25% of men and 27% of women consumed the recommended five or more portions of fruit and vegetables daily in 2010 (HSCIC, 2012). Clearly then encouraging healthier behaviours is a major focus for health promotion activity but so too is encouraging a healthier environment that makes it easier for people to buy healthy food and to be more active.

There are some medical reasons for obesity, such as hypothyroidism and adrenal disorders and some antidepressants and other medications can contribute to increased weight gain. Genetic disorders such as Prader-Willis syndrome are rare. There is some evidence that a high BMI is hereditary in about 50% of cases but the relative contribution of nature and the environment is complex to disentangle.

Obesity as a public health priority

Obesity has differing consequences for both individuals and communities such as:

- *Health* – obesity is a risk factor for other conditions.
- *Social* – obese individuals often face discrimination and stigma.
- *Psychosocial* – obese individuals often have lowered self-esteem, depression or anxiety.
- *Economic* – direct costs to healthcare system and indirect costs to society.

The risk of co-morbidities rises in a linear fashion with increasing BMI. A number of chronic medical conditions are associated with overweight and obesity, including diabetes, hypertension, cardiovascular diseases (CVD) and stroke, metabolic syndrome, osteoarthritis and various cancers (Kopelman, 2007). It is estimated that life expectancy is reduced by an average of 2–4 years for those with a BMI of 30–35 kg/m^2, and 8–10 years for those with a BMI of 40–50 kg/m^2 (Dent and Swanston, 2010).

Policy context

Since the 2001 report *Tackling Obesity in England* (NAO, 2001), there have been a number of key government strategies and initiatives to tackle adult obesity at an individual and population level. *Healthy Weight, Healthy Lives* (DH, 2008) introduced a national strategy for obesity in England. There is currently no National Service Framework (NSF) aimed at tackling obesity in this country, though obesity care is encompassed in the NSF for diabetes, mental health, and coronary heart disease as well as the national stroke strategy. A timeline of some key developments is shown in Table 8.2.

Table 8.2 A timeline of key policy initiatives relating to obesity.

Year	Action
2001	National Audit Office report *Tackling Obesity in England* notes the scope of policy to effect lifestyle change directly is very limited and states that the Department of Health cannot be expected to combat the problem alone.
2004	Based on a House of Commons report, the government identifies obesity as a policy priority and sets the first Public Service Agreement target specifically for obesity, initially focusing on childhood obesity. *Choosing Health: Making Healthy Choices Easier* asserts the importance of informed choice; argues that government should create a "demand for health" (p. 20) through information and marketing, in order to stimulate behaviour change for healthier lifestyles.
2005	*Choosing Activity* and *Choosing a Better Diet* highlight how the Department of Health and the NHS will help more people make healthier choices and reduce health inequalities. The documents call for intersectoral collaboration at regional, local and national level.
2007	The Foresight report, *Tackling Obesities: Future Choices* highlights the need for a comprehensive approach to obesity through cross-governmental initiatives, and recognizes the social and economic costs of obesity in the UK. The report argues that social and environmental factors interplay to create an "obesogenic environment" which promotes weight gain, and local authorities' role in reducing obesity through "place shaping" is stressed.

(*Continued*)

Table 8.2 (*Continued*)

Year	Action
2008	*Healthy Weight, Healthy Lives; A Cross-Government Strategy for England* is published as England's first national obesity strategy. It details the strategy for implementing the public service target ambition to be "the first major nation to reverse the rising tide of obesity and overweight in the population". The National Obesity Observatory (NOO) was established.
2009	*Change 4 Life* established as the social marketing arm of the *Healthy Weight, Healthy Lives* strategy, with an initial focus on families with children of school-going age.
2010	Adult arm of *Change 4 Life* is launched after one-year-on progress report shows evidence of success. *London Health Inequalities Strategy* introduced. Marmot Review *Fair Society, Healthy Lives* published. *Healthy Lives, Healthy People* policy introduced in a White Paper which proposes a new integrated public health service – Public Health England – created to ensure expertise and responsiveness on public health issues, including obesity. The document also sets out local government and local communities' responsibility for improving health and well-being.
2011	*Healthy Lives, Healthy People: A Call to Action on Obesity in England* revises the 2008 *Healthy Weight* ambition to "a downward trend in the level of excess weight averaged across all adults by 2020".
2012	Alcohol awareness component of *Change 4 Life* campaign launched. Public Health Outcomes Framework introduced. NICE guidance to be published on *Preventing Obesity: A Whole System Approach.*

Addressing obesity

Scenario 8.1

Angela is a 45-year-old divorced mother of three children aged 18, 16 and 12 years, of Black Caribbean descent. Angela is classified as obese with a BMI of 30 and a waist circumference measuring 40 inches or 102 cm.

Angela is effectively an unsupported single parent who works as a receptionist in the local authority where she has to face an often hostile public on a daily basis as part of her role, and she lacks confidence especially as sometimes the public make unflattering personal remarks about her appearance.

She desperately wants to lose weight and has struggled for many years with various diets and inconsistent exercise classes, all of which had little success, and worryingly she has steadily gained weight over the years. Over time Angela has suffered from numerous health problems associated with being obese, including hypertension, lower back pain, depression, fatigue and sleep apnoea.

Angela is seen in the outpatients department where she tells the doctor that she wants to have a gastric band fitted as she has seen celebrities on television who have had this procedure and they have reported that they have lost significant amounts of weight. Angela is adamant that this is the only acceptable choice she has as all her previous attempts at weight loss have been unsuccessful and left her with low self-esteem.

What advice would you give to Angela?

Discussion

Most people who are overweight or obese express a desire to lose weight for health or aesthetic reasons and many will have tried on previous occasions usually by dieting or portion control. There is not a strong evidence base to guide the choice of strategies to manage adult obesity and to maintain weight loss in the long term, particularly for men. Interventions in non-clinical settings that are shown to be effective in terms of weight management are likely to demonstrate significant improvements in participants' dietary intakes (usually fat and calorie intake) and/or physical activity levels (Cavill and Ells, 2010).

In 2006, the National Institute for Health and Clinical Excellence (NICE, 2006) published the first national guidance on the prevention, identification, assessment and management of overweight and obesity in adults and children in England and Wales. NICE is currently developing new guidance for whole-system approaches to tackling obesity and lifestyle-based weight management of overweight and obese adults. Multi-component interventions are the first-line option for management of obesity in the clinical setting and patients should discuss all treatment options, including the use of commercial weight loss services. Information on patient support programmes should also be provided. Previous experiences, preferences and social circumstances, as well as level of risk and existing co-morbidities, should all be considered in designing a treatment regimen.

Table 8.3 summarizes some of the evidence for effectiveness of various interventions. Evidence has been drawn from the NICE guidance (2006), unless otherwise stated.

Table 8.3 Interventions for weight management and review of effectiveness, including lifestyle and clinical interventions.

Type of intervention	Is it effective in tackling obesity?
Lifestyle change interventions	
Commercial weight loss services	Some evidence to suggest that a multi-component commercial group programme may be more effective than a standard self-help programme. Weight Watchers is the only programme with good quality data underpinning its effectiveness, thus it remains unclear if it is more effective for weight loss than other branded programmes. The majority of research in this area has been funded by organizations themselves; therefore results must be interpreted with caution.
Meal replacement plans	There is a lack of evidence to support the use of meal replacement products over a standard low-calorie diet.
Calorie or food-controlled diets	Some evidence to suggest low Glycaemic Index (GI) diets may be an effective method of promoting weight loss. The effectiveness of all diets appears to change over time, with a reduction in weight loss in the longer term.
Workplace-based interventions	Limited evidence of effectiveness, although some weight loss may be noted in the short term. Recent reviews of workplace interventions for weight management suggested that studies with an environmental component (e.g. team competitions or management commitment) may be particularly effective. Unlike most research in non-clinical settings, workplace interventions studies predominantly involve men.
Internet-based interventions	Some evidence that the internet may be an effective mode of delivery for weight loss interventions, if combined with ongoing support via email or in person. The majority of research has been carried out in the USA and participants are predominantly white, well-educated women so results may not be generalizable to a UK or low-income setting.
Behavioural interventions	Behavioural and cognitive-behavioural therapies significantly improve weight loss success, especially if combined with dietary and exercise strategies. Cognitive therapy alone (i.e. ignoring behaviour change) is not effective for weight loss. Involving family members (particularly spouses) in behavioural therapies for weight loss can be more effective, though there is some evidence to suggest that this is only true for women, with men doing better when treated individually.

Table 8.3 (*Continued*)

Type of intervention	Is it effective in tackling obesity?
Behavioural interventions	The greatest weight loss occurs when behaviour therapies are combined with active support for a low-calorie or very low calorie diet (VLCD), which are less than 1000 kcal/day.
Brief interventions for physical activity	Evidence of effectiveness in primary care in producing moderate increases in adult populations in the short term, longer term and in the very long term (i.e. one year or more). A minimum level of 30 minutes physical activity three times a week is effective for weight loss, but physical activity alone is less effective than diet alone. NICE noted that the intensity and duration of exercise needed for long term weight loss may be much higher than recommended in most behavioural treatment programmes (2006, p. 579). Both NICE and the Department for Health consider brief physical activity intervention in primary care "exceptional value for money" (DH, 2009, p. 28).
Pedometer-based interventions	Insufficient evidence to make any conclusions about the effects of pedometer interventions, though some evidence suggests short-term benefits, particularly for women. Guidelines on pedometer interventions are currently under development by NICE.
Financial incentives for weight loss	A 2011 systematic review of the literature focusing on obesity treatment generally supported a positive effect of monetary incentives on weight loss, though this may be a premature finding as the body of evidence is still very small (Paloyo *et al.*, 2011).
Clinical interventions	
Weight loss medication	The only pharmaceutical treatment currently recommended by NICE for prescription is Orlistat (marketed as Alli in the UK). A Cochrane review noted Orlistat reduced weight by around 5 kg or less and reduced the number of high-risk patients who developed diabetes (Padwal *et al.*, 2009). The review notes that weight loss with Orlistat is modest, and the additional clinical benefits of the drug for some may be overshadowed by its adverse gastrointestinal effects for many.
Bariatric surgery	There are a number of bariatric surgical procedures available to reduce weight but it remains unclear which are most effective in reducing weight or have the least number of complications. A Cochrane review of the evidence suggests surgery results in greater weight loss than other conventional interventions, but side effects, complications and potentially death may occur (Colquitt *et al.*, 2009).

(*Continued*)

Table 8.3 (*Continued*)

Type of intervention	Is it effective in tackling obesity?
GP referral schemes	Research from referral to weight loss services in England suggests that it may be cheaper and achieve greater weight loss than primary care-provided services. Evidence from randomized controlled trials suggests that exercise referral schemes can have positive effects on physical activity levels in the short term (6–12 weeks), but they are ineffective in increasing activity levels in the longer term or over a timeframe longer than one year. Some research suggesting exercise referral programmes may only be beneficial for those who are overweight but not yet obese, and no more effective than other physical activity interventions or standard care.

Addressing obesity and promoting a healthy diet: health education

Current government recommendations are that everyone should eat plenty of fruit and vegetables (at least 5 of a variety each day), plenty of potatoes, bread, rice and other starchy foods, some milk and dairy foods, meat, fish, eggs, beans and other non-dairy sources of protein. Foods and drinks high in salt, fat and sugar should be consumed infrequently and in small amounts. This is visually represented in the eatwell plate in Figure 8.4, a tool that helps to make healthier eating easier to understand, showing the types and proportions of foods needed for a healthy, balanced diet.

Advice and health education on weight loss demands of the nurse the same practice as for other issues, namely encouragement and empowerment. Some key pointers based on successful weight loss programmes are:

- to support patients to make small sustainable changes in eating behaviour;
- to be positive and focus on the additions patients can make towards a healthy diet, rather than the dietary restrictions;
- to set achievable weight loss goals, e.g. 1–2 lbs per week and also give themselves healthy rewards for weight lost to reinforce change;
- to pre-plan meals to enable healthy eating;
- to encourage patients to evaluate food choices when shopping for food, i.e. reading labels and to write shopping lists before they go shopping;
- to help patients to understand the cues to eating behaviour such as environmental triggers; keep office desks free from food, and the kitchen cabinets free from unhealthy high fat, high sugar, snacks, and replace unhealthy snacks with fruit and nuts.
- to discourage patients from eating while watching television, driving or working on the computer as it may be hard for the patient to keep track of how much they have eaten.

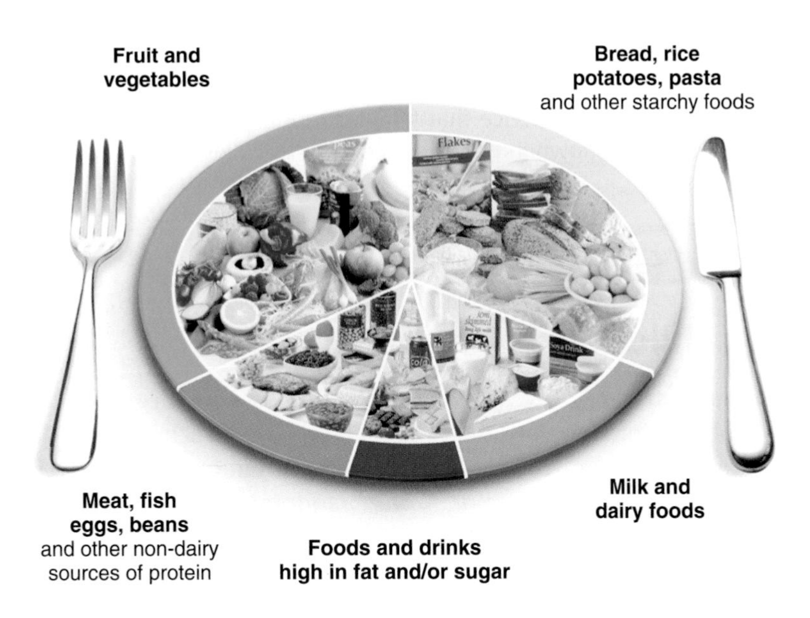

Figure 8.4 Eatwell plate. Source: Public Health England in association with the Welsh Government, the Scottish Government and the Food Standards Agency in Northern Ireland. Reproduced under the Open Government Licence.

- to encourage patients to eat a variety of foods and not to give up all of their favourite foods but to make small changes to how they cook food, e.g. jacket potatoes instead of roast potatoes;
- to help patients to consider appropriate portion sizes, not having more than one portion or serving and always to eat off a plate as opposed to a bag, container or wrapping;
- to encourage patients to consider the healthier options from menus in restaurants and to feel confident to ask for alterations or amendments to their meals such as less sauces;
- to encourage patients to have healthy snack readily available at all times to avoid lapses.

Addressing obesity in children: using social support

Childhood obesity is a serious public health challenge, figures from the National Child Measurement Programme show that about 9.6% of children in the Reception year (aged 4–5 years) and 18.3% in Year 6 (aged 10–11 years) are obese. During these school years children develop potentially life-long patterns of behaviour in relation to diet and activity that will affect their ability to maintain a healthy weight. They are also exposed to an "obesogenic" environment, in other words, an environment at school and in their neighbourhood that contributes to obesity through the provision of fast food and lack of opportunities to exercise or play.

Most of the strategies to promote healthy weight amongt children use a combination of health education, healthy food preparation or cooking classes, and activity groups (Aicken *et al.*, 2008). There is some evidence that family support is key to successful weight loss programmes for children as shown in the evidence from the MEND programme.

Evidence 8.1

Addressing childhood obesity

The Mind, Exercise, Nutrition, Do it (MEND) programme is a multicomponent community-based childhood obesity intervention (www.mendcentral.org) which has been widely adopted in the UK. In a randomized controlled trial to examine its effectiveness, 116 children (BMI > or = 98th percentile, UK 1990 reference data) were randomly assigned to the intervention or a waiting list control group. Parents and children attended eighteen 2-hour group educational and physical activity sessions held twice weekly in sports centres and schools, followed by a 12-week free family swimming pass. Waist circumference, BMI, body composition, physical activity level, sedentary activities, cardiovascular fitness, and self-esteem were assessed at baseline and at 6 months. Participants in the intervention group had a reduced waist circumference and BMI at 6 months when compared to the controls. Significant between-group differences were also observed in cardiovascular fitness, physical activity, sedentary behaviours, and self-esteem. High-attendance rates (86%) suggest that families found this intensive community-based intervention acceptable (Sacher *et al.*, 2010).

Addressing obesity and promoting physical activity: creating a supportive environment

Although the whole population would benefit from increased levels of physical activity, it is especially important for those who live sedentary lifestyles, including most older people. Evidence suggests that low intensity activities such as tai chi and dance classes and walking programmes are effective in reducing the frequency of falls, improving physical functioning and improving balance (see bhfactive.org.uk).

Figure 8.5 illustrates some of the guidance for older people based on the Chief Medical Officer's guidance (CMO, 2011).

Addressing obesity through public policy

Part of the Public Health White Paper, *Healthy Lives, Healthy People* (DH, 2011) was a Public Health Responsibility Deal to encourage businesses and other organiZations to improve public health and tackle health inequalities through their influence over food, alcohol, physical activity

Moderate intensity physical activities will cause older adults to get warmer and breathe harder and their hearts to beat faster, but they should still be able to carry on a conversation.
Examples include:
• Brisk walking • Dancing

Activities to improve balance and co-ordination may include:
• Tai chi • Yoga

Vigorous intensity physical activities will cause older adults to get warmer and breathe much harder and their hearts to beat rapidly, making it more difficult to carry on a conversation.
Examples include:
• Climbing stairs • Running

Minimising sedentary behaviour may include:
• Reducing time spent watching TV
• Taking regular walk breaks around the garden or street
• Breaking up sedentary time such as swapping a long bus or car journey for walking

Physical activities that strengthen muscles involve using body weight or working against a resistance. This should involve using all the major muscle groups. Examples include:
• Carrying or moving heavy loads such as groceries
• Activities that involve stepping and jumping such as dancing

Figure 8.5 Examples of physical activity for older people that meet recommended guidelines.

and health in the workplace. It aimed to deliver voluntary agreements or "pledges" to improve public health through activities such as further reformulation of food; better information for consumers about food; and the promotion of more socially responsible retailing and consumption of alcohol.

Activity 8.5

Do you think that large corporations who sell foodstuffs including confectionary and drinks promote health?

Discussion

There has been concern that the attempt to "nudge" large companies to be more health promoting relies on a voluntary agreement and not regulation. Certain moves may be made to cut salt or sugar but essentially, many popular food and drinks are based on their sugar content. There have been calls by health care professional organizations to tax sugary drinks and thereby reduce demand and to ban vending machines.

The role of the nurse in tackling obesity

In many settings the nurse will be required to take height and weight measurements. This provides an opportunity not only to assess a patient's weight but also to discuss and raise the issue of obesity if relevant and the importance of eating healthily and being active. Rarely, however, do nurses do this and there is some evidence that those who are overweight themselves may be reluctant to raise the issue.

Individuals who are obese or physically inactive are responsive to four simple messages:

- *Benefits*: what they will get from change.
- *Self-efficacy*: reassuring them that they can change and building confidence and experience.
- *Social support*: who can help them.
- *Fitting the change into their everyday life*: e.g. active transport or portion control.

The role of the nurse is to:

- Give advice to enable patients to make an informed choice about treatment options, including safe and effective diet and physical activity and any drug treatments.
- Act as an advocate for patients who feel unable to make choices due to their low self-esteem.
- Make referrals to the most appropriate services and support patients to access these services.
- Mobilize resources so that patients can get the best available treatment given the limited choices that are sometimes available to them.
- Lobby for change in government policies on the pricing of fruit and vegetables; availability of healthy low calorie food; affordable physical activity options and access and availability of physical activity facilities.
- Understand the impact of obesity on patients' self-esteem and self-confidence and subsequently ensure that the care provided is non-judgemental.

The NMC (2012) requirements state that nurses:

- Must give advice based on the best available evidence – this is especially important when new guidance is regularly issued on effective interventions.
- Must recognize and work within the limits of their competence – it is important therefore to be informed about this topic and be able to provide accurate nutritional and activity advice appropriate to the patient.
- Must not discriminate in any way against those in their care – discrimination and prejudice exist against those who are obese who are often perceived to be just lazy and gluttonous. "Blaming the individual" could mean nurses spend less time with obese patients or do not take their problems as seriously. Nurses should also take care not to attribute all of a patient's problems to their obesity – "writing them off" effectively. It is vital not to stigmatize the obese patient, even though their health risks are clear, and to remember that the obesogenic environment shapes behaviour and has a direct impact on people's health.

On placement: checklist

- ❑ What proportion of patients would you say were obese?
- ❑ Was this recorded in their notes?
- ❑ Was the opportunity taken to raise the issue and offer advice or signpost to services?
- ❑ What information was offered to patients about weight management?

Key learning points

1. Obesity is frequently stigmatized. Do not "blame the victim".
2. There are many causes of obesity and the inability to maintain or lose weight, so treatment and management must be personalized.
3. Health education advice must be accurate and tailored to the patient's needs.

Chapter summary

This chapter discussed definitions of obesity and the difficulties of using body weight as a measurement associated with various measures of obesity. The scale of the problem, including the health risks associated with being obese, and economic impact and health risks associated with being obese were also discussed. The chapter emphasizes the importance of health care professionals being able to raise the issue of obesity when appropriate, using non-pejorative language and to adequately refer or signpost patients for further support. Most people want to lose weight and messages should not be patronizing, overwhelming or unrealistic and should be simple and able to be incorporated into everyday life by catering to an individual's needs and circumstances. There are windows of opportunity to intervene at particular life moments such as pregnancy or a diagnosis of diabetes, or after a vascular episode and population groups need specific services for their life stages and psychosocial attitudes.

Further reading and resources

The best source for up-to-date information on the prevalence and causes of obesity is the National Obesity Observatory. Available at: http://www.noo.org.uk.

The National Institute for Health and Clinical Excellence produces clinical guidelines (CG 43), public health guidelines on working with communities (PH 42) and guidelines on prevention, see http://www.nice.org.uk.

References

Aicken, C., Arai, L. and Roberts, H. (2008) *Schemes to Promote Healthy Weight Among Obese and Overweight Children in England. Report.* London: EPPI-Centre, Social Science Research Unit, Institute of Education, University of London. Available at: http://eppi.ioe.ac.uk/mapchildobesityen.

Butland, B. *et al.* (2007) *Foresight Report: Tackling Obesity – Future Choices.* Government Office of Science, London. Available online at: http://www.bis.gov.uk/assets/foresight/docs/obesity/17.pdf.

Cavill, N. and Ells, L. (2010). *Treating Adult Obesity Through Lifestyle Change Interventions. A Briefing Paper for Commissioners.* NOO, London.

Chief Medical Officer (2011) *Start Active, Stay Active: A Report on Physical Activity for Health from the Four Home Countries.* DH, London.

Dent, M. and Swanston, D. (2010) *Briefing Note: Obesity and Life Expectancy.* NOO, London.

Department of Health (2001) *Exercise Referral Systems: A National Quality Assurance Framework.* DH, London.

Department of Health (2004) *Choosing Health: Making Healthy Choices Easier.* DH. London.

Department of Health (2005a) *Choosing a Better Diet: A Food and Health Action Plan.* DH, London.

Department of Health (2005b) *Choosing Activity: A Physical Activity Action Plan.* : DH, London.

Department of Health (2008) *Healthy Weight, Healthy Lives: A Cross-Government Strategy for England.* DH, London.

Department of Health (2011) *Healthy Lives, Healthy People: A Call to Action on Obesity in England.* DH, London.

HSCIC (2012) *Statistics on Obesity, Physical Activity and Diet England 2012.* Available online at http://www.aso.org.uk/wp-content/uploads/downloads/2012/03/2012-Statistics-on-Obesity-Physical-Activity-and-Diet-England.pdf.

Joint Health Surveys Unit (2004) *Health Survey for England 2003:* Vol. 2 *Risk Factors for Cardiovascular Disease.* The Stationery Office, London.

Kopelman, P. (2007) Health risks associated with overweight and obesity. *Obesity Reviews: An Official Journal of the International Association for the Study of Obesity,* **8**, 13–17.

National Audit Office (2001) *Tackling Obesity in England.* HMSO, London.

National Institute for Health and Clinical Excellence, (2006) *Obesity. Guidance on the Prevention, Identification, Assessment and Management of Overweight and Obesity in Adults and Children.* CG 43 NICE, London. Avaialble at: http://www.nice.org.uk/nicemedia/pdf/cg43niceguideline.pdf.

National Institute for Health and Clinical Excellence (2010) *Weight Management Before, During and After Pregnancy.* PH 27. NICE, London. Available at: http://www.nice.org.uk/nicemedia/live/13056/49926/49926.pdf.

National Obesity Observatory (2011) *Obesity and Mental Health.* Available at: http://www.noo.org.uk/uploads/doc/vid_10266_Obesity%20and%20mental%20health_FINAL_070311_MG.pdf.

National Obesity Observatory (2013) *Health Inequalities.* Available at: http://www.noo.org.uk/NOO_about_obesity/inequalities.

NHS Information Centre for Health and Social Care (2012) *Statistics on Obesity, Physical Activity and Diet: England, 2012.* NHSIC, London. Available at: https://catalogue.ic.nhs.uk/publications/public-health/obesity/obes-phys-acti-diet-eng-2012/obes-phys-acti-diet-eng-2012-rep.pdf.

NMC (Nursing and Midwifery Council) (2012) *The Code: Standards of Conduct, Performance and Ethics for Nurses and Midwives.* NMC, London.

Sacher, P.M., Kolotourou, M., Chadwick, P.M., *et al.* (2010) Randomized controlled trial of the MEND program: a family-based community intervention for childhood obesity. *Obesity*, Feb;**18** Suppl. 1:S62–8. DOI: 10.1038/oby.2009.433.
Sport England (2013) *Active People Survey 7*. Available at: http://archive.sportengland.org/research/active_people_survey/active_people_survey_7.aspx.
WHO (2008) *Waist Circumference and Waist–Hip Ratio: Report of a WHO Expert Consultation*. WHO, Geneva.

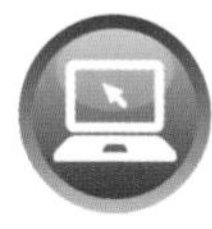

Don't forget to visit the companion website for this book: www.wileyfundamentalseries.com/healthpromotion where you can find self-assessment tests to check your progress.

9

Long-term conditions

Sandie Woods

Senior Lecturer, Occupational Therapy, London South Bank University, London, UK

Learning outcomes

By the end of this chapter you will be able to:

1. Define long-term conditions and their impact on public health
2. Discuss the concepts of self-care, self-management and the benefits of expert patient programmes
3. Identify the ethical and professional issues associated with self-management

Introduction

A long-term condition, sometimes referred to as a chronic condition, has been described as a condition that cannot, at present, be cured but is controlled by medication and/or other treatment/therapies (DH, 2012). Increased life expectancy means the chances increase of developing such a condition and the number of individuals with two or more conditions is set to rise to 2.9 million by 2018, an increase of 1 million since 2008 (DH, 2013). A long-term condition may affect physical health, mental health and well-being and accounts for 70% of the total health and care spend in England including 70% of hospital admissions and 80% of GP consultations (DH, 2012).

This chapter outlines the role of the nurse in promoting health and well-being for individuals with a long-term condition with a focus on self-management and living well. The nurse and other health care professionals have a key role in personalized care planning, providing health information, promoting self-care and supporting individuals to take control of their own health.

Fundamentals of Health Promotion for Nurses, Second Edition. Edited by Jane Wills.

Companion website: www.wileyfundamentalseries.com/healthpromotion

Enabling involves helping individuals who have a long-term condition to do the things they want to do. This may be related to daily activities, caring for a family, undertaking work or studies and maintaining a healthy social life (SCIE, 2013).

In Chapter 3 we considered different approaches to health promotion. What Beattie calls "personal counselling for health" or empowerment is at the heart of self-management that builds the patient's confidence, self-esteem and self-efficacy to take control of their health.

Activity 9.1

What examples of long-term conditions have you come across? Why are they of prolonged duration?

Discussion

Conditions you may have mentioned include: Arthritis, Asthma, Cancer, Chronic Obstructive Pulmonary Disease, Coronary Heart Disease, Dementia, Depression, Diabetes, Multiple Sclerosis, Parkinson's Disease, Schizophrenia, Stroke. These are all conditions that may affect any aspect of life and cannot currently be cured.

Long-term conditions as a public health priority

- 60% of people over 60 years suffer from a long term condition.
- Due to the ageing population, this number is set to rise by 23% over the next 25 years.
- 5% of the patients account for nearly 50% of patient hospital days.
- People with a long-term condition account for nearly 70% of the primary and acute care budget in England (DH, 2008).

These figures illustrate the scale of such conditions and how the likelihood of having a long-term condition increases with age. They also show the huge demand on services. Clearly, then, one of the biggest challenges is the redeployment of resources to manage such conditions whether through self-care and/or through providing sufficient support in the community to enable the individual to manage.

Table 9.1 shows that the most prevalent conditions are hypertension, depression, and asthma. Conditions rising most quickly are cancers, diabetes, and chronic kidney disease.

Table 9.1 The prevalence of long-term conditions in general practice (DH, 2012).

Type of long-term condition	Number affected		% change
	2006–07	2010–11	
Hypertension	6,706,000	7,460,000	11
Depression	0	4,878,000	N/A
Asthma	3,100,000	3,273,000	6
Diabetes	1,962,000	2,456,000	25
Coronary Heart Disease	1,899,000	1,878,000	−1
Chronic Kidney Disease	1,279,000	1,855,000	45
Hypothyroidism	1,367,000	1,667,000	22
Stroke or Transient Ischaemic Attacks (TI)	863,000	944,000	9
Chronic Obstructive Pulmonary Disease	766,000	899,000	17
Cancer	489,000	876,000	79
Atrial Fibrillation	692,000	791,000	14
Mental Health	380,000	438,000	15
Heart Failure	420,000	393,000	−6
Epilepsy	321,000	337,000	5
Dementia	213,000	267,000	25

Source: Long Term Conditions Team (2012), Table 1, p. 5. Reproduced under the Open Government Licence.

Activity 9.2

From your experience, what are the impacts of a long-term condition on a patient's quality of life?

Discussion

Every long-term condition will affect different people in different ways. However, there are some common issues that can affect a lot of people living with long-term conditions. These are summarized by NHSInform, Scotland's information service (www.nhsinform.co.uk) *as:*

- *Shock when a person is initially diagnosed with a condition as they may have difficulty coming to terms with the implications this might have for them, e.g. having to take daily medication, make lifestyle changes or the realization that there may be no cure.*

- *Social exclusion if their condition leads them to lose contact with their social networks or they have to give up work.*
- *Strong emotions including frustration, anger and resentment and loss of self-esteem because they are more reliant on other people, because the condition changes their view of themselves or the way others see them. People who have experienced a stroke may experience intense feelings that they unable to control.*
- *Problems accessing appropriate treatment, support and information to manage their condition. Moving between services or dealing with different professionals and departments can be stressful and often requires a lot of coordination.*
- *Difficulties dealing with the day-to-day symptoms of particular conditions. Symptoms might include chronic pain, fatigue, allergic reactions, mobility problems, bowel problems, sleep problems and personality changes.*
- *Depression which is very common in those who have experienced a stroke or heart attack, and there are much higher rates of depression and suicide in people with epilepsy than in the general population.*

Long-term conditions are more common in people from lower socio-economic groups. General Household Survey data (2006) analysed by the Department of Health, shows those from unskilled occupations (52%) suffer from long-term conditions more than groups from professional occupations (33%). Those from lower socio-economic groups are less likely to use health services and more likely to be admitted as an emergency. Figure 9.1, adapted from analysis by the London School of Economics of multiple studies, shows that in part this may be due to:

- differences in recognition or acceptance of the need for services;
- differences in awareness and knowledge about the availability of services;
- differences in ability to make themselves heard and to navigate service systems.

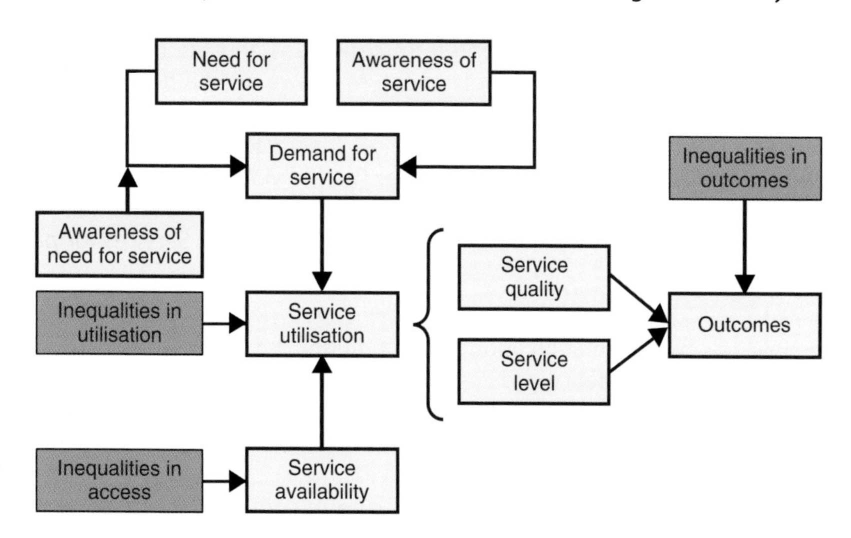

Figure 9.1 Inequalities in the use of, and access to, services by older people. Source: *Just ageing?* 2009, Appendix 2, p. 25. Reproduced with permission from the Equality and Human Rights Commission.

Health policy context

Various documents have set out the framework for and guidance on how to accomplish the shift towards a patient-centred NHS that focuses not just on the treatment of disease but also encourages self-management (DH, 2009, 2010b). The National Service Framework for Long-Term Conditions (DH, 2005) set out quality standards that individuals with a long-term condition should expect to receive.

This section will focus on what is meant by a person-centred service. Recent policy in the NHS over the past decade has emphasized the need for patient- centredness and patient involvement (DH, 2006). The term "co-production" is increasingly being used to describe the approach applied to public service delivery in which patients and service users become active participants in their own care rather than passive recipients of services designed and delivered by someone else. It emphasizes that the people who use services have assets (skills, knowledge) that can help to improve those services, rather than simply needs which must be met. The Health and Social Care Act (DH, 2012) reinforced the importance of improving quality and choice of care for patients and increasing transparency. A key phrase within the Act, "No decision about me without me" emphasizes the importance of the service user in the process.

Managing a long-term condition will require integrating self-management into health care planning in a holistic and patient-centred way. For the nurse, the challenge is to support the patient so that they do not feel they are alone with their condition(s) and also for them to feel they have some control. This entails several basic principles:

- collaborative approach with the patient;
- multidisciplinary working among different services with clear signposting;
- clear goals and personalized planning tailored for the individual;
- self-management that enables patients to be confident and active in their own care.

The demands placed by the rise in long-term conditions and the need to re-orientate care towards patient responsibility and involvement, mean we need a new health care system in which health care professionals and patients collaborate to enable people to live better with their conditions. A collaborative approach requires shared agreement about the priorities and confidence in the individual's ability to change. The individual with a long-term condition is encouraged to play an active role and is supported to define goals and make decisions with the correct information and support (Entwistle and Cribb, 2013). Services for patients should include:

- accessible, reliable information about the condition;
- skills to develop competence and confidence in living well with the condition;
- support networks including local and national groups for individuals and carers;
- signposting to appropriate technology and devices to support self-care (DH, 2006).

An individual may have been living with a long-term condition for many years and having a co-ordinated approach among different services can be helpful to reduce duplication.

Activity 9.3

What do you think a patient or service user with a long-term condition wants from health and social care services?

Discussion

- *They want to be involved in decisions about their care.*
- *They want to be listened to and have access to information to help to make decisions.*
- *They want support and confidence to support self-care.*
- *They want joined-up seamless services and proactive care.*
- *They do not want to be in hospital unless it is absolutely necessary and part of a planned approach.*
- *They want to be treated as a whole person and for the NHS to act as a team (DH, 2012).*

Scenario 9.1

Dan started to experience stomach pain and blood in his stool when he was 15. He was eventually diagnosed with Crohn's Disease just as he was about to start his GCSE exams. He was very frightened and unclear what would happen to him. The chronic pain and diarrohea meant that he was reluctant to eat and had to rely on liquid supplements. He is now 20 and at university. He has had colonoscopies twice a year which have revealed that his bowel is damaged and it is possible he will require surgery. At present, he manages pain, mostly with paracetamol and receives antibiotic therapy.

Which health care professionals would you expect to be involved in Dan's care?

Discussion

You may have included the following: Gastroenterologist, Colorectal Surgeon, Clinical Nurse Specialist, Dietitian, Histopathologist, Psychologist, Radiologist.

Approaches to long-term conditions: developing personal skills and self-management

Self-care involves the individual taking responsibility for their own health and well-being to maintain physical and mental health, meet social and psychological needs, prevent illness or accidents and care for long-term conditions. To do this, the patient needs to feel confident in their knowledge and skills to be able to take control.

Self-management is related to living with a long-term condition including the person's ability to manage symptoms, treatment, physical and psychological consequences and lifestyle changes (DH, 2011).

The Department of Health (2010c) identified five Es to self-management to help change behaviour and improve outcomes for people with a long-term condition:

- **E**ducate
- **E**nthuse
- **E**nable
- **E**mpower
- **E**mbed.

Individuals with a long-term condition may feel it is too late to make a change, may feel it is beyond their control or find it difficult to look at a new lifestyle or behaviour. Listening to the individual and encouraging them to discuss beliefs, concerns and behaviours can help promote self-care. Hope is an important concept when facing the challenges of living with a long-term condition and staff values, attitudes and behaviours can all influence hope for the future. Valuing the person as unique and accepting them for who they are, believing in their potential and accepting relapse as part of recovery, having a genuine concern and helping the person find meaning in their lives are all strategies for promoting hope. The transition may be gradual and involve coaching and motivational techniques (see Chapter 12) to promote active involvement in their health and care.

A person with a long-term condition may have to review their life and what they wish to achieve. Personal goals may be approached from the perspective of how life has changed and how it could be different. Assessment should include consideration of important activities (e.g. self-care, productivity, leisure), desirable but not essential activities, and those activities that the patient may feel happy to delegate to others.

Facing a long-term condition can involve physical and psychological adaptation and changes in lifestyle. During an acute phase, for example following a stroke or myocardial infarction (heart attack), the individual with a long-term condition and the family may require greater levels of support and guidance as well as information to make sense of what has happened. Active listening skills are important to hear an individual's story, finding out what matters to them, showing awareness and empathy of the situation being faced and flexibility to provide the right level of support and guidance. It may not be a smooth transition, each person's journey will be different, and individuals need to know that there is access to a professional when needed. The "life thread model" (Ellis- Hill *et al.*, 2008) focuses on the importance of the interpersonal relationship, including a positive view of self, being with someone as well as doing things for them and recognizing transition rather than simply loss.

Observation skills are essential to identify with the individual and professional team whether difficulties in self-care are due to physical changes, psychological changes or the environment. Encouragement, shared goal-setting, decision-making, discussion about the costs and understanding the benefits of action or intervention can all help with motivation and adherence. This may relate to medication, exercise, diet or other behaviour change. The individual who is low in mood or is in pain may not recognize their own progress and encouragement and monitoring is important whether related to performance, confidence or sense of control over health and well-being.

The Department of Health (2001) recognized that the knowledge and expertise held by the person living with a long-term condition was an untapped resource and called for action to create expert patients with the confidence, skills, information and knowledge to play a role in their own self-management and to share their expertise with professionals and other people living with a long-term condition. Expert patient programmes and self-management have become an important and established part of primary and secondary health promotion. Attending self-management programmes or becoming an expert patient can enable individuals not only to share their expert knowledge of living with the condition but also can provide psychological and social support to those newly diagnosed.

The nurse can help the individual consider their readiness to undertake training to become an expert patient. It requires a range of interpersonal skills, including being a good listener, motivation, the ability to build rapport and personal adaptation including exploring their own feelings. Other skills include being able to commit to training sessions and be adaptable to working with different people (Amro *et al.*, 2012). The design, length and frequency of programmes will vary but may include areas such as communication, healthy lifestyle, pain management, positive thinking, fatigue management, problem solving and accessing information (Arthritis UK, 2012). Chaplin *et al.* (2012) outline a programme for individuals with Parkinson's disease, including understanding the condition, exercise, daily living, medication management, communication and swallowing, psychological aspects, nutrition and self-management tools.

Scenario 9.2

Millie was diagnosed with relapsing remitting multiple sclerosis 12 years ago at the age of 28. She lives with her husband and two children in a ground floor flat.

Multiple sclerosis (MS) is a disease of the central nervous system (CNS) the brain and spinal cord. MS is an auto-immune disease, where the immune system gets confused and instead of attacking an infection or virus, it turns on itself and attacks nerve cells. The CNS cells are covered in a protective layer of fatty protein called the myelin sheath (a bit like insulation on an electrical cable). It is these cells that are attacked by the faulty immune system and the damage that results is called demyelination. During demyelination, messages from the brain are disrupted causing them to slow down, become distorted or not get through (MS Society, 2013).

Millie recently had a relapse and although physically she has improved, she describes feelings of exhaustion, anxiety and isolation. Millie has been invited to attend a self-management programme.

What might be an approach to self-management for Millie and what might be the challenges?

Discussion

Table 9.2 outlines difficulties associated with MS as well as the self-management themes and programmes that need to be considered when looking at Millie's case.

(Continued)

Scenario 9.2 *(Continued)*

Table 9.2 Areas to consider when dealing with the self-management of a patient with MS.

Difficulties associated with MS	Self-management themes	Self-management programme
Anxiety Balance Bladder and bowel Cognitive problems Depression Fatigue Heat intolerance Mobility Mood swings Muscular weakness Pain Sensory disturbance Sexual problems Spasticity and spasm Speech problems Swallowing difficulty Tremor Visual disturbance	Dealing with symptoms and relapse Making informed choices about medication Making the best use of available resources Being a partner with health professionals in making decisions about treatment Living well and the accommodation of MS into everyday life	Symptom management Diet Exercise Activity Pain management Medication management Fatigue management

Approaches to long-term conditions: developing personal skills: telehealth and telecare

Telehealth and telecare involve the use of technology to help people with a long-term condition maintain their independence, to feel in control of their health and promote health and safety. Telehealth has been described as equipment to monitor people's health in their own home. It may include a small device that can take readings such as blood pressure, oxygen levels, weight and temperature via a telephone line to a monitoring centre. If the condition gets worse, it is picked up by the health care professional who contacts the person and take appropriate action (DH, 2012). The equipment can be used in or out of the home, reducing the number of visits to the GP or clinics. A change or risks can be identified quickly, potentially reducing serious incidents and the need for emergency admissions.

Telecare includes a system of alarms, sensors and other equipment around the home that detects risks, for example, fire, floods and falls. Types of telecare include movement detectors, enuresis sensors, alarms, environmental sensors such as carbon monoxide or detecting gas, sensory impairment alarms for those with visual or hearing impairment, carer alerts, location sensors and activity monitors (Independent Age, 2011). When a risk is detected, an alert goes to the monitoring centre to summon help. The person may activate the system themselves through the use of a pendant or it will identify a change in normal action, for example, if a person gets up from bed during the night but does not return in a reasonable period of time signifying that there could be a problem (DH, 2012).

Technology can provide valuable information to enable the individual to monitor their health and take appropriate action and can also give greater freedom to enable the person to continue with everyday community life. Technology can also be beneficial in allaying fears and anxieties, for example, individuals living with coronary heart disease, chronic obstructive pulmonary disease or stroke. Living with a long-term condition can increase anxiety for carers, for example, where a family member has been falling or where there has been cognitive changes, resulting in not remembering to take medication, leaving the front door open or going out in the middle of the night. Carers can receive comfort and support, knowing that they will be contacted via a pager alert if an incident occurs. It is also cost effective, reducing the need for 24-hour care and enabling carers to continue with employment.

Evidence 9.1

Telehealth

While telehealth for chronic conditions is strongly supported by the Department of Health, the evidence for its effectiveness and cost effectiveness is limited. The Department of Health-commissioned Whole System Demonstrator programme assessed the impact of telehealth on hospital use by patients with long-term conditions (diabetes, COPD or heart failure) between May 2008 and November 2009 (Steventon *et al.*, 2012). Patients were randomly split into two groups:

1. an intervention group of 1570 people, who were given devices and taught how to monitor their condition at home and transmit the data to health professionals;
2. a control group of 1584 people, who received usual care, excluding telehealth.

The results showed that 43% of people in the intervention group were admitted to hospital during the study period compared with 48% of patients in the control group. Of the intervention group, 5% died compared with 8% of controls.There were also statistically significant differences in the mean number of emergency hospital admissions per head (0.54 for patients in the intervention group compared with 0.68 for those in the control group) and the mean hospital stay per head (4.87 days for patients in the intervention group compared with 5.68 days for those in the control group). Other measures of hospital use (elective admissions, outpatient attendances and emergency department visits) were not significantly different between the groups, nor were the differences in notional hospital costs.

Many telecare or telehealth users are likely to continue using the equipment for periods longer than 12 months, and patterns of telecare and telehealth equipment use may change over time – both of which will affect health and social care outcomes. A review by the Centre for Reviews and Dissemination (2013, p. 11) concluded that:

> *although there is a large amount of evidence evaluating the effects of telehealth interventions, much of it is weak and/or contradictory. However, there is good evidence that telehealth monitoring can reduce mortality in patients with heart failure, particularly those recently discharged from hospital.*

Approaches to long-term conditions: developing personal skills and health education

People with a long-term condition need support to understand their conditions and to understand the services available. When first diagnosed, people are often not given much information about their condition. There is some evidence that people with low health literacy manage their condition less well. Health literacy is a term used to describe the ability to do the following:

- know when and where to seek information;
- have the verbal communication skills needed to describe one's health issues and understand health professionals' responses;
- show assertiveness (linked to successful communication);
- retain and process information;
- have skills in applying information.

Activity 9.4

What might a newly diagnosed patient with type2 diabetes want to know?

Discussion

- ❑ *Understand blood glucose and optimal blood glucose parameters.*
- ❑ *Understand the physiological interactions from food, exercise, stress.*
- ❑ *Understand diabetes complications.*
- ❑ *Understand the medication including different types, dosage, why it is required.*

As one participant in Sturt et al.'s study (2005) put it:

I've picked up the different leaflets. I keep reading them from time to time and suddenly it struck me that they keep going on about your feet and having them examined. Nobody anywhere has ever told me to have my feet examined and why you have them examined.

Structured education programmes may be set up for patients with particular conditions and their carers e.g. DESMOND (Diabetes Education and Self Management for Ongoing and Newly Diagnosed) is a programme which aims to help people with type 2 diabetes to self-manage their condition effectively and includes medical management of the condition, emotional management, and managing the condition in the context of everyday life.

Approaches to long-term conditions: creating a supportive environment

The Equality Act (DH, 2010a) applies to everyone in Britain and sets out the personal characteristics that are protected by the law and the behaviour that is unlawful. These include age, disability, gender reassignment, religion and belief, pregnancy/maternity, race, gender and sexual orientation. All service providers have a responsibility to treat their service users fairly. Treating fairly involves understanding the needs of different groups, awareness of how an individual with a long-term condition may face discrimination and action to promote inclusion and equality.

Scenario 9.3

Consider the patients described in Table 9.3 and identify action(s) to promote inclusion and equality.

Table 9.3 Patient scenarios.

Difficulty	Action
Mary has a visual loss and is unable to read the appointment letters. She is not happy that she has to rely on neighbours to provide information	
Sebastian wants to attend an expert patient programme but is unable to access the venue in his wheelchair	
Caroline finds it difficult to take time off work to go to the surgery to get her blood pressure checked	
Raveena wants to join the cooking group at the community centre following her heart attack but finds that the meals are not suitable for her low salt and low cholesterol diet	
Brian has diabetes. He wants to lose weight but works as a long-distance lorry driver and cannot commit to a set time and place to exercise	
Deidre is recovering from depression and wants to join an art group but feels anxious about talking to new people	

On placement: checklist

1. Have you taken time to listen to the person and hear their concerns?
2. Have you worked in partnership with the person in setting goals? How was this done?
3. Have you worked in partnership with the person in identifying an appropriate intervention?
4. Have you provided health information to empower the person to manage their condition more confidently? What was this information and who produced it?
5. Is support given to help the person achieve the best possible outcome from their medicines? Who does this and how?
6. Is information provided about support and services available?
7. What skills or strategies are used to help the person manage their condition more confidently?
8. What is done to support carers in their role?

Key learning points

1. The majority of people over the age of 60 will be living with one or more long-term conditions.
2. Living with a long-term condition may affect many aspects of life, including emotions, confidence, sexual life, cognitive abilities, as well as physical ability.
3. The aim of health promotion with a person with a long-term condition is to encourage self-management.
4. Self-management means helping the patient find the knowledge that they need to manage symptoms, treatment, physical and psychological consequences and lifestyle changes.
5. Self-management means working in co-production with the patient. This means working in an equal and reciprocal relationship with the patient and their family.

Chapter summary

This chapter has discussed the prevalence of long-term conditions and the particular demands posed to working practice by the shift to self management. The nurse can be a tool in creating a framework to engage, encourage, enable, equip and empower the individual with a long-term condition to manage the different stages in living with a long-term condition and take an active role in their health and well-being.

Further reading and resources

Diabetes is a condition for which there are numerous patient education resources, e.g. http://nhsdiabetes.healthcareea.co.uk/scotland.

For other conditions such as arthritis, specialists may develop their own, e.g. http://www.enherts-tr.nhs.uk/patients-visitors/our-services/rheumatology/information-for-patients/.

The NHS Information Centre has information on many health conditions including, for example, asthma, http://www.nhs.uk/conditions/asthma/Pages/Introduction.aspx.

There are numerous NICE guidelines for professionals on the clinical management of long-term conditions that include how these can be self-managed e.g. Clinical management of primary hypertension in adults, available at: http://www.nice.org.uk/nicemedia/live/13561/56015/56015.pdf.

Structured education programmes include diabetes education, available at: www.desmond-project.org.uk and www.dafne.uk.com.

References

Amro, R., Cox, C.L., Waddington, K. and Siriwardena, D. (2012) Glaucoma expert patient programme. *International Journal of Ophthalmic Practice*, **2** (1), 32–38.

Arthritis Research UK (2012) *Living with Long-Term Pain: A Guide to Self-Management*. Arthritis Research UK, Derbyshire. Available at: www.arthritisresearchuk.org.

Centre for Reviews and Dissemination (2013) *Telehealth for People with Long-Term Conditions*. CRD, York. Available at: http://www.york.ac.uk/inst/crd/pdf/Telehealth.pdf.

Chaplin, H., Hazan, J. and Wilson, P. (2012) Self- management for people with long- term neurological conditions. *British Journal of Community Nursing*, **17** (6), 250–257.

DH (Department of Health) (2001) *The Expert Patient: A New Approach to Chronic Disease Management for the 21s Century*. TSO, London.

DH (Department of Health) (2005) *National Service Framework for Long-Term Conditions*. TSO, London.

DH (Department of Health) (2006) *Self-Care for People with Long-Term Conditions*. TSO, London. Available at: www.dh.gov.uk/longtermconditions.

DH (Department of Health) (2008) *Ten Things You Should Know about Long-Term Conditions*. Available at: http://webarchive.nationalarchives.gov.uk/20080906003929/http://dh.gov.uk/en/Healthcare/Longtermconditions/DH_084294.

DH (Department of Health) (2009) *Your Health, Your Way: A Guide to Long-Term Conditions and Self-Care*. DH, London.

DH (Department of Health) (2010a) *Equality Act*. TSO, London.

DH (Department of Health) (2010b) *Improving the Health and Well-Being of People with Long-Term Conditions*. DH, London.

DH (Department of Health) (2010c) *The E's of Self Management for Long-Term Conditions*. TSO, London. Available at: http://www.uhsm.nhs.uk/community/EPP/Esofselfmanagement.pdf.

DH (Department of Health) (2011) *What Motivates People to Self-Care*. TSO, London.

DH (Department of Health) (2012) *Health and Social Care Act*. TSO, London

DH (Department of Health) (2013) *Improving the Quality of Life for People with Long-Term Conditions*.TSO, London.

Ellis-Hill, C., Payne, S. and Ward, C. (2008) Using stroke to explore the Life Thread Model: an alternative approach to rehabilitation. *Disability and Rehabilitation*, **30** (2), 150–159.

Entwistle, V.A. and Cribb, A. (2013) *Enabling People to Live Well*. Health Foundation, London.

Equality and Human Rights Commission (2009) *Just Ageing*? Available at: http://justageing.equalityhumanrights.com/wp-content/uploads/2009/08/Socio-economic-inequalities-in-the-older-population-of-the-United-Kingdom-Just-Ageing-Public-Service-report.pdf.

Independent Age (2011) *Telecare and Telehealth: What It Is and How to Get it*, Independent Age, London. www.independence.org.

Long Term Conditions Team (2012). *Long-Term Conditions Compendium of Information*, 3rd edn. Department of Health, London.

MS Society (2011) *Multiple Sclerosis: Information for Health and Social Care Professionals,* 4th edn. Multiple Sclerosis Trust, Letchworth. Available at: www.mstrust.org.uk.

MS Society (2013) *Diet and Nutrition (MS Essentials 11),* MS Society, London.

Social Care Institute for Excellence (2013) *Maximising the Potential of Reablement*. SCIE, London. Available at: www.scie.org.uk.

Steventon, A., Bardsley, M., Billings, J.,, *et al*. (2012) Effect of telehealth on use of secondary care and mortality: findings from the Whole System Demonstrator cluster randomised trial. *BMJ*, **344**, e3874.

Sturt, J., Hearnshaw, H., Barlow, J.H., *et al*. (2005) Education for people with type 2 diabetes: what do patients want? *Journal of Diabetes Nursing*, **9** (4), 145–150.

Don't forget to visit the companion website for this book: www.wileyfundamentalseries.com/healthpromotion where you can find self-assessment tests to check your progress.

Part Three

Skills for Health Promotion

Introduction

The next chapters in the book, Chapters 10–13, discuss the key strategies involved in promoting health: using information and data, being evidence-informed in practice, infection control and health protection; and promoting healthy lifestyles through behavioural change

While nurses may see practice as focusing on individuals and families, many recognise the need for a wider understanding of the health of local populations or communities and a service directed towards those with greatest needs. This book emphasizes throughout that the NHS is often too medically-focused and that patients may need support or a different service in health, social care or the wider public service system, and nurses need to know how to help people to access it.

Using existing information to identify the main issues, the contributory factors and who is affected will help identify the most appropriate interventions. Morris (2007) describes epidemiology as "*completing the clinical picture*", with its methods therefore being an important tool of nursing practice in helping to plan and determine health policy. Despite this, according to Whitehead (2000), it seems to be poorly understood and greatly underused by the nursing profession. Chapter 10 outlines some of the key concepts associated with using existing data sources to describe a population's health. As a lone practitioner or with others, the nurse may need to gather and generate data from a variety of sources to assess health needs and then to agree priorities for action and local health plans. This information will also help influence resource allocation to areas of greatest health and social need

Research evidence provides a knowledge base for public health and health promotion practice and ensures care is clinically and cost effective, and based on the best evidence of what works to achieve the best outcomes. Chapter 11 explores the concept of evidence-based practice and how nurses can find evidence quickly and easily.

Chapter 12 focuses on health education and how to promote healthy lifestyles. There are numerous opportunities for the nurse to encourage behaviour change and underpinning such an approach are the objectives of increasing awareness of health information, developing self-efficacy through better decision-making, assertiveness and interpersonal skills. Nurses' communication skills are paramount so they can engage with individuals and communities to understand the attitudes and behaviours that underpin their health and the influence of factors like family and culture. In addition, they need to be able to explain complex information and work with a patient to motivate them to take control over their health. For all nurses having a clear values base and skills in communication, critical thinking and problem solving are key to delivering high quality, evidenced-based care.

Disease surveillance, particularly of communicable disease, is a core public health function and Chapter 13 outlines the principles of screening and vaccination programmes. A major hazard associated with hospital admission is the risk of acquiring an infection. Whilst the challenge of monitoring, controlling and treating methicillin-resistant *Staphylococcus aureus* (MRSA) may lie with a specialist infection control nurse, all health professionals in secondary care are responsible for the basic aspect of their role – hygiene. Hand washing is the single most important action a nurse can take which can reduce the spread of disease. Chapter 13 also discusses the key role for the nurse in communicating about risk. Sometimes a nurse wishes to convey to a patient the risk associated with their behaviour or they may wish to discuss the risks associated with a particular intervention. Increasingly, understanding the role of gene mutations has led to the development of targeted risk management and preventative strategies. For example, familial breast cancer clinics have been set up to address the needs of women concerned about their perceived risk of developing breast cancer because they have a relative with the disease.

References

Morris, J.N. (2007) Uses of epidemiology. *International Journal of Epidemiology*, **36** (6): 1165-1172.
Whitehead D. (2000) Is there a place for epidemiology in nursing?, *Nursing Standard*, **14**, 42, 35–39.

10

Using health information and epidemiology

Amanda Hesman

Senior Lecturer, Adult Nursing, London South Bank University, London, UK

Learning outcomes

By the end of this chapter you will be able to:

1. Describe how health can be measured
2. Describe common sources of health information and their limitations
3. Understand how to use health information to describe health needs
4. Explain frequently used epidemiological terms
5. Consider how epidemiological studies contribute to our understanding of health inequalities
6. Demonstrate how health information informs public health policy
7. Relate public health information accurately to your client group and translate how this information can be used to assist individuals in order to improve their health

Introduction

This chapter considers how health information and epidemiological knowledge are relevant to nursing and how they can be used by nurses when caring for clients and groups of patients. Health information, including demographic and epidemiological information, underpins the

Fundamentals of Health Promotion for Nurses, Second Edition. Edited by Jane Wills.

Companion website: www.wileyfundamentalseries.com/healthpromotion

body of nursing theory by increasing knowledge about health. In clinical practice, this knowledge includes knowing:

- "who" is most likely to be affected by a disease or condition;
- "why" a disease or condition is more likely to occur;
- "what" steps are necessary in order to alleviate or prevent the condition;
- "how" to best care for the client or patient with that condition.

Health information and epidemiology can contribute to our understanding of health by identifying:

- the natural history of a disease or a condition and predisposing characteristics for ill health;
- the best strategies to prevent ill health;
- the best treatment and management of a condition.

The focus is on populations and why some populations are healthier than others. Epidemiological study can also be used to orientate public services to promote health, manage chronic conditions and contribute to the evaluation of service quality. Primarily, in order to use health and epidemiological information, it is necessary to be able to articulate what it is and why it is useful. Thereafter, health information needs to be located and retrieved and, finally, health information needs to be applied to practice in order to promote health and prevent ill health.

Health information

Demography

Demographic information includes the basic characteristics of the population and includes:

- age
- gender
- ethnicity
- mobility
- morbidity
- population growth and fertility.

This information gives a picture of the size and structure of the population, e.g. the percentage of those over 75 years. Information is also collected from the following routine data sources:

- the census of the population;
- birth and abortion notifications;
- disease registers;
- mortality registers.

The census is coordinated from the Office for National Statistics (ONS, 2013) and provides a detailed "snapshot" of the resident population in the UK and occurs every ten years. In 2011, each person in the household was asked to rate their health in general; the possible responses were "Very good", "Good", "Fair", "Bad" and "Very bad". Unlike simple indicators based on the

Activity 10.1

The population pyramid (Figure 10.1) shows the age distribution in the population of Lewisham, South London, compared to the age distribution in the population of England, as at Census Day 2011 (Public Health Lewisham, 2013). How would you describe the age profile of Lewisham?

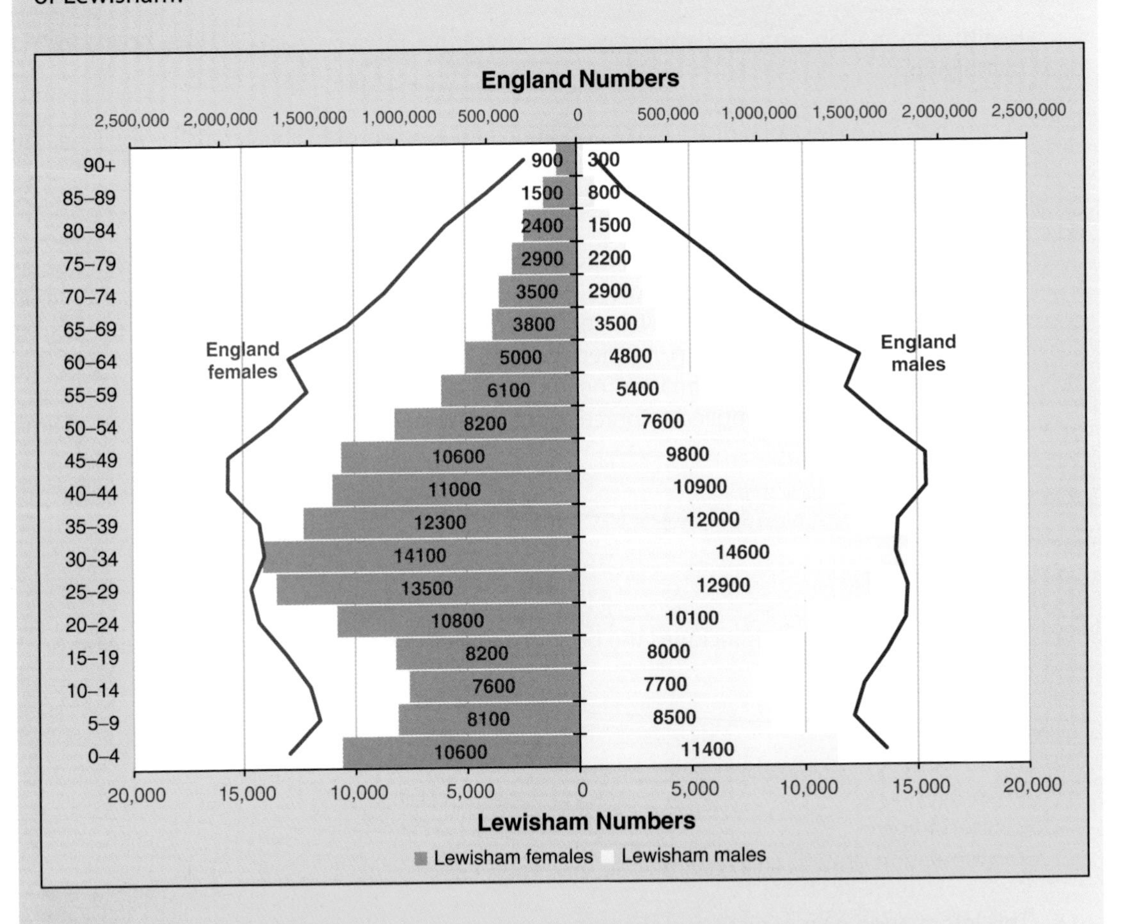

Figure 10.1 Age-sex population pyramid counts for Lewisham and England by 5-year age bands. Source: Lewisham's Public Health Information Team, 2013; data from ONS/ Census 2011.

Discussion

Compared to England and Wales which have 16.4% of the population over 65 years, London has 11.1% of the population over 65 years and Lewisham has a younger population with only 5.4% aged over 65 years.

presence or absence of disease, an important aspect of the general health status indicator is that it includes the entire spectrum of health states, ranging from "Good" to "Not good" health. People living in London and the South-east England region had the highest percentages of "Very good" or "Good" general health, and Wales and the North-east region had the lowest. Within a comparison of local authorities in England, Blackpool is ranked as having the least "good health", in Wales, it was Caerphilly, and in Scotland, it was Glasgow (ONS, 2013).

The data from the census is used to allocate resources in order to plan public services, including health, education, transport and determining fitness for work. Asking an individual a general health question means that health and social services need is identified at a local level. Self-reported measures of illness may not always be accurate, however, as people perceive symptoms differently, some may not consider their long-term condition serious enough to report and others may over-emphasize symptoms.

The fertility rate peaked in 2010 with the highest total fertility rate since 1973. The total fertility rate (TFR) in England and Wales saw a steady decline during the 1990s, to a low of 1.63 in 2001 and then gradually increased between 2001 and 2008. From 2008, the TFR has remained relatively stable, fluctuating between 1.90 and 1.94 children per woman and peaking in 2010. Possible causes may include:

- More women currently in their twenties having children.
- More women having children at older ages.
- Increases in the numbers of foreign-born women who tend to have higher fertility than UK-born women.
- Government policy and the economic climate indirectly influencing individuals' decisions on childbearing.

It is possible to find out about the health profile of any neighbourhood by using the Health Profile and interactive map found at the Association of Public Health Observatories website at: www.apho.org.uk.

Activity 10.2

Go to the Northern Ireland Public Health profile (NIPHA) at http://www.nisra.gov.uk/.

- What does this Health Profile for Northern Ireland tell you about the incidence, prevalence and duration of breastfeeding?
- Now find the 'Health Profile' for Haringey, North London, on the APHO website at www.apho.org.uk. What is the rate per 1000 for breastfeeding in that borough?
- How do ethnicity and education impact on breastfeeding?

Discussion

Breastfeeding is more common in mothers over 30, minority ethnic groups, those who left education over 18 and in managerial and professional occupations. Mothers who left full-time education over the age of 18 are nearly twice as likely to be breastfeeding at 6 weeks compared with mothers who left education aged 16 or under (HSCIC, 2012).

Social classification

As we saw in Chapter 2, inequalities in health and life expectancy can be observed between groups of people from different social groups. In order to compare groups, people are placed in categories according to occupation, which is meant to reflect their social status within society, including their education and income. Inequalities in health can then be assessed using this information on social class together with other information on ill health collected from disease registers and health surveys. Most ill health demonstrates a positive social class gradient with a higher incidence in manual groups of most conditions, including coronary heart disease (CHD), mental health, cancer and injuries.

The most commonly used classification to date is the Registrar General's social class classification which classifies jobs into six "social classes" based on occupation. The assigning of jobs to each of these bands has been criticized because dissimilar jobs have been assigned to the same group. As a result, a more recent classification system is now used (Table 10.1).

Deprivation measures

Inequalities in health and life expectancy are also evident between affluent and deprived geographic areas. It is possible to obtain a measure of deprivation for specific geographical areas which can then be compared with other geographical areas and importantly, linked to morbidity and mortality data. Frequently used deprivation indices include the Jarman Underprivileged Area Score, the Townsend Material Deprivation Score, the SCOTDEP index for Scotland, and the Index of Multiple Deprivation for England.

The Jarman Underprivileged Area Score (Jarman, 1993) is based upon eight factors that are used to measure potential General Practice workload. The Townsend Material Deprivation Score measures include unemployment (lack of material resources and insecurity), overcrowding (material living conditions), and lack of car ownership (a proxy indicator of income). SCOTDEP replaces rented housing with low social class on the grounds that the proportion of social rented

Table 10.1 Revised social classifications.

(1)	Higher managerial and professional occupations
(2)	Lower managerial and professional occupations
(3)	Intermediate occupations
(4)	Small employers and own account workers
(5)	Lower supervisory, craft and related occupations
(6)	Employees in semi-routine occupations
(7)	Employees in routine occupations
(8)	Never worked and long-term unemployed

Source: Office for National Statistics (2010).

housing in Scotland was sufficiently high to blunt its effectiveness as a measure of deprivation. The Index of Multiple Deprivation for England has seven domains with indicators designed to directly measure particular aspects of deprivation. The seven deprivation domains are:

1. income
2. employment
3. health and disability
4. education, skills and training
5. barriers to housing and services
6. crime
7. living environment deprivation.

Ethnicity

The 1991 census was the first census to include a question on ethnicity with 3.3 million people describing themselves as non-White. The 2011 census shows that England and Wales have become more ethnically diverse with rising numbers of people identifying with minority ethnic groups. Despite the White ethnic group decreasing in size, it is still the majority ethnic group that people identify with at 86.0%. London was the most ethnically diverse area, with the highest proportion of minority ethnic groups and the lowest proportion of the White ethnic group at 59.8%. Belonging to certain ethnic groups is associated with poorer health due to the relationship with deprivation markers such as poverty, unemployment and poor housing (see Chapter 2). The collection of ethnic data also plays an important role in monitoring access to, and uptake of, public services. Ethnicity and implicitly cultural difference will also have an effect on illness presentation, health beliefs, lifestyle and cultural practice.

Definitions and uses of epidemiology

Traditionally epidemiology studied illness in groups of people, i.e. who becomes ill and why they fall ill. However, a contemporary definition is more inclusive: the study of the distribution and determinants of health and illness in populations. To prevent ill health and to improve health, it is necessary to identify why diseases and particular conditions occur in one population and why they do not occur in another population.

Our understanding needs to be informed by four important domains:

- the biological;
- the physical environment;
- the social environment;
- attitudinal and behavioural factors (lifestyle).

Studying the features of a population who will develop a disease or a condition, will make visible risk factors in that population that increase the likelihood of that condition developing. By studying an individual patient these risk factors remain invisible. The focus of public health enquiry is always the community or population and never the individual. Using the four domains as headings, Table 10.2 lists some "characteristics" that could be studied in a population or community in order to identify risk factors that may be present.

Table 10.2 Describing a population.

Biological	Physical environment	Social environment	Attitude and behaviour
Gender Age Ethnicity Genetic markers	Rural Green space Transport Access to food Dwellings	Social networks Occupation Income Education	Exercise Diet Sexual Smoking Alcohol Addiction

Measuring health and disease in populations

Prevalence is the total number of individuals with a disease or a condition in a defined population in a defined period of time and is usually expressed by the term "cases". Prevalence may be measured: at a single point in time (point prevalence); over a defined period of time (period prevalence); or over an individual's entire lifetime (lifetime prevalence).

Case study 10.1

The global prevalence of asthma

The WHO (2013) estimates that 235 million people currently suffer from asthma with asthma being the most common chronic disease among children. Asthma occurs in all countries regardless of the level of development with most asthma-related deaths occurring in low- and lower-middle income countries.

Figure 10.2 is a map to demonstrate the global prevalence of asthma and highlights some of the difficulties encountered when collecting health information. This prevalence information has been collected from self-reports of "wheezing in the last 12 months" and is used to indicate the prevalence of asthma symptoms. The limitations of collecting information on asthma in this way are that self-reported wheezing is not diagnostic of asthma and no single objective test to measure the frequency or severity of wheezing exists. This means that the prevalence of current asthma symptoms is not the same as the prevalence of clinical asthma. Difficulties are also encountered when comparing health information internationally as some languages do not have a colloquial term for wheezing. In an attempt to counteract this, a video questionnaire was used which showed, rather than described, the signs and symptoms of asthma. The influence of raised public and professional awareness on asthma may also impact on the reporting of symptoms, making it difficult to establish the true prevalence of asthma.

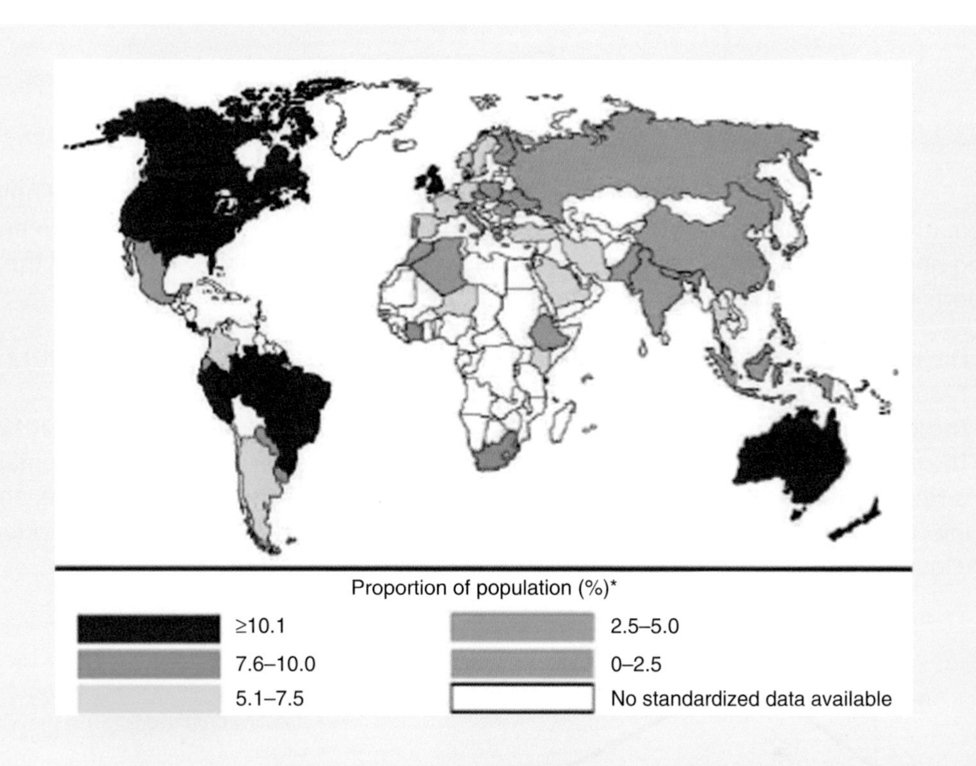

Figure 10.2 World map of the prevalence of clinical asthma. Source: Masoli *et al.*, 2004, Figure 4, p. 472. Reproduced with permission from John Wiley & Sons Ltd.

The limitations that need to be considered when interpreting health information include the limitations of:

- self-reporting;
- definitions and interpretations of signs and symptoms;
- the presence or otherwise of a single diagnostic test;
- language barriers;
- increased awareness of the disease or condition.

The incidence of a disease or a condition is the number of new cases of a disease or condition that occur during a defined period in a specific population. For example, the numbers of new cases of human immunodeficiency virus (HIV) are reported in confidence to the Communicable Disease Surveillance Centre (CDSC PHLS) of the Health Protection Agency (HPA).

Case study 10.2

HIV/AIDS monitoring

The Centre for Infectious Disease Surveillance and Control (CIDSC) of Public Health England currently collects information on the incidence and prevalence of HIV which has been measured since the HIV antibody test was developed in 1985. The information contained in the HIV reports to CIDSC includes routes of probable acquisition.

- The total number of HIV cases diagnosed in the UK up to and including those in 2012 is 128681 (period prevalence). This figure includes deaths of people with HIV/AIDS.
- The incidence of newly diagnosed HIV in 2012 was 5916 (PHE HIV/STI Department, 2012).
- The three major risk groups for HIV acquisition are: sex between men if the sexual contact is HIV positive; sex between men and women if the sexual contact is HIV positive; and injecting drug use when needles and syringes are shared with an HIV positive individual (Figure 10.3).

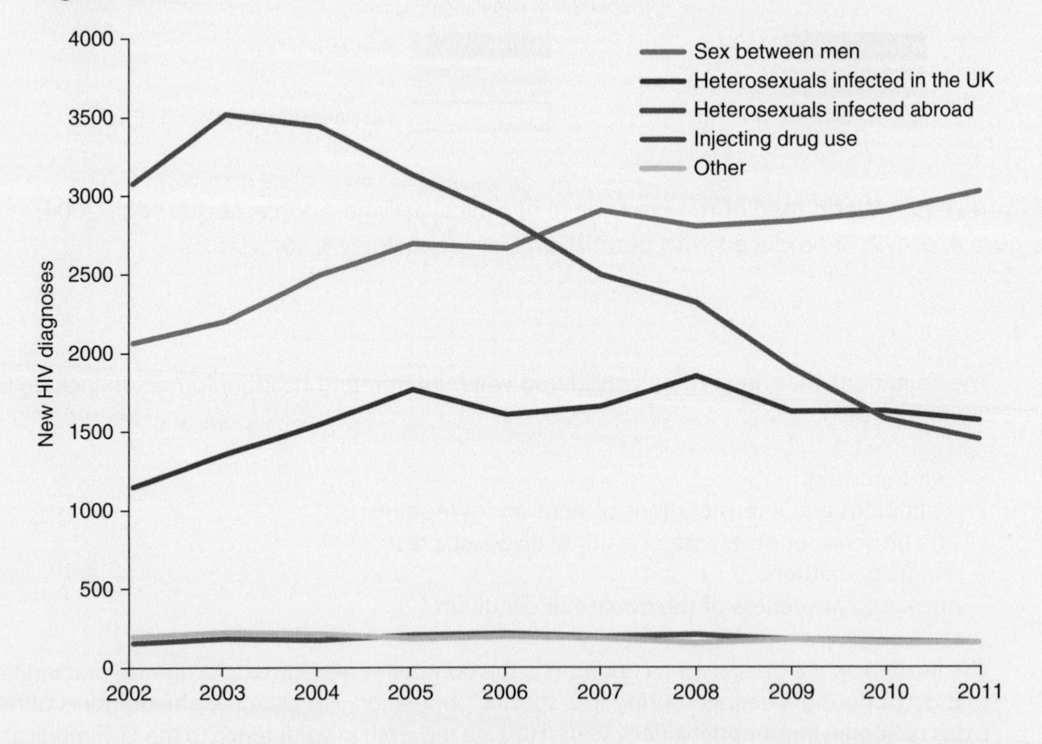

Figure 10.3 New HIV diagnoses by exposure group, 2002–2011[1]. Source: Health Protection Agency, 2012, p. 5. Reproduced under the Open Government Licence and with permission from Public Health England.

[1]Data adjusted for missing exposure group information

- By the end of 2011 there were 96000 individuals in the UK living with HIV, with 24% of this population living with HIV being unaware of their infection (HPA, 2012).
- Overall prevalence rate in 2011 was: 1.5 per 1000 population in the UK; 47 per 1000 men who have sex with men (MSM); 37 per 1,000 the Black African community.
- For the first time in 1999 the incidence of HIV was higher in heterosexuals than in men who have sex with men. However, the greatest prevalence was still in the risk group of men who have sex with men.
- Intravenous drug users account for the lowest incidence and period prevalence of HIV. In 2011, this group accounted for only 2% of the total number of new HIV cases.
- In areas with a high prevalence of diagnosed HIV infection (>2 per 1,000 population aged 15–59 years), UK national guidelines recommend expanding HIV testing among people admitted to hospital and new registrants to General Practice. In 2011, 58 English local authorities had a diagnosed prevalence above 2 per 1000, of which 30 were in London.

Although this data tells us about risk, it also highlights one of the limitations of epidemiology, i.e. that it simply tells us about the scale of the problem and risk factors but not how these should be tackled as demonstrated by the sustained growth in HIV incidence.

In order for the nurse to begin to understand their role as health promoter the numbers and characteristics of people at risk of ill health or death need to be known. The most common means of measuring the health status of the population is actually by the number of people who die!

Mortality rates

Mortality data for England and Wales can be obtained from the Office for National Statistics (ONS) and in their journal the *Health Statistics Quarterly*. For Northern Ireland, this information is published in the *Annual Report of the Registrar General for Northern Ireland* and for Scotland in the *Annual Report of the Registrar General for Scotland*. Not all countries have robust systems for death registration or population counting, both of which are necessary to obtain a death rate, but in the UK this information is routinely collected. All deaths must be registered by a medical practitioner within five days of the date of death. These deaths are then coded according to the International Classification of Diseases (ICD). A common problem is identifying the direct cause of death as distinct from contributory causes.

Mortality information is data that counts the number of deaths, e.g. in 2012 there were 499331deaths registered in England and Wales (ONS, 2013). A number like this is not, however, very helpful as it does not allow any comparison across populations. To do this, we need a rate. A rate has three components:

- the numerator – the number of the population who have died;
- the denominator – the total number of the people in the population;
- the time period in which the deaths took place.

The crude death rate

This is the total number of deaths in a population in a year expressed as a rate per 1000 of the population and does not consider the age at which death occurred. The crude death rate in 2008 for England and Wales was 9.4 (ONS, 2008).

The age-specific death rate

This refers to deaths in an identified age group of a population expressed as a rate per 1000. In England and Wales in 2011 the age-specific death rate for females aged 35–39 years was 0.7 and for males aged 35–39 was 1.2 (ONS, 2013).

The perinatal mortality rate (PMR)

This is the number of still-births and deaths within the first week of life per 1000 total births. In 2011, England and Wales had a rate of 7.5 per1000 (ONS, 2012).

The infant mortality rate (IMR)

This is the number of infants dead within 12 months of birth per 1000. In 2011, England and Wales had a rate of 4.2 per 1000 (ONS, 2013b).

Activity 10.3

The highest infant mortality rate (infant deaths aged less than 1 year) in England and Wales in 2008–2010 was in Newcastle-under-Lyme, Staffordshire, at 9.3 per 1000 live births. The lowest at 1.2 per 1000 live births was in Tonbridge and Malling in Kent.

Why do you think that Tonbridge and Malling have the lowest infant mortality rate?

Discussion

Infant mortality is an indicator of the general health of an entire population. It reflects the relationship between causes of infant mortality and upstream determinants of population health such as economic, social and environmental conditions. The following women have the lowest infant mortality rate:

- *women having their first child;*
- *women aged 20–29 years;*
- *women who have a gap between their children of between 18–35 months.*

The PMR is higher for illegitimate births than it is for legitimate births and there is a positive social class gradient with social class V having the highest PMR. Low birth weight is correlated with perinatal mortality. Factors associated with a high PMR include: hypertension; poorly controlled diabetes; renal disease; infections that cause foetal abnormalities; severe malnutrition; smoking and alcohol.

The cause-specific death rate

This is the number of people who have died from a particular condition compared to the total number of cases of that condition.

Epidemiological studies

Epidemiological studies that use death rates may hope to identify specific characteristics and behaviours in that population that could be modified in order to reduce premature deaths. Descriptive studies make use of routinely collected data such as death certification data or infectious disease notification and may give a general indication into the aetiology or cause of a disease or condition. There are certain categories that need to be analysed when using descriptive studies:

- when
- where
- who.

Case study 10.3

Using epidemiological data to identify cause

Excess winter deaths are calculated by comparing the number of deaths in winter months (December to March) with the expected number of deaths (average non-winter deaths). It is possible to express the above value as an index (Excess Winter Death (EWD) Index) by dividing the average winter deaths per year by the average non-winter deaths. Generally speaking, excess winter deaths tend to increase with age and are due to CVD and respiratory disease. Low-income families spend less on heating, on average indicating that they live at colder temperature levels.

Winter deaths in Portsmouth are higher than average with a local EWD value of 24.7 compared to the average for England which is 15.6. Most deaths occurred in those aged over 65 and who died as a result of respiratory conditions such as bronchitis and circulatory conditions such as coronary heart disease.

As part of the "Keep Warm and Carry On" campaign in 2012, offers of grant or loan to help with central heating installation or new double glazing and free cavity wall and loft insulation were available. Flu vaccinations were encouraged for those at risk and practical advice was given on how to maintain body temperature such as having hot drinks, not sitting down for too long, getting up and moving around in order to stay active and generate heat, and using an electric blanket or hot water bottle to warm the bed.

The standardized mortality rate

The standardized mortality rate is used to compare death rates between different populations. Standardization will identify the ratio between the actual number of deaths to the expected number of deaths in a specific population. When comparing two populations that have large differences in the proportions of the very old and very young, it is necessary to alter the data to take account of this difference – this alteration is known as standardization. In 2011, the age standardized death rate for all causes per 100000 population for Scotland using the European Standard Population was for males 766 per 100000 and for females 540 per 100000 population.

Life expectancy

Life expectancy at birth is an estimate of the average number of years a newborn baby would survive if they experienced the designated areas' age-specific mortality rates for that time period throughout his life.

Expectation of life at birth is used as an index of mortality and reflects both childhood and adult mortality. Differences in life expectancy are evident between countries with a high income and low income and even within countries differences can exist (Table 10.3).

In countries with a low income it is not always possible to collect robust and accurate health information on life expectancy. In these countries the infant mortality rate (IMR) is often used as it is easier to collect this information. Life expectancy and infant mortality information give a proxy measure of the socio-economic status of the country, with the IMR being particularly sensitive to poverty. The population of a poorer country can have a shorter life expectancy and higher infant mortality rate than the population of wealthier countries.

Another way of measuring health is to measure the number of healthy years at birth that can be expected. Once we know the life expectancy and healthy life expectancy (HALE) of a population, we can think about the number of years that a population will be living in ill health or with a long-term and chronic condition. Table 10.4 lists the HALE years for females and males born in 2011 in selected European countries.

Years life lost (YLL) denotes the number of years lost due to deaths at a premature age. To calculate this, it is assumed that everyone may live to some arbitrarily chosen age based on life expectancy, and that death at a younger age means that some future life years have been lost. When reading research papers that use YLL as a marker of ill health, it is important to know what was the chosen age of life expectancy for that population.

Table 10.3 Local authorities with the highest and lowest life expectancy at birth in the England and Wales, 2009–2011.

Male's life expectancy		Female's life expectancy	
East Dorset	83.0 years	East Dorset	86.4 years
Blackpool	73.8 years	Manchester	79.3 years

Source: Office for National Statistics (2013).

Table 10.4 Healthy life expectancy (HALE) years for females and males born in 2011 in selected European countries.

	Women	Men
Switzerland	74.4	71.1
France	73.5	69.0
UK	70.9	68.4
Poland	66.6	62.1
Latvia	64.9	55.2

Source: Data from Eurostat (2013).

Activity 10.4

The following are measures used to describe the health of populations. Which of these is a good indicator of health?

- ❑ standardized mortality rate
- ❑ infant mortality rate
- ❑ life expectancy
- ❑ hospital episodes
- ❑ GCSE rates
- ❑ childhood obesity
- ❑ smoking prevalence
- ❑ depression rates
- ❑ happiness

Discussion

A good indicator is one that accurately and reliably describes an aspect of health of the population. Infant mortality and life expectancy are used to compare populations internationally and were both used to set targets to reduce inequalities in England. GCSE rates are used in the Marmot review (2010) as an indicator of social disadvantage. Childhood obesity is measured through the National Child Measurement Programme but smoking prevalence rates are estimates based on national surveys. Depression rates depend on the condition being identified as such and recorded by the clinician. Happiness is being measured as part of the National Wellbeing measurement that includes indicators on relationships, job satisfaction, economic security, education, environmental conditions as well individuals' assessment of their own well-being.

Morbidity

Mortality data alone does not adequately represent the health or ill health of the population. Morbidity data measures the psychological and physical health illness and disability experienced by a population. Chronic conditions such as degenerative joint diseases like arthritis and

Activity 10.5

182

Look at Figure 10.4 that comes from the WHO report on the Global Burden of Disease, 2010. The shaded portion of each bar represents the specific disease attributable to that risk factor while the bar size represents the percentage of DALYS linked to specific risk factors. What are the biggest risk factors for disease in the UK?

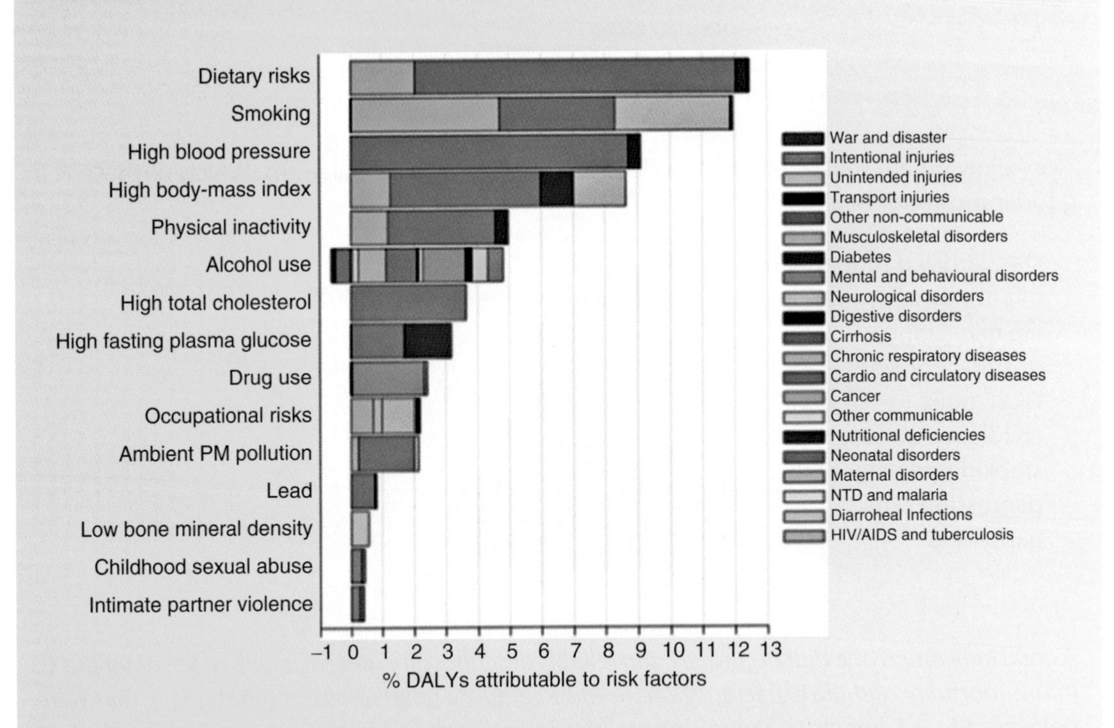

Figure 10.4 The global burden of disease: United Kingdom 2011. Source: Murray *et al.*, 2013, Figure 7, p. 1015. Reproduced with permission from Elsevier.

Discussion

The three risk factors that account for the most burden from disease in the UK are dietary risks, tobacco smoking and hypertension. In 2010, the leading risk factor for both children under 5 and adults aged 15–49 years was tobacco smoking, for children, this risk is due to second-hand smoke exposure.

mental health illnesses like depression may not be the primary cause of death but can cause severe disability. Morbidity data can be used to describe the experience and impact that a health problem may have and measures the burden of a disease or condition. Other methods that measure the burden of disease include "disability-free life expectancy" and "disability adjusted life years" (DALYs). DALYs combine years of life lost from premature death with loss of healthy life from disability. Premature death is the difference between the age at death and life expectancy at that age in a population with a low mortality.

Surveillance of health and the collection of health information

There are two distinct types of surveillance: surveillance to assess acute health trends such as communicable diseases, which is explored in greater detail in Chapter 13, and surveillance of longer health trends which are assessed with the use of disease registers. The purpose of surveillance is to follow rates of disease and illness within a population (such as the information collected about HIV/AIDS that is described in Case study 10.2) in order to better plan the actions that might be needed to control the risks of that disease. A wide diversity of data has been collected which can provide us with a large amount of information about the population. Some examples are given in Table 10.5.

Table 10.5 Sources of data and health information.

Routine registration and notification: birth, death, marriage
Cancer registry
Communicable diseases
International Classification of Disease (ICD)
National Health Service (NHS): statistics – waiting lists, length of bed stay, completed consultant episodes
Service uptake and utilization
Census
Measures of deprivation
Health and disease scales
Quality of life surveys
General household survey
Social information: benefit levels, crime statistics, unemployment, class classification
Smoking and food surveys

(Continued)

Table 10.5 (*Continued*)

Breastfeeding
Vaccination and immunization
Teenage (under 18) conceptions
Sexual health data
Terminations
Smoking cessation
Hospital activity
Prescribing

Information is collected at many different stages of life as routine data. Mortality from all causes is a good indicator of the general death rate. When using SMRs as a measurement, deaths below the age of 75 years are deemed premature based on the assumption that this is average life expectancy. For some diseases, there is the potential for health care service to prevent almost all deaths, at least within certain age groups, and so such deaths, suicide and road traffic deaths, for example, may be considered preventable through public health policies, wider social interventions, or a combination of these.

There are several reasons for health information being incomplete in a population, ranging from an "unwell" person feeling healthy and therefore not presenting at their general practitioner (GP) practice to poor service orientation that deters presentation. The accurate recording of health information relies on the following:

- an "unwell" person presenting to a GP surgery;
- the GP making a correct presumptive diagnosis;
- the GP requesting the correct investigations;
- the accuracy of the test result also called the positive predictive value;
- the documentation of the correct diagnosis in the patient's notes which is normally done by using ICD10 classification code;
- the entry of that code into the appropriate health database.

Activity 10.6

Mary is a 7-year-old child with severe abdominal pain who arrives in A&E with her mother, Rebecca, a 24-year-old prima gravida of Afro Caribbean descent. What information will already be available about her?

Discussion

During her pregnancy the following information will be recorded:

- *Height and weight*
- *Blood pressure*
- *Smoking status*
- *Weekly alcohol consumption and any drug use past and current*
- *Results of tests for HIV, Hepatitis B and C, syphilis, rubella, sickle cell, thalassemia, foetal anomaly, blood glucose.*

The following demographic information is recorded:

- *The postcode will indicate in which lower super output area (area of about 1000 households) she resides which can give an indication of socio-economic status.*
- *Ethnicity.*
- *Current employment or unemployment of Rebecca and any partner is also noted (giving information on potential maternity benefits in addition to information on her social situation).*
- *Marital status or civil partnership.*
- *From birth bloodspot: congenital hypothroidism, phenylketonuria, sickle cell disease disorders, cystic fibrosis and medium-chain acyl-CoA dehydrogenase deficiency.*

At birth, the child will have been registered (civil registration) showing parents or sole registration and place and date of birth. An NHS number is created and the child added to the local child health system and GP clinical system.

In the first two years, the following information will be recorded on the Child Health Information System (CHIS) about the baby:

- *breastfeeding initiation;*
- *the baby's weight trajectory;*
- *head circumference and body length;*
- *vaccinations;*
- *hearing;*
- *sight for congenital cataracts*

While at school her child will be able to have their weight recorded as part of the National Child Measurement Programme.

Mary's radial fracture at age 5 and her referral to ophthalmology for a squint will all be recorded when admitted to hospital. The date of admission and discharge, and a diagnosis/results will be sent to the GP and added to the medical records.

It is possible to link various sources of routine data from education, housing and social circumstances and clinical in order to build a complete picture of a patient.

Many conditions are under-reported and so a proportion of the population may be ill but not seeking help. Morbidity data from those receiving or awaiting care thus represent just the tip of the iceberg. Research into the experiences of men and women with CHD by Tod *et al.* (2001) identified six categories that hinder the full use of primary and secondary health services:

- structural factors;
- personal factors;
- social and cultural factors;
- past experiences and expectations;
- diagnostic confusion and knowledge;
- awareness.

Delay, denial and self-management by individuals mean that the full extent of symptoms often remained hidden from GPs. It is also known that more women remain under-represented and undiagnosed with CHD when compared with men.

Activity 10.7

Find out some statistics about your local area using the profile at www.apho.org.uk.

- What are the main causes of death? What is the standardized mortality rate (SMR) of the population of the electoral ward that that you live in?
- What does it tell you about the social determinants of health in the area?
- Does the profile indicate any particular need?

Annual Public Health reports are produced by local public health departments and these highlight the main priorities for the area (see, for example, the report of the financial crisis on the health of people in Lewisham, South London, at http://www.instituteofhealthequity.org/projects/lewisham-annual-public-health-report-2011–2012 or the report from a rural area such as Cornwall http://www.cornwall.gov.uk/default.aspx?page=29523).

How would you summarize the health needs of your area (in 100 words)?

Health outcomes

Increasingly, patients want to know about the "success rate" of the services they use. Dr Foster is an independent agency that analyses mortality data for hospitals and surgeons and can expose anomalies or poor health care delivery. The Francis Inquiry was an independent inquiry set up by the government that reported in 2013 on the raised mortality rates compared to other areas at the Mid-Staffordshire NHS Foundation Trust (Francis, 2013). It found poor standards of care, a lack of attention to complaints and concerns and a disengaged leadership.

Other outcomes include the Quality and Outcomes Framework (QOF) which is a voluntary annual reward and incentive programme for all GP surgeries in England. The QOF clinical register on obesity was started in 2006/7 and is based on patients aged 16 and over with a BMI greater or equal to 30 recorded in the previous 15 months.

The Public Health Outcomes Framework (see Chapter 1) includes two outcomes to measure public health progress:

- increased healthy life expectancy;
- reduced differences in life expectancy and healthy life expectancy between communities.

It also includes a range of indicators grouped into four domains that are deemed to be available and reliable (https://www.gov.uk/government/uploads/system/uploads/attachment_data/file/216159/dh_132362.pdf).

Needs assessment

The Health and Social Care Act 2012 established Health and Well-being boards to oversee the health planning for local populations. In the Act, the government also devolved power and responsibility for commissioning services to groups of GPs, these groups are called Clinical Commissioning Groups (CCG). The Health and Well-being Boards will bring together Clinical Commissioning Groups (CCG) and local authorities in order to conduct a Joint Strategic Needs Assessment (JSNA). This integrated approach to health care delivery is needed to reduce health inequalities and care for the increasing prevalence of people with long-term conditions and co-morbidities and therefore complex health needs. JSNAs will put emphasis on integrated health and social care services being organized around people in way that is seamless in order to maximize health and well-being. Health information from local Health Profiles and public consultations are essential to the JSNA in order to plan what the priorities and needs of communities are and to identify the wider public health issues (see Figure 10.5). They will include information on issues such as housing, safety and crime, education as well as health status.

The role of the nurse in using health information

In order to be able to promote the health of patients and clients and contribute to preventing further ill health, the nurse needs to understand how common the condition is and what the risk factors for a condition or disease are. Epidemiological studies highlight risk factors, for example, we know that elderly people from nursing homes with repeated hospital admissions are likely to have methicillin-resistant *Staphylococcus aureus* (MRSA) cultures. For the nurse, epidemiological studies may also show what information the nurse may need to decide upon appropriate intervention, for example, we know that referral to a community exercise programme sustains longer change in physical activity when compared to written information and brief advice from a health professional. To enable the nurse to practise evidence-based nursing, the following skills need to be developed: seeking information; appraising information; extracting findings; synthesizing information; and applying this new information to the clinical context (see Chapter 11).

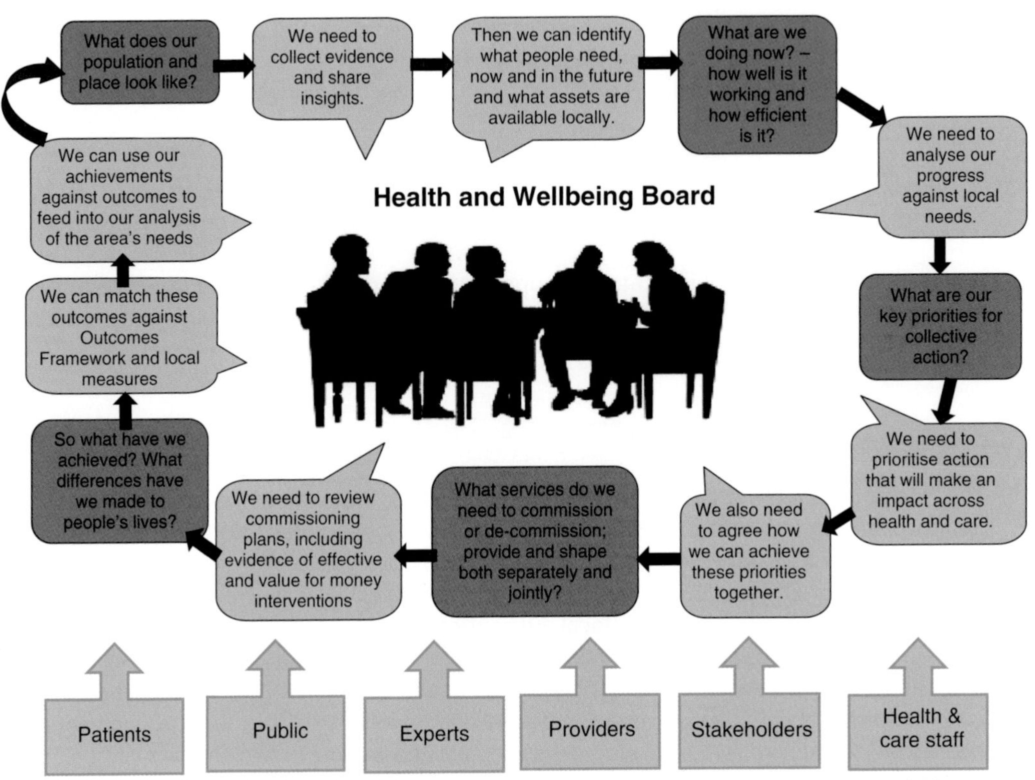

Figure 10.5 The link between health information and planning. Source: Department of Health, 2013. Reproduced under the Open Government Licence.

On placement: checklist

- ❑ What information is collected to assess the wider determinants of health?
- ❑ Are local prevalence and incidence rates of relevant conditions known?
- ❑ Is existing data used? How?
- ❑ Are health needs assessed?
- ❑ How are health outcomes measured?
- ❑ How do nurses contribute to the JSNA and other population health assessments?

Key learning points

1. Different measures and indicators are used to measure the population's health.
2. The Joint Strategic Needs Assessment has a role in planning services.
3. There is a range of outcomes that may be used to assess public health progress.

Further reading and resources

Health profiles can be used by local authorities and the health service to highlight the health issues for their local authority area and to compare them with other areas. The profiles are designed to show where there are important problems with health or health inequalities. They can be accessed from the Association of Public Health Observatories at http://www.apho.org.uk.

There are many accessible textbooks providing introductions to epidemiology. The following chapters provide shorter overviews and examples of how the nurse can use health information:

Carr, S., Unwin, N. and Pless-Mulloli, T. (2007) *An Introduction to Public Health and Epidemiology*, 2nd edn. Open University, Buckingham.

Crichton, N. (2008) Epidemiology, in *Health Studies: An Introduction* (eds J. Naidoo and J. Wills), Palgrave Macmillan, Basingstoke.

Jones, L. and Douglas, J. (eds) (2012) *Public Health: Building Innovative Practice*. Sage, London.

This book contains a useful section on techniques in statistics and epidemiology that allows the student to use data with confidence and how to use research techniques to identify needs and set priorities.

Harvey, J. and Taylor, V. (eds) (2013) *Measuring Health and Wellbeing*. Sage, London.

This very useful book provides an introduction to the health surveillance competences for public health practitioners.

National Institute for Clinical Excellence: http://www.publichealth.nice.org.uk.

Chapter summary

This chapter has demonstrated how epidemiology and health information can be used to describe populations and their health and assist the nurse in understanding how the individual is part of a bigger picture. Knowing and being able to apply the "when", "where" and "who" alerts the nurse to consider potential threats to health and well-being for the individual, and should inform nursing practice. Challenges for the nurse include understanding frequently used epidemiological terms and understanding how population-based information is relevant to care delivery. Additionally, the nurse needs to be able to identify the necessary health information to be able to deliver effective and efficient nursing care. This nursing care may be therapeutic, palliative or preventative. In order to do this, the nurse needs to know how to do this and to have the information technology skills to access relevant health information from credible sources.

References

Arowobusoye, N. (2004) *Lewisham Health Profile 2004.* Lewisham PCT, London.

British HIV Association, British Association for Sexual Health and HIV, British Infection Society, UK (2008) *National Guidelines for HIV Testing 2008*. British HIV Association, London.

Department of Health (2001) *The National Service Framework for Diabetes.* DH, London.

Department of Health (2003) *Health Survey for England.* DH, London.

Department of Health (2005) *Improving Diabetes Services: The NSF Two Years On.* DH, London.

Farmer, R. and Lawrenson, R. (2004) *Epidemiology and Public Health Medicine*. Blackwell Science, Oxford.

Francis, R. (2013) *Report of the Mid Staffordshire NHS Foundation Trust Public Inquiry*. TSO, London. Available at: http://www.midstaffspublicinquiry.com/sites/default/files/report/Executive%20summary.pdf.

General Register Office for Scotland (2004) *Table 5.1 Death Rates by Sex and Age, Scotland, 1946 to 2003.* Available at: http://www.gro-scotland.gov.uk/files/04t5-1.pdf.

General Register Office for Scotland (2005) *Table 4.2 Stillbirth, Perinatal, Postneonatal and Death Rates, Scotland, 1946 to 2004*. Available at: http://www.gro-scotland.gov.uk/files/04t4-2.xls.

Griffiths, C. (2003) The impact of Harold Shipman's unlawful killings on mortality statistics by cause in England and Wales, *Health Statistics Quarterly*, **19**, 5–10.

HPA (Health Protection Agency) (2012) *HIV in the United Kingdom: 2012 Report*. HPA, London.

HSCIC (Health and Social Care Information Centre) (2010) *Infant Feeding Survey UK 2010*. DH, London.

Jarman B. (1993) Identification of underprivileged areas, *BMJ*, **286**, 1705–1709.

Masoli, M., Fabian, D., Holt, S., Beasley, R. and GINA Program (2004) The global burden of asthma: executive summary of the GINA Dissemination Committee Report, *Allergy*, **595**, 469–478.

ONS (Office for National Statistics) (2001a) *Census 2001: Ethnicity and Religion in England and Wales*. Available at: http://www.statistics.gov.uk/census2001/profiles/commentaries/ethnicity.asp.

ONS (Office for National Statistics) (2001b) *Census 2001: The Most Comprehensive Survey of the UK Population.* Available at: http://www.statistics.gov.uk/census2001/census2001.asp.

ONS (Office for National Statistics) (2003a) *Annual Public Health Report: Excess Winter Deaths: Lambeth, Southwark, Lewisham and London 1996–2002.* ONS, London.

ONS (Office for National Statistics) (2003b) *Table 2 Births, Perinatal and Infant Mortality Statistics 2003*. Available at: http://www.statistics.gov.uk/StatBase/Expodata/Spreadsheets/D8518.xls.

ONS (Office for National Statistics) (2004) *Geographic Inequalities in Life Expectancy Persist across the United Kingdom*. Office for National Statistics, London.

ONS (Office for National Statistics) (2005a) *2003 Mortality Statistics: Cause, England and Wales.* Available at: http://www.statistics.gov.uk/downloads/theme_health/HSQ25.pdf.

ONS (Office for National Statistics) (2005b) *Infant and Perinatal Mortality by Social and Biological Factors, 2004.* Available at: http://www.statistics.gov.uk/downloads/theme_health/HSQ28.pdf.

ONS (Office for National Statistics) (2008) *Birth Statistics: Births and Patterns of Family Building England and Wales (FM1); Mortality Statistics: Deaths Registered in England and Wales in 2008*, (DR_08), Office for National Statistics, London.

ONS (Office for National Statistics) (2010) *Standard Occupational Classification 2010*, (SOC2010). Office for National Statistics, London.

ONS (Office for National Statistics) (2012) *Deaths Registered in England and Wales*, (Series DR) 2011. Office for National Statistics, London.

ONS (Office for National Statistics) (2013a) *General Health in England and Wales, 2011 and Comparison with 2001 Coverage: England and Wales: 30 January 2013*. Office for National Statistics, London.

ONS (Office for National Statistics) (2013b) *Childhood, Infant and Perinatal Mortality in England and Wales, 2011*. Office for National Statistics, London.

ONS (2013c) *Statistical Bulletin: Life Expectancy at Birth and at Age 65 for Local Areas in England and Wales, 2009–11*. Available at: http://www.ons.gov.uk/ons/dcp171778_320078.pdf.

PHE HIV/STI Department (2012) *United Kingdom New HIV Diagnoses to End of December 2012*. No. 2:2012. Available at: www.hpa.org.uk.

Public Health Lewisham (2013) *A Picture of Lewisham*. Available at: www.lewishamjsna.org.uk.

Tod, D., Read, C., Lacey, A. and Abbot, J. (2001) Barriers to uptake of services for coronary heart disease: qualitative study, *British Medical Journal*, **323**, 1–6.

UK Collaborative Group for HIV and STI Surveillance (2005) *Mapping the Issues: HIV and Other Sexually Transmitted Infections in the United Kingdom: 2005*. Health Protection Agency Centre for Infections, London.

WHO (World Health Organization) (2002) *The World Health Report 2002: Reducing Risks, Promoting Healthy Life*. WHO, Geneva.

WHO (World Health Organization) (2013) *Asthma Fact Sheet*. Available at: http://www.who.int/mediacentre/factsheets/fs307/en/.

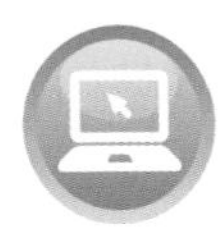

Don't forget to visit the companion website for this book: www.wileyfundamentalseries.com/healthpromotion where you can find self-assessment tests to check your progress.

11

Evidence-based practice

Jane Wills

Professor, Health Promotion, London South Bank University, London, UK

Pat England

Faculty Information Adviser, Health and Social Care, London South Bank University, London, UK

Learning outcomes

By the end of this chapter you will be able to:

1. Understand what is meant by evidence-based practice
2. Examine what types of information and evidence are available and the different purposes for which each may be used
3. Understand how to search for information

Introduction

This chapter discusses the different types of evidence and information that may be used when deciding what is done to promote health with patients. There are a number of considerations that should underpin practice, including effectiveness and cost effectiveness and the acceptability of an intervention to a patient. Evidence-based practice (EBP) claims to provide an objective and rational basis for practice by evaluating available evidence about what works to determine current and future practice. As such, it is clearly differentiated from:

- tradition ('this is what we've always done');
- practical experience and wisdom ('in my experience, this approach is the most effective one');

Fundamentals of Health Promotion for Nurses, Second Edition. Edited by Jane Wills.

Companion website: www.wileyfundamentalseries.com/healthpromotion

- values ('this is what we should do');
- economic considerations ('this is what we can afford').

Chapter 10 explored the nature of the information available on a particular problem or need and how to identify a community or locality that is targeted. This chapter considers what is known about the success or failure of interventions aiming to tackle the problem and where this information can be obtained. There are countless examples of therapies that have proved effective in clinical practice, such as aspirin and thrombolytic therapy for acute myocardial infarction in the 1970s, yet their uptake into routine practice has been slow. Similarly, there are assumptions about what works to promote health such as shock-horror campaigns to dissuade people from smoking, that have been continued until rigorous and appropriate evaluations revealed that the results were not as intended.

Practice and decision-making

Any decision about what to do is made up of:

- a balanced consideration of what we know;
- what we think might plausibly work;
- what we think we ought to do;
- what we think we can do.

In other words, when we make a decision, we use information in the form of data about the issue, theories based on information about why things are the way they are, values and opinions about what we should do, and all set in a context of limited resources and practical constraints of what people want.

In the 1970s, Archie Cochrane, a physician, became aware that there were substantial variations in practice on a range of issues and many practices were unsubstantiated. He instituted the drive to use research evidence to inform what was done and after his death, the first repository for evidence was named after him in 1993– the Cochrane Collaboration. It is also important when there are limited resources to identify interventions that are of best value. A lack of transparency in how decisions are made about how to tackle an issue can be reduced by providing a framework for decision-making.

Nurses may need information about:

- the need for something to be done;
- the relative effectiveness of specific interventions aimed at addressing the problem and what should be done;
- the design and implementation of an intervention, the context in which an intervention is carried out and how it has been received – in other words, information about how something should be done.

Activity 11.1

Consider the following health promotion issues that have arisen in practice:

- the best way of addressing maternal obesity;
- how to encourage diabetic patients to look after their feet;
- how to offer an HIV test to a heterosexual woman.

Where would you go to find out what to do?

Discussion

Practitioners most frequently base what they do on what their colleagues suggest. Yet all of these questions will have been widely researched and there are also guidelines from the National Institute of Health and Clinical Excellence on these issues that advise on the most effective and acceptable interventions.

What do we need to know?

Public health and health promotion interventions are intended to promote or protect health or prevent ill health. Because health promotion may involve many different interventions, over a period of time and different levels and across different sectors, it can be hard to determine its effectiveness.

Activity 11.2

How do we know if health promotion works?

Discussion

This is a major question. When deciding whether an intervention is successful or effective, we look at its outcomes. Traditionally, these are final outcomes such as life years gained or an improvement in health status. Many public health or health promotion programmes, however, seek a change in the health or behaviour of an individual or group. This might relate to their knowledge, attitudes, skills, service utilisation, participation and involvement, self-esteem or self-confidence which may best be measured by qualitative data (information that is more concerned with people's meanings or accounts).

The simplest strategy to identify if an intervention works is to identify a target population and compare measurements of change (effect) made before the intervention to those made afterwards.

Activity 11.3

A study suggests that exercise can improve the self-esteem of children(Ekeland *et al.*, 2005). What problems might there be in determining effect in such a study?

Discussion

In addition to the variation in measures of self-esteem, there are other questions that might be important to answer before deciding whether to introduce an exercise intervention as part of a positive mental health programme:

- *Is an effect sustained over the long term?*
- *Which exercise interventions are most effective?*
- *Do all interventions have an equal effect?*
- *How much activity needs to be completed before an increase in self-esteem can be measured?*
- *Is the participation in any activity the key variable rather than the specific exercise?*

Experimental studies are the only design capable of establishing if an intervention works because they set out to establish the relationship between intervention and effect. The experiment sets out to exclude the effect of any other factors that might influence the outcome. For example, if you wanted to see if a school-based nutrition education programme was effective in encouraging children to eat more fruit and vegetables, it would be important to ensure that other factors that might influence this such as a national television programme were not influencing the results. The only way to limit this sort of potential bias is to set up an experiment in which there are two comparable groups at the same time – one receiving the intervention and one not receiving it. It would be assumed that the extraneous variable (the television programme) affects both groups in the same way. Any differences between the two groups must therefore be attributed to the intervention. The experiment thus has two key features:

- There is an intervention and at least one comparison group.
- Outcomes are compared after the intervention.

The "gold standard" design for attributing observed outcomes to planned interventions is the randomized control trial (RCT). Given a sufficiently large sample size and efforts to ensure a comparable distribution of key subgroups, (e.g., age, gender), randomly allocating participants ensures that the intervention and control groups will be comparable.

A major challenge for public health and health promotion is to identify which elements of a programme lead to change. Demonstrating the outcomes of a health promotion intervention may be difficult to identify or detect:

- Change may not be able to be attributed to the intervention. For example, a decline in change may not be apparent for several years, for example, reduction in smoking-related deaths.
- Change in mortality or morbidity rates may be very small.

For an intervention to claim to be effective, it needs to show some change has occurred. But how much of a change is necessary? For example, if the number of children eating fruit and vegetables following a nutrition education programme increases from 20% to 21%, can the intervention be said to be effective? This will partly depend on the size of the sample and the number of children involved and the statistical significance of the change (whether it could have happened by chance or reflects a pattern).

The evidence-based practice movement has relied on the RCT study design as providing credibility to evidence, and evidence briefings, guidelines and syntheses often only include evidence gathered from RCTs. However, these are difficult to set up to evaluate public health and health promotion interventions which may not be discrete single interventions, standardized or simple to measure and control.

Activity 11.4

In addition to evidence of effectiveness, what other evidence might be needed in relation to public health and health promotion?

Discussion

You might consider some of the following:

- *whether a change in practice would be acceptable to service users;*
- *whether a service or intervention reduces health inequalities;*
- *whether a service or intervention offers "value for money".*

Information from studies and evaluations can help to answer these questions.

The Picker Institute has produced a summary based on an analysis of over 50 systematic reviews of the health promotion interventions that are shown to improve patient outcomes, available at: http://www.investinengagement.info/HealthPromotionWhatWorks.

- There is good evidence that well-designed, carefully targeted interventions can reduce health risks among disadvantaged groups. The extent to which they reduce inequalities *between* socio-economic groups has not been well studied.
- A variety of methods – reminders, educational programmes, mass media campaigns and routine health checks – can help to increase uptake of screening, immunization and other preventive procedures.
- There is some evidence that proactive telephone counselling using motivational techniques can reduce health risks among disadvantaged groups.
- There is good evidence that parenting programmes and home visits can help to reduce health risks among children. They can also help to reduce substance misuse among adolescents.
- There is good evidence that opportunistic advice from health professionals (in primary care, hospital and workplace) can help to reduce risk factors (smoking, exercise, diet, alcohol).
- There is some evidence that self-help programmes, including those that are internet-based, can help some smokers to quit.

- There is reasonably good evidence that well-designed mass media campaigns and banning tobacco advertising can help to reduce smoking rates.
- Coordinated sexual health strategies including one-to-one counselling can help to reduce sexually transmitted infections and teenage pregnancies.
- Exercise programmes can help to enhance older people's mental well-being.

The rise of evidence-based practice

Policy and professional drivers are making practitioners more accountable for the decisions they make and for the processes by which they reach those decisions to be more transparent. The NHS reforms of the late twentieth century focused on quality, audit and clinical governance as providing the framework through which NHS organizations would be accountable for continuously improving the quality of their services. In addition, for many professions, but especially nursing, practice guidance in the past has been focused on ethical issues and the scope of the role. As nursing has become increasingly autonomous and self-regulating, it demands much greater accountability. One way of enhancing professional credibility is by claiming that practice is research-based.

So, in part, evidence-based health promotion is about being research-minded and instead of taking practice for granted, asking repeatedly, "How do we know this is the right thing to do?" and "Who says so?" This questioning approach to practice is similar to the reflective practice that is expected of all nurses.

Activity 11.5

- What do you understand by evidence-based practice?
- Is this something you are encouraged to be?
- Why do you think this is?

Discussion

Nurse education is taught by practitioners who may have a particular view on how things are or should be done. Many interventions are carried out with little thought as to why they are done that way. As Bertrand Russell is supposed to have remarked: "The fact that an opinion has been widely held is no evidence whatever that it is not utterly absurd." Being an evidence-based practitioner ensures that practice is up to date and based on the best available information on effectiveness and means that nurses can confidently support their actions.

Many nurses will probably be used to finding evidence from two main sources: more experienced colleagues and textbooks. But in both cases:

- How can you be sure that the information they give you is reliable?
- Where have they obtained their opinions?
- Is their knowledge up to date?

There are many factors that have given rise to the concern for practice to be based on research and evidence and proven interventions:

- a need to prioritize expenditure when treatment costs are spiralling;
- the introduction of new technologies or treatments which need to be assessed;
- consumer awareness of rights and choices of service and programme;
- increased availability of IT, making access to range of information easier.

Evidence-based practice: what it is and what it isn't

Activity 11.6

Sackett and colleagues (1996) defined evidence-based medicine as

the conscientious, explicit, and judicious use of current best evidence in making decisions about the care of individual patients based on skills which allow the doctor to evaluate both personal experience and external evidence in a systematic and objective manner.

Does this match your own definition?

Being evidence-based thus means seeking out as much information as possible. The principles of EBP suggest this must be done in a transparent and systematic way so that someone else could follow what was done. Before information is used in a decision, an assessment should be made of the accuracy of the information and the applicability of the evidence to the decision in question.

Written reports of primary research (original studies) are what is normally considered to be evidence – information that demonstrates whether something is true or not. Evidence comes in various forms:

- published in academic and professional journals;
- commercially produced in academic and professional texts;
- independently published reports;
- unpublished reports which are known as grey literature.

The conventional approach to finding, reviewing and assessing evidence has been imported from medicine and clinical decision-making. It has established a "gold standard" of evidence that privileges systematic reviews of randomized controlled trials.

A systematic review is a review of literature, which identifies, appraises and synthesizes all the empirical evidence that meets pre-specified eligibility criteria to answer a given research question. Increasingly, organizations such as the National Institute of Health and Clinical Excellence (NICE, 2009) are translating systematic reviews of research evidence into practice in a clear, up-to-date summary. Guidelines are systematically developed statements to assist decisions about appropriate health care for specific circumstances. They translate evidence into recommendations that can be implemented. For example, NICE Pathways (https://www.evidence.nhs.uk/nhs-evidence-content/public-health) bring together all NICE recommendations on topics such as diet, physical activity, smoking, alcohol use, needle and syringe programmes and social and emotional well-being.

Evidence 11.1

Here are some examples of public health (PH) guidance from NICE for a range of problems.

Smoking cessation

- PH1 Brief interventions and referral for smoking cessation
- PH5 Workplace interventions to promote smoking cessation
- PH10 Smoking cessation services
- PH26 Quitting smoking in pregnancy and following childbirth
- PH39 Smokeless tobacco cessation: South Asian communities

Alcohol and drugs interventions

- PH4 Interventions to reduce substance misuse among vulnerable young people
- PH7 School based interventions on alcohol
- PH24 Alcohol use disorders

Physical activity

- PH2 Commonly used methods to increase physical activity
- PH13 Promoting physical activity in the workplace
- PH17 Promoting physical activity for children and young people

Nutrition/weight management

- PH11 Maternal and child nutrition
- PH27 Weight management before during and after pregnancy

There are many organizations that are repositories of evidence reviews:

- http://www.campbellcollaboration.org/ (for social care reviews)
- http://www.cochrane.org/
- http://www.eppi.ioe.ac.uk/cms/ (major centre for health promotion reviews and methodologies)
- http://www.nice.org.uk/
- http://www.vichealth.vic.gov.au/cochrane/ (the public health review group)
- http://www.york.ac.uk/inst/crd/

Doing a review

Although practitioners do not normally do reviews themselves, they may identify an issue or need for which they wish to find information. That will mean being able to find the information and be sure that what they have found is comprehensive and reliable and not simply an arbitrary selection of information, possibly to support what they already thought. Figure 11.1 identifies the steps involved in doing a review.

Doing an evidence review is not the same as a literature review which will be an overview of what is known about a topic and may also include how it has been studied. A systematic review is:

- comprehensive: it attempts to identify and review all relevant evidence;
- systematic: it clearly describes the process of searching, selecting, appraising and extracting evidence;
- question-focused: it focuses on a specific question;
- replicable: replication of the process should produce the same results.

Conventionally, an evidence review uses a PICO question, based on a clear framework:

- **P**opulation
- **I**ntervention
- **C**omparison
- **O**utcome

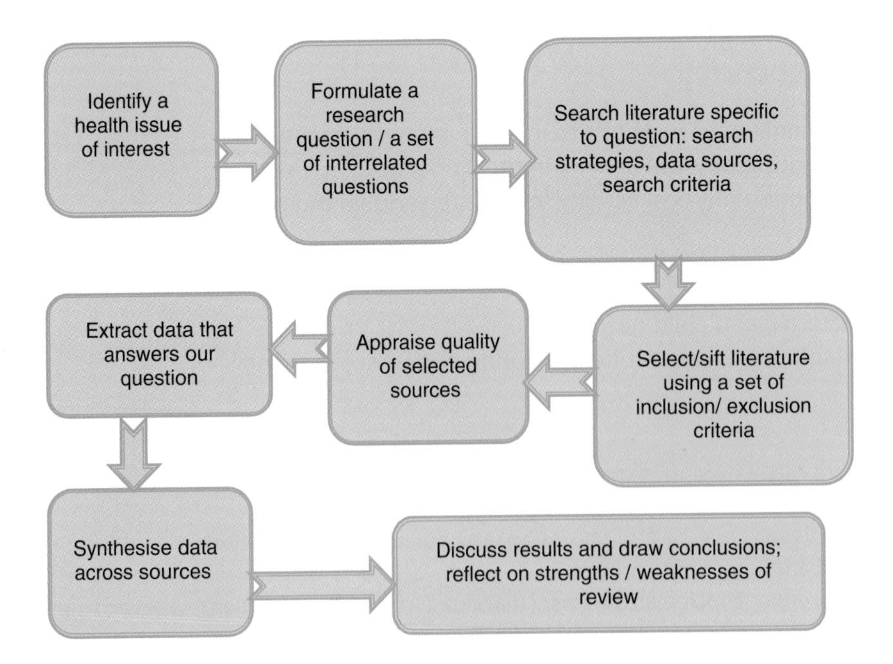

Figure 11.1 The stages of an evidence-based review.

In public health, the focus of interest is often whether an intervention is effective but review questions can also focus on other issues such as risk factors or health actions.

Activity 11.7

Identify in the following typical questions what is the population of focus, the intervention, the comparator and the outcome that would be measured to demonstrate success.

- Are bottle-fed babies more likely to be obese in adulthood than breast-fed babies?
- Do financial incentives work to increase levels of physical activity among people over 40?
- Is peer-education or counselling effective to increase uptake of HIV testing in men who have sex with men?

Discussion

See Table 11.1, a summary of the population of focus, the intervention, the comparator and the outcome for each question.

Table 11.1 The populations, interventions, comparators and outcomes for each scenario.

Population	Intervention	Comparator	Outcome
Bottle-fed babies	Feeding	Breast-fed	Obesity
People over 40	Financial incentive	No incentive/ standard advice	Increased activity in amount and/or frequency
MSM	Peer education	Counselling	HIV testing uptake

Finding evidence

For many new nurses there may appear to be an overwhelming amount of information and it may be hard to find the information needed. Finding information on any topic is a skill and depends on a systematic and logical approach, and competency in information literacy is a key task for the student nurse.

Finding evidence demands:

- time;
- access to facilities;
- computer skills;
- a fast internet connection.

Literature to be searched is diverse and may cover numerous sources. There are a variety of tactics that can be used to access information:

- Searching online databases of secondary or 'appraised' research.
- Searching online databases of primary research.
- Searching the web with search engines such as Google and Google Scholar.
- Contacting acknowledged experts.
- Hand-searching professional and academic journals.
- Hand-searching theses and independently published reports by organizations, for example, Alcohol Concern, Terrence Higgins Trust, Cancer UK.

Activity 11.8

Think of an occasion when you tried to find something out. Reflect on what helped and what hindered your search.

Discussion

Being clear about what information you need, where to look and how to organize the information you find are all likely to help when you are looking for information.

Being systematic about how a search is done will make it less likely that key information is missed and it will save time in the long run as it will be less likely that the student will have to go back and repeat the search. So practitioners carrying out reviews or just looking for evidence develop a search strategy which is the formal statement of how the search was carried out.

Before conducting a literature search, it is important to take time to think about what you need to find out. This involves planning the process of the inquiry and will ultimately save time when sifting through the results. This stage mainly involves thinking carefully about the topic and taking some time to define and clarify it clearly.

Keywords

Before starting a search, whether in an internet search engine such as Google or a database, take some time to consider the scope of the question. What exactly are you looking for? Try to define your ideas: it is harder to search for a "soft" concept like "attitudes to obesity" than it is to find research relating to a particular drug.

The topic will need to be summarized into keywords or phrases – not sentences. Although internet engines such as Google will accept whole sentences, most of the databases that include primary research will expect subjects or concepts to be broken down into keywords. It can help to use a dictionary or thesaurus to help define the subject and think of alternative terms. Because many resources include international coverage, differences and spelling or terminology need to be considered. So, for example, the term "occupational therapy" is not recognised in the USA and the term "physical therapy" would be used. In public health and health promotion, terminology may be less standardized and so it is often necessary to use variant and related terms.

Activity 11.9

If you wanted to find information on reducing teenage pregnancy, what keywords might you use?

Discussion

- *Alternatives or synonyms to pregnancy might be: conception, motherhood – and, even though it may seem counter-intuitive – fathers!*
- *Alternatives for teenage might be: adolescent, young people, young women, teen.*

When thinking about keywords, a useful tip is to think of how the concept is likely to be expressed in the literature you are searching, rather than how you would express it. In the same way, be careful about using keywords such as "effectiveness" – an article may just describe an intervention and leave it up to the reader to judge whether it was effective or not.

The search strategy is a formal statement of how a literature search was carried out. It should contain the keywords, how they were combined, which databases were used, and any subject headings for each one. It will develop and be refined as the search proceeds, but it is an important part of the transparency of the review, as it will enable a reader to replicate your results.

Using databases

Internet search engines such as Google are useful in the early stages of finding literature but it is likely that the major part of an inquiry will be in online databases. These act as indexes to published (and sometimes unpublished) literature. Such databases tend to be organized around the literature of a particular subject:

- *Medline* covers medicine, dentistry, and veterinary science.
- *Cinahl* covers nursing and allied health.
- *PsycInfo* covers psychology literature.
- *ASSIA* covers social sciences.

Medline is the world's largest database and includes nearly 5000 journals worldwide. Although searching on Medline could therefore give access to thousands of articles, major journals are indexed in more than one place and so you may need to run your search on any relevant indexes to be sure of picking up the research you need.

The profusion of online databases may be confusing, especially to the novice searcher. They will have different interfaces (what you see on the screen) depending on the company that provides them, for example, *Medline* may also be searched online as *PubMed*, which is freely available.

The databases that a student is able to use will depend on their home institution: a large university library will give access to a wider range of databases in different subjects than an NHS Trust library. The means of gaining access to the databases may vary. Many databases include access to the full text of journal articles, and this can cause confusion when articles are not instantly available. A database should give a list of titles and abstracts of articles; anything more (at the present time) is a bonus. It is worth discussing the search with a qualified librarian, who will be able to give advice on what to expect from the library.

There are different ways of indexing information:

- title
- source, i.e. journal title
- authors
- abstract or summary of main points.

Online search engines employ sophisticated software to interpret natural language so that it can be understood by a computer. The database will require a more controlled vocabulary than might be used in everyday language or even using a search engine such as Google. This means that searching for all keywords and their synonyms in all their forms – singular, plural, British and American spelling, and so on. Most databases provide tools to make this easier, such as truncation symbols – where a word is shortened to its stem, enabling a search for all variants with a minimum of typing, or wild card symbols which enable the substituting of one letter for another. It is usually possible to search for a phrase by enclosing it in speech marks e.g. "National Health Service". The Help pages provided by the database will show all these tools.

There are two main ways of searching a database – using free text or subject headings. Using free text means that the database searches for the words that are typed in and gathers up all the articles that mention the words typed. Normally the best way of searching is using the database's own subject headings which is like a dictionary that collects all the articles that are ABOUT a specific topic. These terms can be used to extend the search so that rather than asking the database software to find every occurrence of the word typed in (which is what happens in a keyword search), it is asked to find articles which are *about* that topic.

Scenario 11.1

Finding evidence on women and smoking cessation

This search is on interventions to help women stop smoking. The student decided to use as keywords "women", "smoking cessation". They decided to use the Cinahl database selecting all years (Cinahl goes back to 1982).

Using free text searching

- Decide to search for records for last ten years. Click on "set other limits" and type in 2000–2010.
- In search screen, type in "women" and "smoking cessation". Result is over 800 records so need to refine.
- In search screen, type in "women" and "smoking cessation" and intervention* (* is the truncation symbol in the database).Result is 304 records so still need further refinement.

- Go back to search screen and type in "women" and "smoking cessation intervention?" Result is just over 90 records which is manageable and some of the results look useful but I realize that intervention(s) may not cover all possibilities.

Using subject headings

The student decided to check terminology in the thesaurus. Click on the thesaurus option.

- Type in "smoking cessation" – main headings used are smoking cessation, smoking cessation programs (there is another heading for smoking cessation assistance but that is a specialist heading for one record only). Smoking cessation programs seems to be most relevant.
- Check "women" – that is in the thesaurus but also "women's health" which might also be relevant. Decide also to check "female" which is also in the thesaurus.
- Check "interventions".
- Go back to the search screen and still searching from 2000–2010, select the subject heading option above the find box (as having checked the thesaurus terms it is possible to now limit the search to subject heading field) and search "women" or "women's health" or "female" and "smoking cessation programs". Result is 274 records.
- Look through all of these and mark those that seem most useful. Despite search terms, the search still brought up articles whose titles or abstracts showed they were not specifically about women so these are not included. Also excluded are any that were about pregnant smokers.
- Click on the show marked records button on the right-hand side to bring all the marked ones together and then save to disk.
- As the database only provides results in the form of a reference – a title and an abstract, to read the article, the search needs to be recorded accurately so that it is possible to go back later and locate and download the relevant articles.

Recording a search

Being systematic will enable the search to be as thorough as possible in each database used, and help prevent having to re-do work. It is essential to document the search as far as possible: keep a list of all the relevant literature found, and record the search technique for each database as you search it. It is usually possible to set up an account with a database that will enable searches to be saved and re-run.

By describing a search, a "map" of the evidence available is produced. A search entails:

- the topic – inclusion and exclusion criteria and keywords;
- the search terms used;
- the source and methods – which databases and/or journals and reports;
- the date accessed (especially important when referencing electronic sources);
- the results – numbers found and those included/excluded;
- the results – the types of evidence included.

For the search on "women and smoking cessation" described by the practitioner above written out formally, the search strategies would look like this:

Cinahl free text search strategy

1. "Women"
2. "Smoking cessation"
3. Intervention*
4. 1 and 2 and 3
5. "Smoking cessation intervention*"
6. 1 and 2 and 5
7. 20000101–20101231 (limit to articles published 1 January 2000 to 31 December 2010)

Cinahl thesaurus search strategy

1. MH "Smoking cessation programs"
2. MH "Women+"
3. MH "Women's health"
4. MH "Female"
5. 2 or 3 or 4
6. 1 and 5
7. 20000101–20101231

Activity 11.10

Try replicating these searches, using this template. How many articles can you find?

Looking for other information to help decision-making

Comprehensive search strategies should include other sources of information. This might include:

- hand-searching relevant journals to the topic;
- government reports;
- expert advice.

"Grey literature" is the term used to describe any literature that is hard to find. It includes conference proceedings, unpublished dissertations, policy documents, internal reports and blog entries. The internet has made the task of searching for grey literature much easier, as well as increasing its quantity. Many organizations (and individuals) publish research findings on their websites or support online journals. It is easy to use a search engine such as Google to find government reports. It is possible to apply the same techniques that are used for the database search to search the web.

Tracking down grey literature may be through reading or colleagues or a specialist library collection. There is little primary research on many public health topics and in these circumstances expert opinion may provide guidance as to how proceed with decision-making. The *British Medical Journal*, for example, frequently includes opinion pieces from physicians and the World Health Organization also makes considered statements on public health actions.

Activity 11.11

If you wanted to find evidence on effective interventions to support prisoners to stop smoking:

- What keywords would you use?
- What databases would you search?
- How would you decide which papers (articles) to exclude?

Discussion

Keywords are likely to include smoking (or a truncated term smok which would also access other words associated such as smoker or smoking) OR tobacco and prison (or truncated term prison*) OR correctional (a US term for prison) OR offend*.*

Databases such as Medline, Cinahl and PsychInfo would capture papers on smoking cessation in the medical journals but also papers focusing on specific characteristics of prisoners which may be more likely to be published in social policy or psychology journals.

Searching across all these databases is likely to result in lots of duplicates. It may also result in papers that do not report primary research. Despite these clear keywords a search may still result in finding papers that are not about smoking cessation interventions or not about prisoners! There may also be papers that do not report quit rates as an outcome and so make it difficult to determine their effectiveness.

Appraising evidence

Having found some evidence, this now needs to be assessed or appraised. Being able to judge the usefulness of information is a key task for practitioners. It is also a skill used every day in decision-making – Does this information help to answer my questions? Is the information detailed enough? To determine what is the best evidence means having critical appraisal skills that help to decide if information is good enough to be used in decision-making.

All information that is used goes through an initial sifting process. Individuals decide whether a piece of information, whether a journal article or written report, is worth reading and whether or not what it says is to be trusted. In that sifting we look for information that is:

- relevant
- trustworthy
- believable.

Decisions on relevance are made all the time. When searching for information on the internet, for example, it is common to get thousands of "hits". Rapid judgements are made on relevance according to words used, or the source of the information. When looking for journal articles, the sifting process may examine:

- The topic and subject matter: is this evident in the title or abstract?
- The type of information: can the study design and data collected answer your question?
- The similarity of the setting to the one you are working in: are the findings applicable?
- The similarity of the population group to the ones you work with: are the findings applicable?

The abstract, which is retrievable on the database, will give you more information. The abstract summarizes the research and includes the objectives, the study design, important findings and conclusions. It is therefore very helpful in determining initial relevance.

Trustworthiness depends on efforts having been made to reduce any possible bias. Initial sifting questions may include:

- Who wrote the paper? Consider their expertise, experience, particular professional/disciplinary stance.
- Source of funding? Is there any potential for bias?
- Journal quality? How rigorously has the study report been reviewed, if at all?
- Up-to-date? How relevant is the work to current circumstances?

It is also important that published research is believable and dependable. Believability may relate to how transparent the means are by which conclusions were made. This relates to the design, methods, and procedure, how the conclusions were reached, and whether there is an audit trail of actions and decisions.

So there are many ways in which we exercise critical thinking in relation to information. Discounting information is easy either in picking holes in the quality and/or because a study might not be relevant and transferable. There is a huge amount of information available and if some kind of sifting process is necessary to avoid getting overwhelmed and being unable to weigh one piece of evidence against another. The advantage of critical appraisal is that it offers a consistent approach to screening out information that should not inform decisions.

Critical appraisal is a formal process using a structured systematic approach, often using a detailed series of questions. Critical appraisal tools (e.g. those of the Critical Appraisal Skills Programme: http://www.casp-uk.net/) often take the form of a questionnaire containing questions about the article being critically appraised that aims to systematically evaluate articles. They consider the following:

- In/exclude evidence that is on/off the topic.
- In/exclude evidence collected in/appropriately.
- Filtering out evidence from studies that are not reported in sufficient detail to judge quality.
- Filtering out evidence from studies that are not methodologically sound.

Acting on evidence

Once a decision has been made as to the quality of the evidence, a nurse will need to draw on expertise, experience and knowledge of the unique patient and clinical setting to help decide whether the evidence should be incorporated into clinical practice. There are benefits and risks of implementing any change, as well as benefits and risks of not making changes. This is why evidence should support decision-making.

On placement: checklist

- ❑ What reasons do nurses give for the way things are done?
- ❑ Do they claim this is based on evidence?
- ❑ What evidence sources are used?
- ❑ Is research conducted in the department?
- ❑ Is that research disseminated?
- ❑ Is there a journal club or any sharing of new knowledge?

Key learning points

1. Evidence-based practice is about using the best available evidence to support your practice.
2. Nurses should be constantly seeking this evidence to improve and innovate.
3. Being evidence-informed means the nurse can justify why they are doing things in the way they are.
4. Being evidence-based means the nurse needs to be computer-literate.

Chapter summary

Nurses work in environments that are constantly changing and evolving and need to ensure their practice is current and that they are equipped with the necessary skills to be flexible and adaptive. The complexity of the issues to be addressed in public health and health promotion makes searching for information a challenging task. Being confined to primary research in databases that is easy to find and complies with an accepted methodological approach may not help to answer the questions that are needed for local decision-making. Evidence-based practice relies on the premise that to make well-informed decisions about practice, nurses need not only to access the best evidence about interventions but also must have the skills to appraise it and judge its relevance. They will also integrate their own expertise and experience, and patients'/clients' values and situation and their views.

Further reading and resources

A good place to gain an overview of understanding and appraising research studies is the book by Tricia Greenhalgh (2000) *How to Read a Paper: The Basics of Evidence-Based Medicine*. BMJ Publishing Group, London.

There are several guides to evidence-based practice for nurses. These take a step-by-step practical approach showing how to identify and evaluate the different types of evidence available and to critically appraise the studies that lie behind them. They also look at the ways in which findings are integrated into practice, showing how research evidence can be applied to clinical-decision making and the delivery of patient care.

Barker, J.L. (2010) *Evidence Based Practice for Nurses*. Sage, London.

Craig, J.V. and Smyth, R.L. (2012) *Evidence Based Manual for Nurses*, 3rd edn. Churchill Livingstone/Elsevier, London.

NHS Evidence covers a wide range of information of interest to those working to improve the health of the population. This includes guidance, systematic reviews of research, implementation tools and practical examples from people working in the field. Available at: https://www.evidence.nhs.uk/nhs-evidence-content/public-health.

References

Ekeland, E.F., Heian, F. and Hagen, K.B. (2005) Can exercise improve self esteem in children and young people? A systematic review of randomised controlled trials. *Br J Sports Med*, **39**, 792–798.

NICE (2009) *The NICE Public Health Guidance Development Process An Overview for Stakeholders, Including Public Health Practitioners, Policy Makers and the Public*, 2nd edn. NICE, London. Available at: http://www.nice.org.uk/media/F19/70/PHProcessGuide2009.pdf (accessed 24 August 2010).

Sackett, D., Rosenberg, W., Muir Gray, J.A. *et al*. (1996) Evidence based medicine: what it is and what it isn't. *BMJ*, 312, 71.

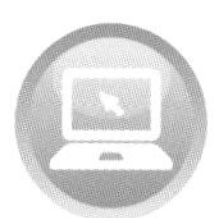

Don't forget to visit the companion website for this book: www.wileyfundamentalseries.com/healthpromotion where you can find self-assessment tests to check your progress.

12

Health education and communication

Jane Wills

Professor, Health Promotion, London South Bank University, London, UK

Learning outcomes

By the end of this chapter you will be able to:

1. Recognize different kinds of communication and how they can be used in health promotion
2. Understand the elements of effective group education and support
3. Identify effective resources and materials to support health education
4. Plan an effective health education strategy
5. Understand the principles of motivational interviewing
6. Discuss the role of the nurse in encouraging and supporting people to change

Introduction

Previous chapters have shown how health and disease are determined by many factors that interact together, yet health behaviours and lifestyles are responsible for a considerable burden of ill health and disease. Because treatment has become expensive and often of questionable efficacy in health improvement and because genetic factors are largely unalterable, the focus has shifted to encouraging changes to individual lifestyles. This chapter explores the ways in

Fundamentals of Health Promotion for Nurses, Second Edition. Edited by Jane Wills.

Companion website: www.wileyfundamentalseries.com/healthpromotion

which nurses may help individuals to learn and understand their condition and change their behaviour through advice and information, counselling and through education and teaching. This is a vital competence for nurses who must use the full range of communication methods to support person-centred care.

Part of the nurse's health promotion role is to encourage people to adopt healthier lifestyles. To do this, it is important to think through what influences whether or not people make changes to their health and health behaviour. A key element in people's behaviour is their attitude to that behaviour. People's attitudes are made up of two components:

- *cognitive* – the knowledge and information which contribute to their beliefs about the behaviour;
- *affective* – their emotions and values about what is of importance.

A person's attitudes will also be influenced by:

- their past experiences of and attitudes towards health and social care provision;
- their previous successes or failures to change their behaviour and lifestyle and self-confidence;
- the support they received from both their family and friends and health and social care providers;
- their perceptions of, or health beliefs about, their illness or disease;
- their gender, age, culture and socio-economic group.

Activity 12.1

Think of a health behaviour that you may want to change. What knowledge or information may influence you? How does your attitude to the behaviour influence what you do?

Discussion

A patient's knowledge will influence their ability to change their behaviour and lifestyle. For example, a patient may wish to change their eating patterns and adopt a healthier way of eating. However, they may be unsure of the healthy eating messages in terms of frequency, amount and types of healthy foods and therefore may feel too overwhelmed to change their current eating patterns.

The extent to which a person perceives the harm or risks from behaving in a certain way as dangerous will also influence them. But as we know, simply being aware of risks does not necessarily change behaviour, as people may simply deny the relevance of such information to them.

A person's skills will also influence their ability and desire to change their health behaviour and lifestyle. If, for example, the individual wants to change their level of physical activity and starts off by participating in a high impact, vigorous activity which requires a high level of skill, after previously leading a sedentary lifestyle, their lack of skill may result in injury and therefore prevent them from any future involvement in that or any other activity.

One way of understanding how people make decisions about their health behaviour and lifestyle is to use a model of health behaviour. Becker's Health Belief Model (1974) (Figure 12.1) suggests that a person will weigh up pros and cons of making a change and choose the action that seems to provide the greatest benefits without costs, such as time or money. An individual may take a protective health action if they believe themselves to be:

- susceptible or at risk;
- at a severe health risk because the consequences of not taking action would be severe;
- capable of taking action.

Perceived susceptibility

This is based on the subjective perception of the risk of developing a condition, illness or disease, i.e. does the individual believe that they are at real risk of developing an illness? Most people think they are less likely to get a problem than other people and nurses may hear patients say things like "People like me don't get that."

Perceived severity

This relates to feelings about the seriousness of contracting an illness or leaving an illness untreated, i.e. is leaving the illness untreated worse than the illness itself? People will not consider the consequences as serious if they believe it can be prevented by taking action at some

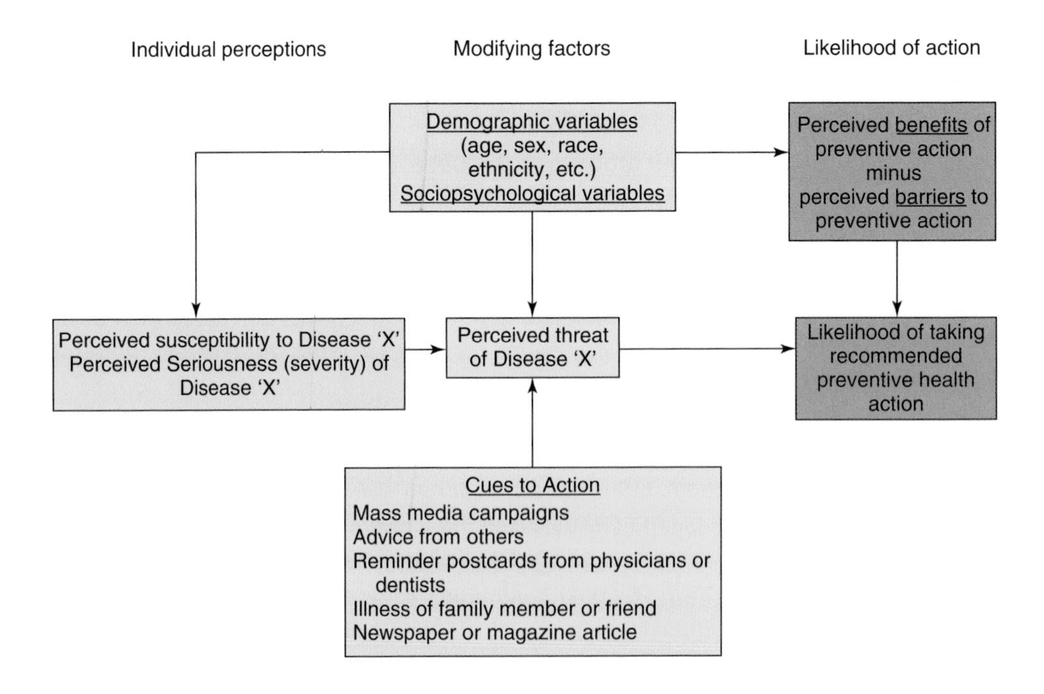

Figure 12.1 The Health Belief Model.

point in the future or if any outcomes are likely to be some time ahead. Nurses may hear patients say "you've got to die some time" or "I'll worry when the time comes."

Perceived benefits

An individual must believe that an action will be effective in reducing the severity of the illness and that there are definite benefits in taking that action, e.g. having a child immunized. Nurses may hear patients say "I would rather stop my child getting one of those awful diseases."

Perceived barriers

An individual may cite a lack of time, lack of access, costs or negative perceptions associated with the behaviour that will deter them from embarking on a health behaviour change. Nurses may hear patients say "If I give up smoking, I'll put on weight" or "I won't be able to cope with stress if I stop smoking."

A person may also need some sort of push or incentive to start thinking about making a change. This might be:

- a change in circumstances, e.g. a pregnancy might prompt a reduction in drinking;
- new information, e.g. a doctor performing a liver function test might prompt a reduction in drinking;
- the passage of time, e.g. older people feeling less mobile might be prompted to be more active;
- a significant other may develop an illness related to their health behaviour which may trigger a patient to take stock of their own health behaviour.

Some people find it easier to make a change than others. The concept of a health locus of control distinguishes between those with an internal or external locus of control:

- *Internal locus of control* – people who see their health as largely within their own control. These people are more likely to adopt activities to enhance their health.
- *External locus of control* – people who see their health as a matter of chance and so outside their control. These people are more likely to adopt health-damaging behaviours than those with an internal locus of control.

People are motivated to take action when they feel the outcome is likely to be valuable or beneficial and when they feel they can do it effectively. Several factors affect people's feelings of self-efficacy and whether they think they can change:

- perceptions of their own will power;
- whether they have enough relevant information;
- perceptions of their own coping skills;
- whether they feel supported by family and friends.

Social networks are also a major influencing factor in prompting a person to change, providing emotional or practical support or as sources of information.

Activity 12.2

Think back to a time in your life when you wanted to change your health behaviour/lifestyle, e.g. giving up smoking, increasing your levels of physical activity, eating more healthily, decreasing your alcohol consumption.

- Did you consider your risk of developing an illness or disease?
- Did you consider the seriousness of the illness or disease?
- Did you weigh up the pros and cons of making a change, e.g. what were the benefits? What were the costs?
- Did you succeed in making the change? What helped you?

Approaches to changing lifestyles

Health promotion is everybody's business and can have a positive impact on the work of the nurse and their patient's health. For example, during a routine contact with a patient the nurse can use this time to discuss:

- any concerns the patient may have with their health;
- what needs the patient has;
- what other influences there are on the patient's health;
- what behaviour changes they may wish to make.

The nurse can use this time to give brief health promotion interventions. This may result not only in the patient feeling valued and listened to, but also give the patient a feeling of control over their own health. If patients feel more in control of their life, they are more likely to feel enabled to make health choices and feel empowered to take part in their own care planning. A range of activities can be used by the nurse to promote health. Such examples include:

- *One-to-one discussions* – these can be carried out by the nurse at the patient's bedside; during outpatients appointments; during primary care appointments; in the patient's home. For example, the student nurse gives advice on healthy eating to a patient while discharging the patient from hospital who had been admitted with unstable diabetes mellitus.
- *Group discussions* – these can be carried out by the nurse during in-patient stays in hospital; during health promotion groups such as antenatal classes; or during primary care clinics. For example, the student nurse helps to facilitate an antenatal class with the community nurse as part of her maternity placement and gives advice on healthy eating in pregnancy.
- *Telephone contacts* – these can be carried out by the nurse from the ward or community setting as a means of making contact or keeping in contact with patients. For example, the student nurse on community placement follows up patients who have attended the health promotion group on healthy eating to offer support and encouragement.

- *Disseminating information and explanation leaflets* – this can be carried out by the nurse during in-patient episodes; while discharging patients; during health promotion groups and health fairs; and in the community. For example, the student nurse gives patients health education leaflets and gives health education advice as part of their discharge information in order to encourage patients to change their health behaviour.
- *Health stalls* – these can be carried out by the student nurse as part of community placement. For example, a student nurse sets up a health stall in the hospital foyer to provide information on smoking cessation groups as part of National No Smoking Day.

In order to be able to carry out health promotion interventions, key skills are required in:

- information giving;
- communication;
- counselling and motivational interviewing;
- education and teaching.

Information giving

It is often forgotten how much information people need to grasp as a patient. Increasingly, there is recognition of the skills, including the ability to perform basic reading and numerical tasks, that are needed to function in the health care environment. Health literacy is the term used to describe the understanding of health information. Numerous studies have shown the association between low levels of functional literacy (reading and numeracy) and poor health outcomes (Berkman *et al.*, 2011).

Activity 12.3

Why might low levels of literacy affect health?

Discussion

A patient may not be able to read medication information, may not be able to access information, e.g. on managing a condition such as how to use an asthma inhaler, may not be able to assess risk, e.g. judge a fever in a child, may not be able to read information about screening, may not give informed consent.

Explaining is a core skill that is often challenging for the nurse and poor information giving is a common source of patient dissatisfaction. As well as giving information about treatments and procedures, the nurse may need to give information about behaviour changes such as healthy eating or reducing alcohol consumption. The nurse has to be able to give information in a manner that is acceptable, understandable, coherent, safe and appropriate. The nurse should also give advice that is contemporaneous and evidence-based. The key features of effective information giving are:

- Tailor information to what a patient needs to know.
- Limit the information to a small number of key messages.
- Present the important information first.
- Explain any technical terms.
- Check the patient's understanding.
- Elicit reactions to the information.

Written information may be used to reinforce verbal information either in a consultation or by being available on a display for patients to read at leisure. Leaflets may be produced by a manufacturer, by a charity or support group, or may be produced by a clinical team. Any information needs to do the following:

- be suitable for its target audience, e.g. culturally sensitive;
- be available in different formats, e.g. braille, pictorial;
- use appropriate language, not medical terms or jargon;
- have an effective design and structure that attract and interest the reader.

Activity 12.4

How would you judge the quality of written information if you were deciding whether to use it in a patient context?

Discussion

The presentation of health information should be appropriate, understandable, accurate, acceptable (as much as possible), visually appealing, clear and precise. Again this should be based on contemporaneous and evidence-based information.

There are numerous guides on producing patient information produced by charities such as Mind and Mencap and also by the Department of Health. Such guides also can be used to analyse existing leaflets:

- Content
  - Is the leaflet brief and to the point?
  - Is it up to date?
  - Does the leaflet emphasize the key points?
  - Is it overly prescriptive?
  - Does the leaflet use language that is easy to understand?

- Does it explain any medical terms?
- Is there a commercial bias (e.g. logo, brand name)?
- Is it acceptable?

- Presentation
  - Are the words and images easy to see?
  - Is the design of the leaflet visually appealing, e.g. colour, images and size?
  - Are the typeface and lettering easy to read, e.g. Arial and size 12 point or bigger?
  - Do the colours make it easy to read (is there a contrast between the text and the background)?
  - How could you use the leaflet to make an effective display?

- Audience
  - How would it make the reader feel: shocked? Disturbed? Offended?
  - Are the images representative of the diversity of communities?
  - Is there any stereotyping of people in the images?
  - Is the language appropriate for the audience?

Displays should be well put together with all materials in good condition, be current and well positioned to attract attention. They should invite the patient to read the information by being well lit, at reading height and creatively put together.

Communication

Good communication in health promotion is important because it enables the nurse to successfully deliver clear, concise, unmistakable health promotion messages. Health promotion communication can take place in any setting and at any time, such as:

- on the ward during admission or discharge of the patient;
- before a procedure, such as changing a dressing;
- during visiting time when the nurse discusses the patient's care with their relatives;
- as part of the rehabilitation process for patients with long-term conditions such as diabetes mellitus.

Communication can be difficult at times for a number of reasons such as:

- The first language of patient and nurse differ.
- The patient is hard of hearing or deaf.
- The patient has a number of presenting problems and may be unable to take on new information.
- Pain, tiredness or fear stop the patient paying attention.
- The patient believes that they are being judged.

- The nurses are busy and therefore do not convey messages effectively.
- Nurses use jargon.
- The health information is unrealistic or appears to be irrelevant.

There are many ways in which health promotion encounters could be improved by better communication skills. Because this is such a core competence, we often take for granted communication and forget to pay attention to its core elements such as really listening and attending to what patients say and showing in body language, attention, respect and recognition that the person is unique. Looking at your watch, answering the phone or even reading case notes give the impression that you are not interested. It is all too easy for a patient to feel pressurized by a busy nurse and not ask questions or say they understand something simply to avoid possible offence.

In order to communicate effectively with patients and engage in active listening nurses must use a range of communication skills known collectively as SOLER which means:

- **S**it squarely facing the patient, ideally on the same level.
- **O**pen questions are used.
- **L**isten actively to the patient.
- **E**ye contact if acceptable to the patient.
- **R**eflection, i.e. repeat the wishes expressed by the patient back to them to clarify that the nurse has heard and understood the patient's expressed needs.

Key tips for active listening

- *Empathy*: Showing you understand how it must be for them "That must be really hard . . ." Acknowledge the individual's problems, issues, and feelings. Listen openly and with empathy, and respond in an interested way, for example, "I appreciate your willingness to talk about such a difficult issue . . ."
- *Paraphrasing*: To show you are listening, repeat every so often what you think the person said — not by parroting, but by paraphrasing what you heard in your own words. For example, "Let's see if I'm clear about this . . ."
- *Summarizing*: Bring together the facts and pieces of the problem to check understanding, for example, "So it sounds to me as if . . ." Or, "Is that it?"
- *Reflecting*: Instead of just repeating, reflect the speaker's words in terms of feelings, for example, "This seems really important to you . . . That must be frustrating." This can prompt the person to explain more or even to challenge you.
- *Probing and clarifying*: Ask questions to draw the person out and get deeper and more meaningful information, for example, "What do you think would happen if you . . .? Would you like to talk about it?"

Activity 12 .5

Ines has been admitted to your ward with an acute asthmatic attack. Ines lives in temporary accommodation and has no relatives in London. She speaks little English and appears frightened and confused.

- What could the nurse do to allay some of Ines' fears?
- What would be the most helpful strategies for the nurse to use in order to assess Ines' needs?
- What would be unhelpful communication strategies?

Discussion

The nurse needs to demonstrate respect for the individual and maintenance of the patient's dignity at all times. As a nurse, it is important to take into account the cultural and social needs of your patients and take on board the impact this may have on their ability to accept and/or interpret the health information you give them. Some possible solutions that may address Ines' fears include providing information in a format that she is able to understand and that she finds acceptable. This health information should include advice that takes into account her social and psychological health as well as her physical health needs.

Some useful strategies that the nurse could employ include using interpreting and advocacy services; the former will translate information from the nurse to the patient and vice versa; the latter will act on Ines' behalf to ensure that doctors and nurses and other health and social care providers meet Ines' needs and enable her to make informed health choices. Nurses should ensure that their communication with patients whose first language is not English is not unhelpful and disempowering, such as:

- *speaking very loudly in order to be understood;*
- *using inappropriate interpreters such as ancillary staff from similar ethnic backgrounds;*
- *making health decisions on behalf of their patients without involving the patient in the process;*
- *disseminating written health promotion literature in a language that the patient is unable to understand;*
- *failing to make any attempt to communicate with their patient because they do not speak the same language.*

Counselling and motivational interviewing

Counselling approaches aim to work with the patient in relation to their own health agenda. They place the patient at the centre of the intervention and the nurse takes on the role of facilitator and empowerer. For example, the nurse will enable the patient to decide on their own course of health action and support them in this, rather than setting the health agenda.

A patient who does not express a wish to change any aspect of their health behaviour would have the right to be respected in their health decision.

Motivational interviewing (MI) is a specific technique, originally developed in the USA for use with people with addictive behaviours when it was realized that trying to persuade problem drinkers to change their behaviour through direct persuasion or confrontation was unproductive and led to denial and resistance. MI is a style of client-centred counselling developed to facilitate health-related behaviours by resolving clients' lack of motivation, which is said to comprise three elements:

- readiness
- willingness
- ability.

MI is different from simply talking to a patient, however advanced a practitioner's communication skills. The methods of motivational interviewing involve exploration more than exhortation, and support rather than persuasion or argument. Nor is MI about imparting information, rather it is about finding out from the person and drawing them out. Although intended to encourage change, any responsibility for change is left with the person, no matter what the views of professionals. It is the client or patient rather than the counsellor who should ultimately present arguments for change. In this way, MI is a big shift in practice for nurses and does require training.

The nurse would use open questions and interventions borrowed from counselling techniques to encourage the patient to develop these elements, often in brief interventions of 5–10 minutes. The intervention would follow a series of stages:

1. *Establishing rapport*. The nurse would use questions that would encourage the patient to examine their knowledge about their health behaviour and the extent to which the patient wants and desires to change. There may be many issues related to the patient's condition and the nurse will need to work to focus an agenda. There may be a discrepancy between what is happening at present and what the patient values for the future and the importance of a change can then be emphasized.
2. *Assessing the patient's readiness to change*. The technique of scaling questions is used in MI and is very successful in prompting the client or patient to reveal a great deal of information about their motivation, e.g. on a scale of 1 to 10, how certain (sure) are you that you want to change this behaviour /how important is it to you to make this change/how confident are you in making this change?

   1 = Not certain at all 10 = Very certain
   Not certain at all 1—2—3—4—5—6—7—8—9—10 Very certain
   Why a 6 and not a 2 or 3?
   What would it take for you to reach an 8?

3. *Exploring ambivalence*. Most patients will be ambivalent about change and both want to and not want to do something, e.g. the desire to give up smoking but the desire not to put on weight. Resolving ambivalence can be a key to change. MI will ask the person about the positives about their current behaviour and about the negatives. Attempts to force a patient in a particular direction through direct persuasion or by making them frightened of the

Table 12.1 Ambivalence in a patient's talk.

I don't want to change	I ought to change
I don't want to talk about it	I want to
It's not necessary	I could if I put my mind to it
It's too hard	It would be better for me
I ought to change but …	It's certainly something I should think about

consequences can, however, lead to a paradoxical response and even strengthen the behaviour.

Table 12.1 illustrates the difference between the sorts of things a patient might say who is resistant to change.

4. *Developing an action plan*. Even when the patient may see the importance of a change and has the confidence to do so, it may not be top of their priorities: 'I want to, but not now.' Relative priorities are part of normal functioning: low readiness can be viewed as the patient needing information about what the next step is towards change. Motivational interviewing is about negotiation, e.g. the nurse and patient discuss the patient's health and together devise a health action plan if the patient is ready to change.
5. *Setting goals*. Motivational interviewing is about goal setting, which should be realistic, specific and measurable and not too ambitious or have unrealistic outcomes, e.g. the patient's aim may be to drink sensibly; their objectives may be that they reduce the number of times a week that they consume alcohol and the amount of alcohol they drink.

Activity 12.6

A patient on a cardio-thoracic unit has had a myocardial infarction. The patient is a smoker but is completely opposed to trying to quit as he claims it will increase his stress levels and that he has been unsuccessful on previous occasions. Which of the following is your most likely response?

- ❑ Argue and reiterate the rationale for change.
- ❑ Give lots of suggestions of how he could quit.
- ❑ Point out the dangers of continuing to smoke.
- ❑ Suggest that as he has tried to quit before, he must want to be a non-smoker.
- ❑ Listen reflectively to the difficulties the client foresees.
- ❑ Ask him how they see the pros and cons of changing.
- ❑ Acknowledge he has a choice whether to change or not.

(Continued)

Discussion

MI will explore with the patient the benefits of making a change and the disadvantages. Do the advantages outweigh the disadvantages? It will point out the discrepancy in the patient's desire to live long and well to be with his family and his smoking. It will attempt to build the patient's confidence that quitting is possible by pointing out his previous commitments to change. The nurse should also encourage patients to discuss any concerns they may have about becoming a non-smoker and the support networks they may have around them. In terms of evidence of effectiveness, it is important to consider that patients may relapse several times before they become a non-smoker but that support from a GP or nurse is valuable for a successful outcome (see Chapter 5). At no time will the practitioner tell the patient about the health risks (he will probably know these already) or try to persuade.

Scenario 12.1

Florence is 58 years old, married with two adult children, in an outpatient diabetes clinic.

I'm not sure about my weight. I don't really think it's a problem, my mother and sister were much bigger than me. I know I could do with losing some though as it'd be better for my health and it can be quite hard getting about. But at this stage in my life I think I should be enjoying myself and I do like food. I don't eat sweet things though. About five years ago I did lose some, mostly exercise, I think, but it just comes back and I have sort of given up since.

- What would be the nature of a brief intervention with Florence?
- How could you resolve her ambivalence?

Discussion

- *Don't be prescriptive: "This is the best method of xxx."*
- *Don't give too little direction: "There's a diet or a group, which would you like?"*
- *Do emphasize personal control: "You will be the best judge of what works for you. Let's go through the options."*
- *Do build confidence: "I can tell you what's worked for other people."*

The Stages of Change Model devised by Prochaska and DiClemente (1982), shown in Figure 12.2, argues that the patient goes through various stages before they are able to change their health behaviour and these stages are sequential and relevant if the patient is able to achieve sustained behaviour change.

1. *Precontemplation*: The patient is unwilling or not intending to change their current health behaviour for the foreseeable future. It may be because the patient is uninformed, uninterested or they may have tried and failed in the past to change their health behaviour. At this stage, the strategy used by the health promoter or nurse would be to give the patient information, i.e. leaflets, helpline numbers, etc. and then leave the door open for them to come back with questions or concerns.
2. *Contemplation*: The patient is thinking about changing their health behaviour. This could be due to a trigger such as a close relative or a friend becoming ill (someone they can identify with) or due to changed circumstances such as an illness in their own lives. The patient intends to change their health behaviour in the near future and the strategy employed by the nurse or health promoter at this stage would be to encourage the patient to draw up a list of pros and cons of their current health behaviour; to discuss any concerns the patient may have with changing their health behaviour; and to keep a diary to help the patient to document and understand their health behaviour.
3. *Preparing to change*: The patient, with the aid of the nurse/health promoter, would make preparations for their new health behaviour and discuss the details of how to change. For example, if the patient wanted to become more physically active, they would perhaps find out what activities were available in their locality. Or perhaps (if financially viable) they might purchase equipment needed in order to take up a physical activity, such as trainers or a new swimming costume.
4. *Making changes* is the next stage and at this stage the patient would be supported to implement their health behaviour change. The strategy used here by the health promoter or nurse would be to devise an action plan, which has specific objectives; measurable outcomes; is agreed by all parties concerned, i.e. negotiated; has realistic objectives/actions and is time-specific, i.e. will start on a specific date or to be for a specific time span.
5. *Maintaining change* is the next stage and is when most people are working to prevent a relapse or recurrence of their old health behaviour. This may be because of the external pressures on the person. This stage is said to be one of the hardest for the patient and they are said to have succeeded if they can maintain the behaviour for a lengthy period of time, depending on the behaviour. For example, not smoking for six months, being physically active for eight weeks. In other words, the new health behaviour has become habitual. The strategy employed here by the nurse would be to encourage the patient to reward themselves for being able to maintain the new health behaviour (obviously not with a reward that would sabotage their efforts).
6. *Relapse* may be the next stage and is said to occur when the patient is unable to sustain the new health behaviour for numerous reasons, such as: bereavement; stress; changed circumstances; lack of support; boredom; lack of incentives; lack of motivation, etc. Relapse is a normal component of behaviour change and Prochaska and DiClemente (1982) argue that the patient should not think of themselves as a failure. The nurse's strategy here would be to use this opportunity to review with the patient their action plan to see if it was realistic or too over- ambitious. It is important to help the patient to understand that relapse is not failure, but a normal part of the process of change.

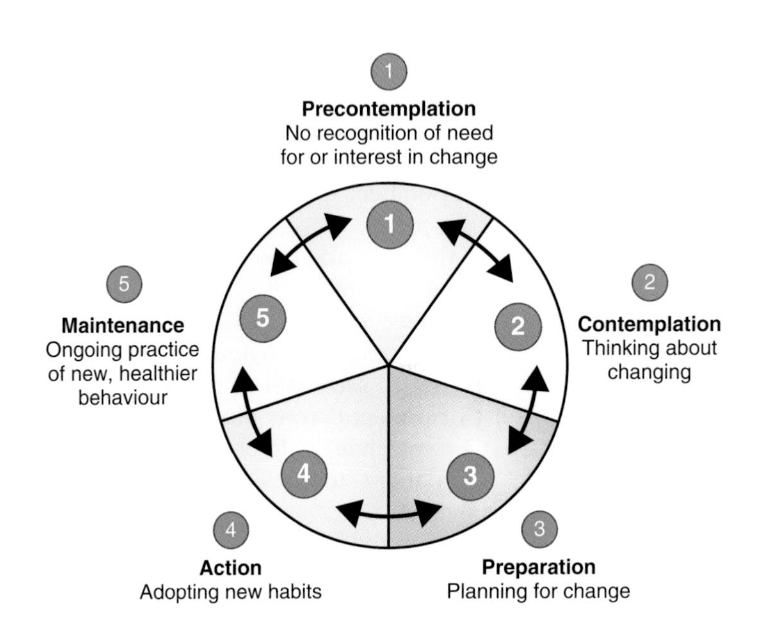

Figure 12.2 The Stages of Change. Source: Prochaska and DiClemente, 1982, Figure 2, p. 83. Copyright © 1982 by the American Psychological Association. Reproduced with permission.

Figure 12.3 shows how these theoretical models on individual behaviour change have been applied to guidance on smoking cessation and recommendations for brief interventions in primary care.

Such client-centred approaches arguably need specific characteristics on the part of the nurse which Carl Rogers (1951) called core qualities. These core qualities help patients in a therapeutic relationship with the nurse and include:

- *Unconditional positive regard* – acceptance of people irrespective of their condition, age, gender, culture, ethnicity, socio-economic background, expressed thoughts, behaviours or beliefs. The patient should not be judged by any set of rules or standards. The nurse must set aside their own values and beliefs, biases and prejudices in order to help their patient. This acceptance should not be confused with liking or approval of the patient.
- *Genuineness or congruence* – this means being oneself or being true and sincere, being non-defensive and free in behaviour and being real. The nurse would therefore use their own language and own behaviour and be genuine.
- *Empathy* – this means being able to appreciate the patient's own meanings and understand the world as seen through the eyes of the patient.

Thus, the focus of the intervention is to take on board the patient's frame of reference and to endeavour to understand the patient and appreciate their circumstances from their perspective; to enable and encourage the patient to take responsibility for their own health decisions and actions. Rogers (1951) argues that if the above is in place, then behaviour change is more likely to happen.

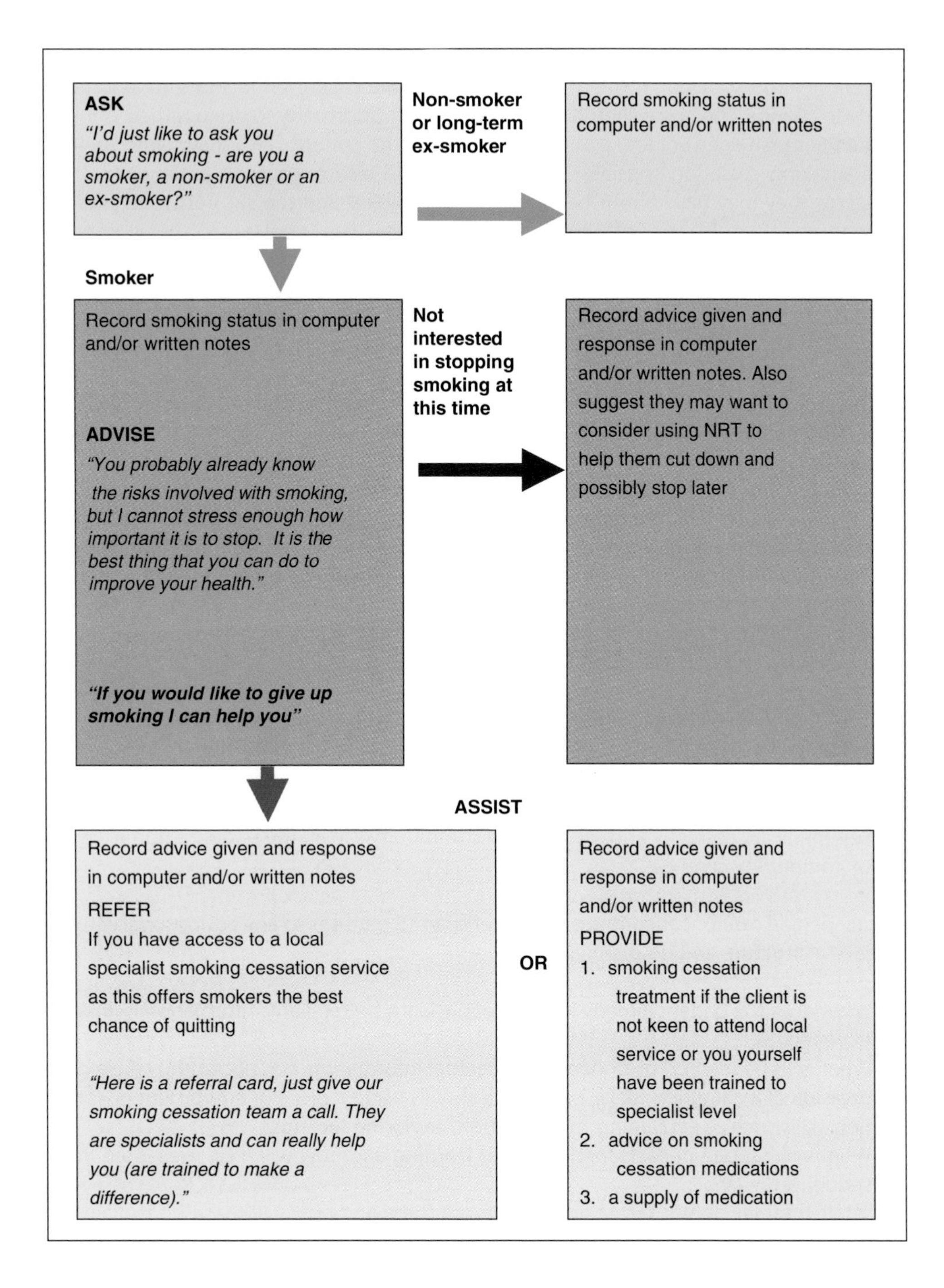

Figure 12.3 Brief advice for smokers. Source: McEwen *et al.*, 2006, Figure 3.1, p. 36. Reproduced with permission from John Wiley & Sons Ltd.

The nurse could ask the patient to consider the benefits and the cost factors related to their current health behaviour; if the benefits outweigh the cost, then it is safe to assume they are ready to change. The nurse should give patients the opportunity to discuss their smoking habit and if the nurse does not feel confident to support the patient, refer them (with their consent) to a smoking cessation specialist. The nurse should also encourage patients to discuss any concerns they may have about becoming a non-smoker and the support networks they may have around them. In terms of evidence of effectiveness, it is important to consider that patients may relapse several times before they become a non-smoker but that support from a GP or nurse is valuable for a successful outcome.

Education and teaching

Educational approaches to health promotion are important because they aim not merely to give people information but to give people an informed choice and to help them to acquire knowledge and skills in order to make that choice. In this approach, education or information is presented and patients are encouraged to explore their own attitudes, skills and knowledge about their health. Patients may also be assisted to help make changes to their lifestyle. For example, a nurse will give patients information on healthy eating; may help the patient to explore their attitudes and knowledge about what constitutes a healthy diet and may escort the patient to a local supermarket to identify healthy food choices.

Educational approaches to health promotion take place in a number of settings, for example:

- health promotion clinics in hospital outpatients departments or GP surgeries;
- on wards when nurses demonstrate to patients how to look after their stomas;
- on wards during admission when a patient is shown how to participate in their care;
- on wards during the patient's discharge from hospital when the patient is shown how to self-medicate correctly and safely in the community, e.g. in the patient's home, GP surgeries or community centres.

Mostly people cannot concentrate for longer than 15 minutes so any educational activity needs to have a structure and be planned.

- What does the patient already know? People learn better if any information is linked to their experiences.
- What is to be learned or understood?: factual information, e.g. about the cause or the progression of a condition; skills, e.g. practical skills using a piece of equipment or communication skills such as explaining the condition, exploring feelings.
- What will happen in each section of the learning and how will it be presented in a logical, sequenced way?
- What complex points, terms or concepts are there and how will these be explained?
- What visual aids will be used?
- How will the patients' understanding, interest, enjoyment be checked?

Activity 12.7

What might be the education plan for the following patients?

- a middle-aged man following a stroke;
- a woman of 65 undergoing a total knee replacement;
- a young man having a retinal replacement following a rugby accident.

Discussion

All the patients will need to know the cause of their condition and may need to see this on a model or diagram, how it is affecting them, what is likely to happen in the future and what they can do to manage the condition such as exercise or weight management and any medication. It may be advisable for family and carers to be present and for some simple do's and don't's regarding rehabilitation and medication. Signposting to support groups particularly the Stroke Association and carers groups for the stroke patient would also be advisable.

Scenario 12.2

A young mothers group

Members of a young mothers group wanted to know about a safe, effective and inexpensive physical activity to help them to lose weight. What might be the content and format of such a group?

Discussion

The community nurse and the group members should draw up a programme together so that it can meet the mothers' needs. It should be planned and structured.

The learning outcomes should be:

- *Know what types of activity are safe and effective.*
- *Explore attitudes and beliefs about different activities.*
- *Know physical activity opportunities available locally.*
- *Consider the gaps in knowledge and skills about physical activity in order to promote activity with their families.*

(Continued)

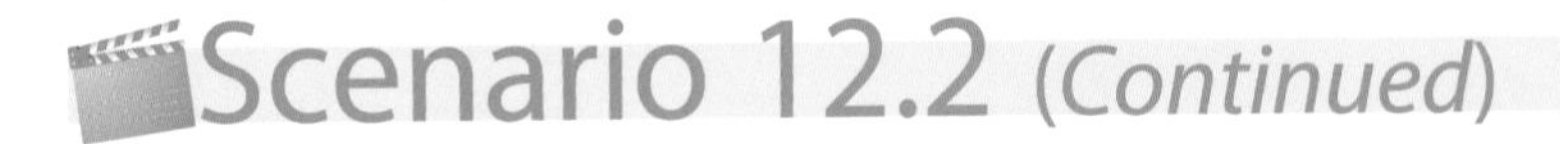

The learning methods are:

- *Keep activity diaries.*
- *Group discussion of experiences, attitudes and beliefs.*
- *The group to disseminate information of opportunities, access and availability of physical activity options.*

Evaluation of objectives would be:

- *The group would be able to describe safe and effective methods of physical activity.*
- *The group would be aware of a range of available options locally.*
- *The group would be participating in physical activity.*
- *The group would feel confident about promoting physical activity with their families.*

Increasingly, the nurse may be involved in running groups, for example, to support patients to manage their condition or to create support in the community. Table 12.2 provides a simple list of things to remember before undertaking this activity.

The role of the nurse in promoting health behaviour and lifestyle change

Changing health behaviour and lifestyles can be a very daunting challenge for the nurse who has to integrate health promotion into their other work. The student nurse has to learn many technical procedures, skills and theoretical concepts and may find health promotion too difficult a concept to apply to their everyday tasks. Although initially the nurse may not see the relevance or importance of health promotion in their work, aiming to change health behaviour can have a much wider impact than on the health of the individual patient. For example, if patients feel enabled and empowered, they may try to influence the health of their families, friends and communities. This knock-on effect could arguably be seen as primary prevention, i.e. addressing the health needs of the population before the onset of disease or illness.

Encouraging people to change their health behaviour and lifestyle can be viewed by the patient and public at large, as interfering and controlling. Victim blaming is unhelpful and nurses could make some people feel that they are being blamed for their ill health and health-damaging lifestyle and that it is their sole responsibility to adopt health-enhancing behaviour. Blaming the victim may encourage people to give up the one coping mechanism they have in their lives, but it may not significantly improve their health; or it may exacerbate the patient's socio-economic situation, by making the patient feel responsible for their ill health and may result in the patient failing to take on board health messages as they may feel unable to change their health behaviour.

Nurses need to be aware of the impact and influence they have on their patients and be careful about how they convey health messages that encourage changes to health behaviour.

Table 12.2 Planning a group activity: checklist.

User group	Checklist
Name of the group	Does it clearly say what it is about and who should attend? The name should be succinct and easy to remember. The title may relate to the medical condition (e.g. Arthritis, Parkinson's Disease, Multiple Sclerosis or include keywords or themes (self-management, exercise group, healthy eating for individuals with diabetes) Does it sound interesting and welcoming? Is it clear who it is aimed at? (e.g. Carers Stroke Support Group)
Location	Is it easily accessible using public transport? Is it suitable for individuals using walking equipment or a wheelchair? Is it easy to find?
Environment	Is it comfortable with enough space and suitable seating for people with a disability? Are the heating and lighting good? Is there a system in place for individuals with hearing loss? Are the toilets nearby and are they accessible for someone with a physical disability?
Staff	Is there a facilitator or co-facilitator? Are other members of the team involved? Will expert patients be involved in the programme? Has a risk assessment been carried out?
Participants	Is it an open group with new members joining or will it be the same group of participants for each programme? Has the criteria for attendance been agreed? How will individuals be prioritized if there are a high number of referrals?
Time of sessions	Have you consulted with users on the most appropriate time? Is it possible for two groups to run at different times to meet different needs?
Number of sessions	What are the key topics and how much time is required?
Topics	What topics do the users want included in the programme? What styles of delivery will be used (face to face, computer, telephone, homework)? Is there sufficient time for individuals to share their experiences and expertise?
Resources	Has money been identified to run the programme and buy resources/ refreshments?

Additionally, nurses need to be aware of the other influences on health that are beyond the reach or control of their patients and aim to address those influences using all the power and influence at their disposal.

On placement: checklist

- Are patient consultations long enough? Do patients ask questions?
- Is the language used appropriate?
- Is key information provided and in what form?
- Is confidentiality observed? How?
- What examples did you observe of active listening?
- What examples did you observe of goal setting? Were these negotiated with the patient?
- Did you observe a health care professional's own beliefs?

Key learning points

1. Health-related decision-making is complex and influenced by many factors including the patient's knowledge, attitudes and the social norms around them. The wider social context in which patients live shapes their ability to make health and lifestyle choices.
2. Health education advice should be safe, evidence-based, appropriate and acceptable to the patients.
3. Health information should be explained and should give opportunities for the patient to ask questions.
4. Empowering patients through education is to enable patients to make health choices; by giving patients the full picture and ensuring that they are aware of their options, the nurse can feel confident that patients are empowered to make an informed health decision. It may also mean acting as an advocate when patients are given health information and feel unable to express their needs or representing patients' needs to health and social service organizations.
5. Core qualities of a counselling approach such as unconditional positive regard, genuineness and empathy make patients feel valued, cared for and understood.

Chapter summary

This chapter discussed influences on lifestyle and health behaviour. Promoting healthy behaviours is a core component of the nurse's role and demands particular skills in information giving, communication, counselling and education. What is evident is that there is no one approach to health behaviour change that could be used in all situations and with all patients to meet their individual needs. The health promotion approach used by nurses must be appropriate, evidence-based, acceptable and patient-centred. Nurses have to develop skills and knowledge in order to use health promotion appropriately to aid health behaviour change.

Further reading and resources

Guidelines on how to develop and present patient information are found at www.nhsidentity.nhs.uk.

The Picker Institute has numerous guides on how to involve patients in health promotion, developing health literacy and self management at http://www.investinengagement.info.

Mason, P. (2010) *Health Behaviour Change*, 2nd edn. Churchill Livingstone, Edinburgh.
This is an excellent practical guide to health behaviour change and motivational interviewing.

Materials on 'Making Every Contact Count', the NHS initiative to systematically use the millions of contacts that people have with providers of health and social care (such as GP, outpatient appointments, etc.) to deliver brief advice using motivational interviewing principles on healthy lifestyle behaviours and to signpost people to appropriate behaviour change services. Available at: http://www.midlandsandeast.nhs.uk/OurAmbitions/Everycontactcounts.aspx.

References

Becker, M.H. (1974) *The Health Belief Model and Personal Health Behaviour*. Slack Thorofare, New Jersey.

Berkman, N.D., Sheridan, S.L., Donahue, K.E. *et al.* (2011) Low health literacy and health outcomes: an updated systematic review. *Ann Intern Med.*, **155** (2), 97–107.

Mason, P. (2010) *Health Behaviour Change*, 2nd edn. Churchill Livingstone, Edinburgh.

McEwen, A., Hajek, P., McRobbie, H. and West, R. (2006) Brief interventions, in *Manual of Smoking Cessation: A Guide for Counsellors and Practitioners* (eds A. McEwen, P. Hajek, H. McRobbie and R.West), Blackwell, Oxford.

Prochaska, J.O. and DiClemente, C.C. (1982) Transtheoretic therapy: toward a more integrative model of change. *Psychotherapy: Theory, Research and Practice*, **19** (3), 276–288.

Prochaska, J.O., DiClemente, C.C. and Worcross, J.C. (1992) In search of how people change: applications to the addictive behaviours, *American Psychologist*, **47**, 9, 1102–1114.

Rogers C. (1951) *Client Centred Therapy*. Houghton Mifflin, Boston.

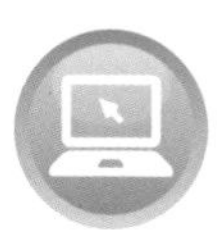

Don't forget to visit the companion website for this book: www.wileyfundamentalseries.com/healthpromotion where you can find self-assessment tests to check your progress.

13

Protecting the health of the population

Amanda Hesman

Senior Lecturer, Adult Nursing, London South Bank University, London, UK

Learning outcomes

By the end of this chapter you will be able to:

1. Demonstrate knowledge of the principles of population-based screening and vaccination programmes in the prevention and control of communicable and non-communicable diseases
2. Describe the principles of surveillance, prevention and control of infectious and communicable diseases
3. Understand the nurse's role in communicating risk and in increasing the uptake of both screening and vaccination programmes

Introduction

Health can be "protected" by preventing disease and illness and be "promoted" by supporting and maintaining a healthier lifestyle. This chapter will focus on the former and introduce the nurse to the concept of health protection and explore the methods used to safeguard the patient and population's health. In Chapter 11 the importance of health information and

Fundamentals of Health Promotion for Nurses, Second Edition. Edited by Jane Wills.

Companion website: www.wileyfundamentalseries.com/healthpromotion

epidemiology was explored and we shall now demonstrate how this data can be used to prevent ill health by informing population strategies that protect health. This chapter will demonstrate how the public's health can be protected through population strategies such as screening and immunization. Within this contemporary context of screening, active immunization and better treatment of acute infections, the shifting pattern of disease and ill health from communicable to non-communicable diseases will be described together with a discussion of current public health threats. The responsibility of the NHS and its public health function will be discussed in relation to its duty for surveillance, infection control and the management of incidents and outbreaks.

The changing pattern of disease and ill health

The communicable disease epidemics of nineteenth-century England – diphtheria, typhus, cholera and tuberculosis – began to be controlled with the introduction of sanitary reform, including the provision of clean water and safer disposal of sewage. In the twentieth century with the development of vaccination programmes and antibiotic therapy, this decline in mortality progressed even further though outbreaks, e.g. influenza, can still occur. With a reduction in absolute poverty and an improvement in nutrition and sanitation, there has been a reduction in the prevalence of communicable disease and a corresponding increase in the prevalence of non-communicable disease. The improvement in bacteriology in the late nineteenth century allowed the development of medical treatments, first, antitoxins and then antibiotics. Despite success in controlling infectious diseases, the UK does face a major problem with health care acquired infections (HCAI) and antibiotic resistance.

Non-communicable disease can include coronary heart disease (CHD), diabetes, osteoarthritis, chronic pain, alcoholism and mental illness. Many non-communicable diseases are preventable and treatable but only in the early stages of development. Whatever proves to be the impact of screening in the control of non-communicable disease, the incidence and prevalence of non-communicable diseases such as cancer and chronic ill-health will only increase with increased life expectancy.

Activity 13.1

Figure 13.1 shows the changing patterns of disease. Are communicable diseases no longer as important a priority as non-communicable lifestyle diseases?

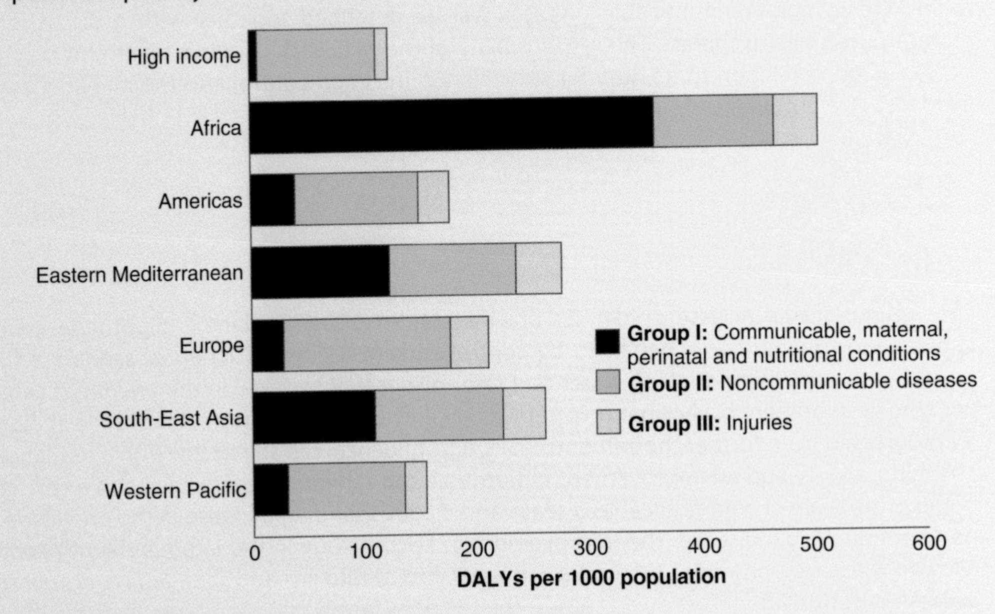

Figure 13.1 The changing pattern of disease. Source: WHO, 2008, Figure 21, p. 41. Reproduced with permission from WHO.

Discussion

Infectious diseases, maternal and child illness, and malnutrition now cause fewer deaths and less illness than they did 20 years ago. As a result, fewer children are dying every year, but more young and middle-aged adults are dying and suffering from disease and injury, as non-communicable diseases, such as cancer and heart disease, become the dominant causes of death and disability worldwide (WHO, 2012).

Globally and nationally the public health picture is quite diverse, with health issues including known "emerging" and "re-emerging threats". The term "emerging" refers to newly identified and previously unknown infectious agents that will have or do have the potential to cause a public health problem. Over the past 30 years, 30 new diseases have emerged and this often starts with a zoonosis mutating to be transmissible to humans such as SARS or HIV. The term "re-emerging" refers to infectious agents that are known with a previously low prevalence but are now causing a public health problem such as dengue fever.

Current public health threats include:

- Known diseases, such as malaria and tuberculosis cause high mortality and morbidity in continents such as Africa and Asia which the Global Health Fund is combating with the "Roll back malaria" and "Stop TB initiative" programmes.
- Newly identified diseases include the hepatitis C virus which was first identified in 1989 and the first cases of variant Creutzfeldt-Jakob disease (vCJD) (a transmissible spongiform encephalitis from cattle) was identified in humans in the UK in 1996.
- Human immunodeficiency virus/acquired immune deficiency syndrome (HIV/AIDS) was first recognized in 1981. In some African countries one in four of the living population have HIV/AIDS and when co-infection occurs with tuberculosis (TB) mortality increases.
- The re-emergence of old diseases in the UK, e.g., the declining trend in TB has been reversed.
- The emergence of CHD as a leading cause of death in poor countries.
- Individual resistance to micro-bacterial drugs due to poor prescribing and poor adherence.
- Mutation and modification of the genetic composition of bacteria and viruses such as HIV and gonorrhoea in order to survive adverse conditions such as antibiotic and viral therapy.
- With increased global travel, population migration and the import and export of food products, disease can travel and developing world viruses can be found in the developed world. For example, in 1999, West Nile Virus was identified for the first time in New York though it had previously only been found in Africa, Asia and Eastern Europe.
- Global epidemics known as pandemics. Experts predict a pandemic of influenza due to the emergence of a new flu virus A/H5N1 (avian influenza).
- The increased potential for the deliberate release of biological and chemical agents. This took place on the Tokyo underground in March 1995 with the release of the nerve gas sarin by terrorists.
- Natural disasters such as the East Asian tsunami in December 2004.
- Manmade disasters such as the Chernobyl nuclear explosion in 1996.

Infection control

A health care associated infection (HCAI) is an infection resulting from medical care or treatment in hospital as an inpatient or outpatient, or even as a result of a health care intervention in the individual's own home. The infectious agent that causes a HCAI is also known as a pathogen, which will be bacterial, viral fungal, parasitic or a prion. *Staphylococcus aureus* is the most prevalent cause of HCAI. An HCAI may infect any part of the body: the urinary system, the skin, a pressure sore, a surgical site, the gastrointestinal system and the bloodstream.

Most patients will recover from a HCAI but an infection can extend hospital duration, cause prolonged illness, disability or even death. Other detrimental effects include anxiety and depression for the patient, family and friends. Some people more than others are more susceptible to acquiring an infection because their immune system may be compromised by illness, e.g. cancer, HIV or diabetes, by medical treatment, e.g. chemotherapy, and by medical intervention and devices, e.g. surgery, IVI , ventilators, catheters, tracheotomies. In these situations even normal body commensal flora such as staphylococcus epidermidis can cause pathology. Some antibiotics harm the body's normal gut flora which can enable other micro-organisms, such as *Clostridium difficile* (c.diff) to multiply, causing diarrhea and vomiting. Furthermore, the widespread misuse of antibiotics has led to resistant strains of bacteria making some HCAI very difficult to treat, such as *methicillin-resistant Staphylococcus aureus* (MRSA), resistant *Streptococcus pneumoniae* and Vancomycin-resistant entrococci (VRE) (The Royal Marsden Hospital, 2005).

Evidence 13.1

Tips to stop a HCAI

- Clean hands in between each patient contact with either soap and water or alcohol hand gel. Remember, soap and water will decontaminate hands from c.diff but alcohol hand gel will not.
- When necessary, wear disposable gloves and aprons to prevent contamination of clothing and skin.
- Maintain asepsis and sterile field when changing dressings
- Adhere to infection control policies.
- Ensure through regular environmental cleaning, that micro-organisms do not build up.
- Develop a good working relationship with the clinical area cleaner and recognize their important contribution to patient health and well-being.
- Isolate patients known to be colonized with a resistant micro-organism to reduce risk of transmission. Ensure these patients and their visitors understand the importance of adhering to infection control policies.
- Administer prescribed antibiotics on time and discuss with patients the importance of completing the full course even if they feel better. Check their understanding.
- If the patient experiences side effects from the antibiotics, inform their doctor quickly so that these may be managed efficiently.

In addition to preventing the ongoing transmission of HCAI in the hospital setting the nurse has a powerful role in educating family and friends on the correct use of antibiotics. When an individual has an illness, such as a cough, cold or flu, it is important not to ask the GP for antibiotics. These are caused by viruses, not bacteria, therefore antibiotics will not help, but may cause other bacteria in your body to become resistant. HCAI is a major concern globally and is increasingly due to antibiotic-resistant strains of infection.

Activity 13.2

The following activity enables you to think about the nurse's role in protecting the health of the hospital population from the on-going transmission of MRSA. You are working in a pre-operative surgical assessment unit. A person attends for a pre-operative assessment which includes a MRSA screen. How will you explain this to the patient?

Discussion

- *The patient needs to know what is going to happen and why: Screening sites include nostrils, axilla and perineum.*

- *A person may be given the opportunity to self-swab: this helps to preserve their dignity and privacy and also involves them in their own care. Answering any questions they have accurately and in an informed manner will help ease anxiety.*
- *If MRSA is found, the operation will be delayed, and an antibacterial wash or powder and cream for the nostrils will be prescribed for 5 days. If the operation is urgent, admission to a side room with immediate MRSA treatment may occur.*

The majority of HCAIs are spread by direct contact, especially via the hands of health care workers.

Evidence 13.2

Hand-washing compliance

The widespread introduction of alcohol hand rubs from 2005 seeks to address the barriers of time and environment where a sink may not be nearby. While alcohol rubs may reduce time for hand hygiene, especially if they are at every patient's bedside, this does not alter the poor technique that some health care workers (HCWs) have adopted when it comes to their hand hygiene routine (Gould *et al.*, 2010). Alcohol rubs may even encourage poor technique as they allow HCWs to walk away while carrying out the procedure, therefore allowing them to become distracted by other tasks without completing all the stages.

Hand-washing practices, both in relation to technique and frequency, have been shown to be poor. Many nurses do not wash their hands as often as they think they do and do not use the appropriate product. A systematic review of compliance studies found compliance was lower in intensive care units (30–40%) than in other settings (50–60%) and lower before (21%) rather than after (47%) patient contact (Erasmus *et al.*, 2010). In other words, nurses are motivated into action in situations where they perceive they may be at risk, thus explaining why hand hygiene is higher after patient contact, rather than beforehand.

Protecting populations: the bigger picture

Health protection is a collective good because the majority of the population will benefit rather than the individual. This raises ethical issues, for example, specific patient consent is not required for public health surveillance programmes that aim to establish prevalence of communicable diseases if the samples are anonymous (HPA, 2004).

Public health is to do with the health of populations and in order to protect and improve the health and well-being of populations, collective action is necessary. This collective action can be mediated by public health regulation. In order to protect the health of populations, it is necessary for public health policy to provide for:

CATCH IT
Germs spread easily. Always carry tissues and use them to catch your cough or sneeze.

BIN IT
Germs can live for several hours on tissues. Dispose of your tissue as soon as possible.

KILL IT
Hands can transfer germs to every surface you touch. Clean your hands as soon as you can.

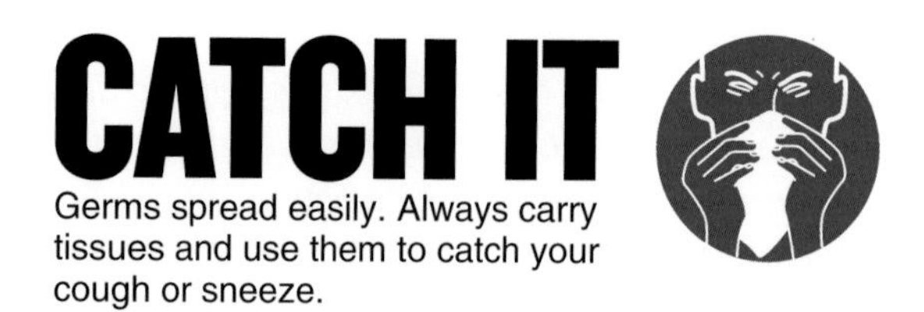

Figure 13.2 Campaign to prevent the spread of flu. Source: Department of Health, 2007. Reproduced under the Open Government Licence.

- surveillance, e.g. of immunization uptake and antenatal screening;
- notification, e.g. of communicable diseases such as TB and measles;
- regulation, e.g. of NHS microbiology laboratories and food standards;
- jurisdiction, e.g. the protection of confidentiality to do with sexually transmitted infections by the NHS (Venereal Diseases) Regulations 1974 and port control that prohibits the movement of animals unvaccinated against rabies into the UK.
- promoting public awareness of ways to limit communicable diseases (see Figure 13.2).

Vaccinations

Vaccinations fall into the category of primary prevention as they aim to prevent the onset of infectious disease that can have serious consequences. Vaccination programmes aim to give lasting active immunity against infection and in the UK there are comprehensive vaccination programmes for the following:

- diphtheria, tetanus, pertussis, polio, Hib, (DTap/IPV/Hib), given at two, three and four months;
- measles, mumps, rubella (MMR) given at 12–15 months;

- seasonal influenza recommended for at-risk groups and those aged over 65 years;
- pneumoccocal infection recommended for at-risk groups and those aged over 65 years.

These vaccination programmes have significantly reduced mortality and morbidity. An immunization programme may be:

- *Selective*: protecting those at highest risk, e.g. BCG for infants in high-risk areas for TB.
- *Universal*: eradicating, eliminating or containing disease, e.g. mass infant immunization for childhood diseases.

Herd immunity is the term given to the resistance of groups of people to infection and is dependent upon the percentage of the population that have been vaccinated. To be effective, herd immunity does not necessarily require 100% of the population to be vaccinated because susceptible people in the population will be shielded from exposure to infected people by immune people in the group. In order to obtain herd immunity for measles, the percentage of the population that require vaccination is 90%.

Activity 13.3

What factors might be associated with low vaccine uptake?

- Health service factors, e.g. poor co-ordination and inaccurate record-keeping or parental attitudes.
- Attitudes to the disease: parents' lack of experience of past common diseases, such as measles, lessens their fears of the disease itself.
- Attitudes to the vaccine: media scares about vaccine safety have resulted in a sub-optimal uptake in some populations.
- Health professionals: health professionals tend to emphasize the benefits of vaccination though parents will be exposed to media scares. Communicating about risk is a key public health competence. The aim is for parents to be able to make an informed decision which is based on knowledge about the risks of the disease, the benefits and risks of vaccinating and the risks of not vaccinating.

Measles is a potentially fatal but entirely preventable disease. In 2012, the total number of confirmed measles cases in England and Wales was 2030, the highest number recorded since 1996. This rise in measles cases can be mostly attributed to the proportion of unprotected 10–16-year-olds who missed out on vaccination in the late 1990s and early 2000s when concern around the discredited link between autism and the vaccine was widespread. At this time measles had been eliminated in the UK, but coverage fell nationally to less than 80% in 2005, with even lower uptake in some parts of the country. After many years of low vaccination uptake, measles became re-established in 2007.

Evidence 13.3

Media publicity and vaccine uptake

Discussion

In November 2012, an outbreak of 700 cases of measles commenced in Wales, at that time 45% of children in the Swansea area had not been vaccinated. A detailed analysis of media coverage of MMR since Dr Wakefield's invalid claims of the link between MMR and autism has shown a clear link with a drop in vaccine coverage (Boyce 2007). In South Wales, adverse publicity in the South Wales Evening Post (SWEP) started in July 1997 and developed into the "MMR Parents' Fight for Facts" campaign. During the period July to September 1997, the newspaper published five front-page main headline articles, three opinions, and at least 18 other articles on the MMR vaccine. Subsequently at least six further front-page main headlines, six opinions, and 22 other articles have been published. A detailed local analysis (Mason and Donnelly, 2000) demonstrates that while a drop-off in uptake of the MMR vaccine occurred in the whole of Wales, there was a statistically significant greater decline in the distribution area of the SWEP.

The following groups are also at risk of low uptake of immunization (DH, 2005):

- children in care;
- young people who missed previous immunizations;
- children with physical or learning difficulties;
- children of lone parents;
- children not registered with a general practitioner (GP);
- children in larger families;
- children who are hospitalized;
- minority ethnic groups;
- vulnerable adults such as asylum seekers and the homeless.

Activity 13.4

Patient advocacy is concerned with providing active support for the patient and most nurses will have been taught that advocacy is a central tenet of nursing. But what happens when the patient's wishes are in conflict with recommended good practice and the behaviour of one individual impacts upon the remainder of the population?

- What do these tensions mean for your practice as a nurse?
- What should you do in these situations?
- Should you use persuasive communication to get patients to follow recommended practice, e.g. should health visitors persuade a new parent to have their infant vaccinated?

Discussion

There is a philosophical tension between doing good for the population, e.g. promoting a screening test or vaccination and acting in a paternalistic manner. At one level, advocacy relates to the concept of informed consent in which the health professional provides information for the individual for them to make a decision. There are inherent power imbalances in the patient/nurse relationship and one way that nurses can use this power is by persuasion (Cribb and Duncan, 2002). Therefore advocacy can be seen as a refined manipulative strategy that ensures that the patient complies with health care requests.

Screening

Screening is used to select people at higher risk of developing a disease and offer an appropriate intervention: primary or secondary.

- Primary prevention: preventing development of disease, e.g., screening for high cholesterol levels.
- Secondary prevention: preventing serious outcomes of existing disease, e.g., breast cancer screening.

It is also used for other purposes:

- Selection of people for a particular job, e.g. health checks for army recruits.
- Containment of infection, e.g., screening new staff for TB, or food handlers for salmonella.

Population screening programmes should contribute to the reduction of disease and disability by identifying those at an early stage of disease progression when treatment is beneficial. Understandably many people will only seek medical advice with the onset of signs and symptoms. Screening aims to identify those individuals who have developed disease pathology before the onset of obvious symptoms.

Screening has been defined as

> *a public health service in which members of a defined population, who do not necessarily perceive they are at risk of, or are already affected by a disease or its complications, are asked a question or offered a test, to identify those individuals who are more likely to be helped than harmed by further tests or treatment to reduce the risk of a disease or its complications.*

(www.screening.nhs.uk)

There are various approaches to population screening: selective, mass, anonymous, routine, genetic testing, or opportunistic.

Selective screening

This is when screening is restricted to identifiable groups identified by behaviour or risk, e.g. hepatitis C screening of intravenous drug users (IVDU). The aim of selective screening is to identify a specific disease or predisposing condition in those with a known risk factor.

Mass screening

This is when everyone is invited, regardless of risk, to attend for testing in a systematic programme which covers the whole population over a defined period of time, e.g. cervical screening. The aim is to test large numbers of people for a predisposing condition without specific regard to their individual risk factors for having or developing a condition or disease.

Anonymous screening

This is when screening is carried out without the individual's knowledge in order to establish the prevalence of a disease or condition in a given population. For example, the Anonymous Prevalence Monitoring Programme (UAPMP) that commenced in 1990 aims to measure the distribution of unrecognized (undiagnosed) infection and associated risk factors for HIV, hepatitis B and hepatitis C.

Routine screening

This is when screening is carried out as pre- and postnatal tests and throughout childhood. For example, pre-natal screening can be used to assess risk and assist in informed decision regarding the continuation of the pregnancy and to help prepare psychologically for any physical and mental limitations that the infant may have.

Genetic testing

This is when screening is carried out to identify individuals at risk of an inheritable condition. Although not strictly speaking population-based screening, genetic screening does have major implications for some groups, such as Ashkenazi Jews among whom 1 in 25 carries Tay-Sachs, a genetic disease that develops progressive neurodegeneration (Kirk, 2005).

Opportunistic screening

Screening can also be opportunistic by offering a screening test for an unsuspected disorder at a time when a person presents to the doctor for another reason. Opportunistic screening can be used as a strategy to maximize participation rates in mass and selective screening programmes. All nurses, having made an assessment of need, have the opportunity to ask patients if they have participated in a relevant screening programme and if not, explore their concerns regarding the test.

Table 13.1 Current national screening programmes.

Name of screening test	Population	Type of screening
Mammography	Women aged 50–70 years	Mass
Cervical screening	Women aged 20–64 years	Mass
Hepatitis B	Selective Health Care Workers (HCW) Men that have sex with men IVDUs (intravenous drug users) Sexual contacts of those with infectious hepatitis B virus (HBV)	Selective
Antenatal HIV	All pregnant women	Mass
Bowel cancer	All men and women aged 60–69 years	Selective
Chlamydia	Men and women aged under 25 years	Selective
Diabetic retinopathy	Diabetics	Selective
Abdominal aortic aneurysm	Men aged 65 yrs and over	Selective
Antenatal and newborn screening programmes, e.g. foetal anomaly, HIV, syphilis and hepatitis B, sickle cell and thalassaemia, newborn and infant physical exam, newborn hearing	Antenatal and newborn	

The UK has several national screening programmes and the UK National Screening Committee regularly reviews whether evidence supports the introduction of new screening, including aortic aneurysms, osteoporosis, cardiomyopathy, ovarian cancer and syphilis. Table 13.1 shows the current national screening programmes and Figure 13.3 shows the range of tests carried out during pregnancy and for the newborn.

A screening test in itself does not reduce the risk or prevent ill health. Screening tests look for signs of possible problems and help identify individuals who have an increased risk of having or developing a health-related problem. Not all screening tests are diagnostic, for example, a nuchal translucency scan, taken between 11 and 13 weeks of pregnancy, measures the risk that the baby has Down's syndrome. The diagnostic test offered to confirm the presence of Down's syndrome is called chorionic villus sampling.

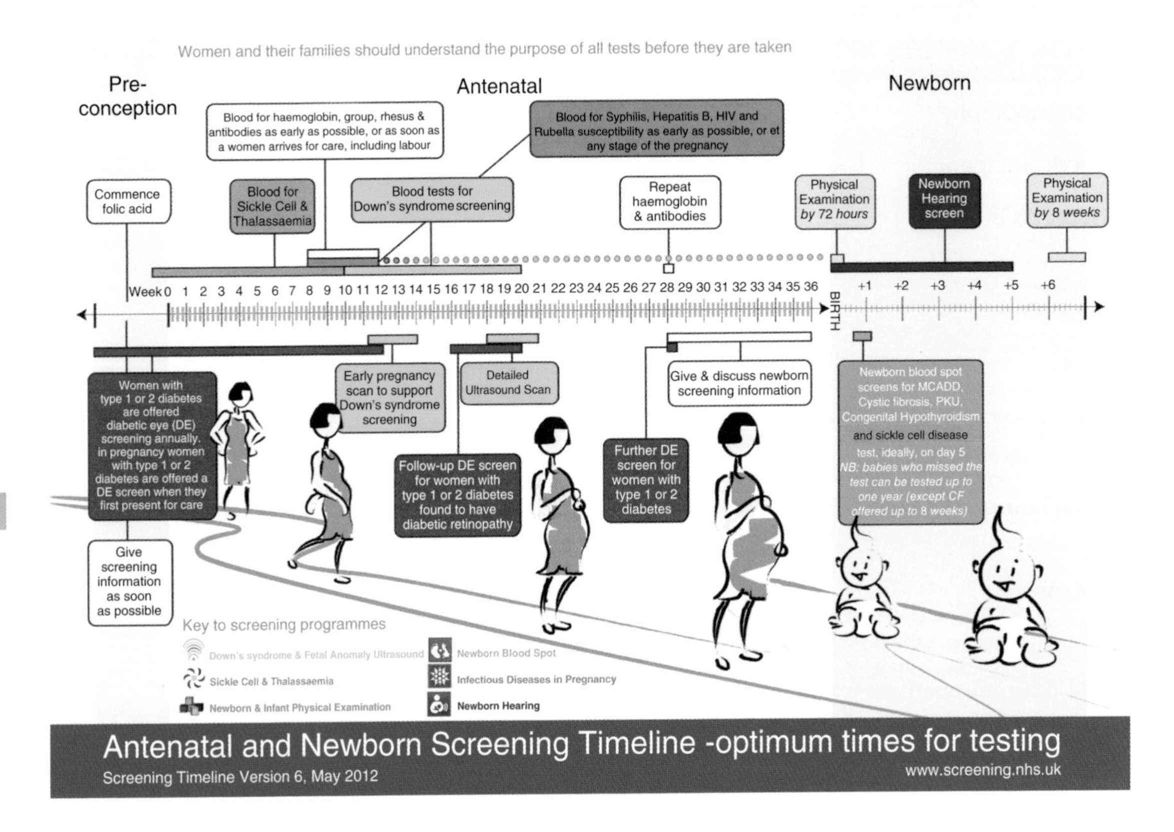

Figure 13.3 Screening timeline for pregnancy and birth. Source: UK National Screening Committee/NHS Screening Programmes, 2012. This information was originally developed by the UK National Screening Committee/NHS Screening Programmes (www.screening.nhs.uk) and is used under the Open Government Licence.

Any screening test with the intention of screening a population needs to be evaluated for efficacy as part of a screening programme. To appraise the viability, effectiveness and appropriateness of a screening programme, the condition, the test, the treatment and the screening programme all need to be scrutinized. The UK National Screening Committee (2000) has adapted Wilson and Junger's classic criteria for evaluation and includes the following:

The condition

- The condition should be an important health problem.
- All cost-effective primary prevention interventions should be implemented as far as practical.
- The epidemiology and natural history of the condition need to be understood with a detectable risk factor or disease marker and a latent period or early symptomatic stage.

The test

- The test should be acceptable to the population.
- There should be an agreed policy on the further diagnostic investigation of individuals with a positive test result and on the choices available to those individuals.
- There should be a simple, safe, precise and validated screening test. The two measures that describe the validity of a screening test include sensitivity and specificity:
    - *sensitivity* is the proportion of people who have the disease and have a positive result. A test that is very sensitive will give a high proportion of false positives.
    - *specificity* is the proportion of people who are free from the disease and have a negative result. A test that is very specific will give a high proportion of false negatives.

The treatment

- There should be agreed evidence-based policies covering which individuals should be offered treatment and the appropriate treatment to be offered.
- There should be effective treatment or intervention for patients identified through early detection, with evidence of early treatment leading to better outcomes than late treatment.

The screening programme

- There is evidence from randomized controlled trials that the screening programme reduces mortality and morbidity. For screening programmes that aim to give informed choice, there must be evidence that the test accurately measures risk.
- The screening programme is clinically, socially and ethically acceptable to the public and health professionals.
- The benefit from the screening programme should outweigh the physical and psychological harm.
- The screening programme needs to offer value for money.

Activity 13.5

If you were to apply Wilson and Junger's classic criteria, would you recommend a national screening programme for the following?:

- asthma
- depression.

Discussion

Asthma would not be recommended for a national screening programme as there is not a phase in which early detection would lead to a better outcome with treatment. Additionally, once

(Continued)

symptoms are apparent, asthma can be readily diagnosed on clinical examination and be adequately managed.

Depression would not be recommended as there is no validated test or assessment for depression at a population level and there is no reliable demarcation of depression from social and situational unhappiness (Summerfield, 2006). Current guidelines (NICE, 2009) do not recommend anti-depressants as the primary intervention for mild/moderate depression which account for the majority of cases. Furthermore, it is most likely that a national screening programme would not be socially acceptable.

Despite rigorous criteria, screening is not foolproof. False positive results can give rise to unnecessary and painful investigations such as biopsies, increase psychological morbidity with needless anxiety, and deter future programme participation. False negative results will give false reassurance of being disease-free and if symptoms do develop, may deter individuals from seeking medical advice. Additionally national screening programmes are more effective at detecting slow-growing cancers as opposed to the more aggressive types of cancer that can progress rapidly in between screening tests.

Activity 13.6

What knowledge does the nurse need to have in order to understand the concepts of sensitivity and specificity and how can this information be best conveyed to the patient concerned?

Discussion

- *The best way to convey this information is as part of a pre-test discussion in order to obtain informed consent. Within this pre-test discussion an explanation of the possible result should be given, be it negative, positive, seen, not seen or inconclusive. The nurse also needs to know how to interpret the result and the likelihood of the result being true. For example, a woman recalled for a repeat cervical cytology may be concerned that she has invasive carcinoma, when in fact her result indicates mild dysplasia (CIN1) which in all probability will resolve without intervention.*
- *The nurse needs to understand whether the screening test is diagnostic or not, and will need to make an assessment of the woman's understanding. For example, mammographies do not give a diagnosis and are very sensitive; this results in a high number of false positives that require invasive investigation for an accurate diagnosis to be made.*
- *The nurse needs to be able to make a judgement as to how and to what extent to best communicate this information.*
- *The nurse needs to know the recommended procedure for establishing a definitive diagnosis.*

Population screening programmes require a high level of participation for three reasons:

1. to be cost effective;
2. to ensure adequate evaluation;
3. to reduce levels of morbidity and mortality.

It is important to consider those populations and groups of people who are less likely to participate in population screening programmes and what measures can be taken to rectify the situation. For example, those not registered with a GP such as travellers, those from a lower socio-economic group, those who are deaf and those with an intellectual impairment are less likely to participate. It is also significant that individuals from the highest risk groups have the highest non-participation rates. For example, those women who are at more risk of developing cervical cancer are those less likely to attend to be screened. The poor response of high risk groups severely compromises the effectiveness of any screening programme.

Surveillance, prevention and control of communicable and non-communicable diseases

The Health Protection Agency (HPA) was established in April 2005 with three separate centres that are responsible for the protection of the public health of the UK:

- the Centre for Infections;
- the Centre for Radiation, Chemical and Environmental Hazards;
- the Centre for Emergency Preparedness and Response.

The HPA Centre for Infections is responsible for the surveillance of infectious diseases, providing specialist microbiology reference services, detailed epidemiological information and coordinating investigations into epidemics and outbreaks of infections. It is now part of Public Health England (www.hpa.org.uk).

The surveillance of a communicable disease is a fundamental activity required for an effective disease prevention and control programme. Surveillance is used for the following reasons:

- to estimate the size of a health problem;
- to detect outbreaks of an infectious disease;
- to characterize disease trends;
- to evaluate interventions and prevention programmes;
- to assist with health planning;
- to identify research needs.

In the UK, a network of Public Health Observatories (PHOs) exist which are now part of Public Health England (www.apho.org.uk). Each regional PHO monitors health and disease trends and works in partnership with local statutory and non-statutory agencies in addressing health inequalities.

The revised International Health Regulations (IHR) and the World Health Organization (WHO) focus on surveillance and management of conditions of global public health concern. There are two important surveillance networks:

1. the Global Public Health Intelligence Network – a computer application that continuously scans the internet for reports of suspicious disease events.
2. the Global Outbreak Alert and Response Network – an operational system for keeping evolving infectious disease threats under close surveillance and facilitating the rapid containment of outbreaks.

Surveillance may be compromised by limited monitoring capacity which may be due to war, natural disaster or poorly funded observational systems. Reporting a disease outbreak may reduce economic viability by impacting on trade, tourism and travel, e.g. in 2003 China delayed reporting the severe acute respiratory syndrome (SARS) outbreak.

Case study 13.1

Seasonal and pandemic influenza surveillance

There are two main types of influenza that cause infection: influenza A and influenza B. Influenza A usually causes a more severe illness than influenza B. Avian influenza (AI), commonly called bird flu, is an infectious viral disease of birds. Most avian influenza viruses do not infect humans; however, some, such as AI/H5N1, have caused serious infections in people. Each year we need a new influenza vaccine to combat the seasonal influenza outbreak as Type A changes its surface antigens in order to produce a different strain of influenza. These minor changes are called *antigenic drift*. A pandemic can occur when there is a major change in surface antigens, resulting in a new influenza strain; this is known as *antigenic shift*. An influenza pandemic can occur at any time of year, may affect all ages and has far higher rates of morbidity and mortality than ordinary seasonal influenza.

Influenza surveillance is a global, European and national activity which entails monitoring the incidence, distribution and genetic changes of influenza. The agencies involved include the WHO National Influenza Centre and the European Reference Laboratory Network for Human Influenza, coordinated by the European Centre for Disease Prevention and Control. Public Health England (PHE) is part of a network that monitors circulating influenza strains in the UK. PHE aims to identify new subtypes of influenza with pandemic potential by collecting health information from GPs on flu-like illness and laboratory reports which are generated from swabs taken from the nose and throat. PHE produces a Weekly National Influenza Report.

Table 13.2 Protection from non-communicable disease: examples of practice.

Surveillance monitoring	Antibiotic resistance to identify emerging strains of antibiotic resistance
	Prescribing habits of GPs in order to ascertain patterns of prescribing drugs
	Long-term conditions in diabetics so that they can be detected and managed at an early stage
Health protection	Fluoridation of water to revent dental decay
	Prohibition of smoking in public places
	Food fortification: there is mandatory fortification of white flour with calcium, iron, vitamins B1 – thiamin and B3 – niacin B1, B2, and margarines with vitamins A and D. Folic acid may be included.
Clinical practice	Folic acid in pregnancy to prevent neural tube defects
	Post-exposure prophylaxis for HIV following sexual exposure to HIV
	Statins for those with increased cholesterol levels or other major risk factors for cardiac disease

In recognition of the changing pattern of disease, measures are also in place to protect populations from non-communicable disease. Table 13.2 gives some examples of how populations can be protected from non-communicable diseases.

The role of the nurse in health protection

A key aspect of the nurse's role in relation to protecting the public is the ability to communicate about risk at an individual and population level. It is necessary to make an assessment of the risk understanding of patients as part of shared decision-making and in order to obtain informed consent. This is because communicating about risk involves making choices, e.g., "Should I have this screening test for cancer?" or "Should I have my child vaccinated?" The manner in which the nurse communicates risk affects the patient's perception of risk.

In order to make an assessment of risk the nurse needs to do the following:

- elicit beliefs;
- understand misperceptions;
- add missing information;
- correct misinformation;
- strengthen correct beliefs;
- de-emphasize unimportant beliefs;
- praise risk perception;
- evaluate their communication.

When discussing risk with either groups or individuals, the focus of the risk communication needs to be clearly defined. For example when informing about sexual health risk, what is the focus?:

- lifestyle risk;
- risk of death;
- risk of acquiring HIV with one episode of unprotected sexual intercourse;
- lifetime risk of, e.g. developing ovarian cancer.

Activity 13.7

- Which is the bigger risk – a 1 in 35 or 1 in 400 chance of developing a disease?
- Which choice is more acceptable from the following estimated probabilities? You have 90 out of 100 chance of dying or 10 out of 100 chance of being cured.

Discussion

Barriers to risk communication occur when there is an ambiguity of risk terms such as "common" and "very rare". Such terms are likely to reflect the speaker's perception rather than being accurate assessments (Paling, 2003). Many people will think that 1 in 400 has a higher probability possibly due to the larger denominator. When giving a probability outcome for different choices you should use the same denominator to lessen confusion. The second question on estimated probability is framed to give the same information positively and negatively, however, the 10 out of 100 probability will be psychologically more acceptable. When seeking informed consent, the nurse should frame probabilities both positively and negatively.

Screening and vaccination are vital public health initiatives and the nurse can support them by doing the following:

- Making time to discuss vaccination and answer questions.
- Being well-informed, confident, empathetic, open and honest, communicating existing knowledge.
- Offering a flexible and accessible service to maximize uptake.
- Recognizing the factors affecting an individual's decision-making and exploring any specific concerns.
- Ensure up-to-date immunization education material is available in places where parents can access them, e.g. playgroups, community centres, schools, etc.
- Identify any groups within the community who are not accessing immunization and work with community leaders to develop strategies to promote immunization within these groups, perhaps offering outreach clinics and opportunistically vaccinating individuals even if they are over the recommended age.

On placement: checklist

- ❑ When immunization or screening are offered, is time taken to explore an individual's concerns?
- ❑ Are written materials available as sources of information?
- ❑ Did you observe good hand hygiene? Did you practise good hand hygiene?

Key learning points

1. Nurses are able to contribute to the lifespan approach to health protection by supporting vaccination and screening.
2. Known health hazards and threats are identified.
3. The mandatory duty of every nurse to maintain high levels of hygiene in person and health care environment is emphasized.

Chapter summary

This chapter has discussed screening and vaccination as part of population initiatives to protect the public's health. The nurse plays a vital role in both by communicating about risk and in promoting their uptake. The importance of being up to date with policy and guidelines has been emphasized. The underpinning principle is that in order to protect the health of populations, individual choice may be eroded and this poses an ethical dilemma for the nurse in practice.

Further reading and resources

The website of the Health Protection Agency contains information about disease trends and health protection interventions: available at: http://www.hpa.org.uk.

Guidance on up-to-date screening is available at: http://cpd.screening.nhs.uk/choicestoolbox/resources/NSCP_link_1.html.

The evidence library of the National Institute of Health and Clinical Excellence (NICE) has a section on the headlines that highlights the most recent media headlines to do with health and should provide up-to-date, clear and evidence-based information on the subject matter. Available at: http://www.library.nhs.uk/rss/newsAndRssArchive.aspx?storyCategory=1.

Department of Health immunization advice is available at: www.immunisation.nhs.uk and at https://www.gov.uk/government/organisations/public-health-england/series/immunisation.

Public Health guidance 21 (2009) *Reducing Differences in the Uptake of Immunisations*. NICE, London. Available online at http://guidance.nice.org.uk/PH21.

NICE (2012) *Infection: Prevention and Control of Healthcare-Associated Infections in Primary and Community Care*, NICE, London. Available at: http://publications.nice.org.uk/infection-cg139.

RCN (2012) *Essential Practice for Infection Prevention and Control: Guidance for Nursing Staff*. RCN, London.

References

Boyce T. (2007) *Health, Risk and the News*. Peter Lang, London.
Cribb, A. and Duncan, P. (2002) *Health Promotion and Professional Ethics*. Blackwell, Oxford.
Department of Health (2005) *Vaccination Services: Reducing Inequalities in Uptake*. DH, London.
Erasmus, V., Daha, T.J., Brug, H. *et al*. (2010) A systematic review of studies on compliance with hand hygiene guidelines in hospital care. *Infection Control and Hospital Epidemiology*, **31** (3), 283–294.
Gould, D., Moralejo, D., Drey, N. and Chudleigh, J.H. (2010) Interventions to improve hand hygiene compliance in patient care. *Cochrane Database of Systematic Review 2010* (9). Art. No.: CD005186. DOI: 10.1002/14651858.CD005186.pub3.
Health Protection Agency (2004) *Supplementary Data Tables of the Unlinked Anonymous Prevalence Monitoring Programme: Data to the End of 2003. Surveillance Update 2004*. HPA, London.
Kirk M. (2005) Tailoring genetic information and services to clients' culture, knowledge and language level, *Nursing Standard*, **20**, 2, 52–56.
Mason, B.W. and Donnelly, P.D. (2000) Impact of a local newspaper campaign on the uptake of the measles mumps and rubella vaccine. *J Epidemiol Community Health*, **54**, 473–474.
National Institute for Clinical Excellence (2009) *Depression: The Treatment and Management of Depression in Adults CG 90*. NICE, London. Available at: http://www.nice.org.uk/cg90.
Paling J. (2003) Strategies to help patients understand risks, *British Medical Journal*, **327**, 745–787.
RCN (2012) *Essential Practice for Infection Prevention and Control: Guidance for Nursing Staff*. RCN, London.
Royal Marsden Hospital (2005) *The Royal Marsden Hospital Manual of Clinical Nursing Procedures*. Blackwell, Oxford.
Summerfield D. (2006) Depression: epidemic or pseudo-epidemic? *Journal of the Royal Society of Medicine*, **99**, 1–2.
World Health Organization (2012) *Global Burden of Disease Report 2010*, WHO, Geneva. Available at: http://www.healthmetricsandevaluation.org/gbd/publications/policy-report/global-burden-disease-generating-evidence-guiding-policy.

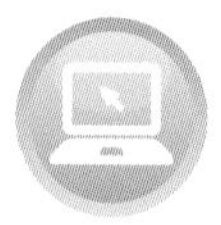

Don't forget to visit the companion website for this book: www.wileyfundamentalseries.com/healthpromotion where you can find self-assessment tests to check your progress.

Part Four

Health Promotion and the Nurse

Introduction

Part four of the book includes chapters from different branches of nursing written by nurse educators. While there is a general recognition that investment in public health and health promotion makes logical sense (prevention being cheaper than cure), health policy is still biased towards the "National Sickness Service" and towards a medical model of avoiding ill health and disease, rather than maintaining and promoting good health and quality of life. These chapters all share a holistic vision of care that moves beyond the signs and symptoms to the social, psychological and environmental factors that influence the patient's health. Health promotion is about challenging the inequalities and discrimination that contribute to the ill health experienced by people with learning disabilities, older people or people with mental health issues.

For most people health promotion is synonymous with health education and the role of the nurse is seen as enabling people to make healthier choices in their lives. This is important at every stage of the lifespan, whether the baby affected in utero by the mother's nutritional status or the older person who can maintain their independence by exercise that improves balance and strength. But health promotion is more than health education. Developing the capacity and confidence of individuals, groups, families and communities (empowering people) to influence and use services and take control over the factors influencing their health, be these informational, behavioural or environmental factors, is at the heart of health promotion work. It is also about community development and community action as resources shift to primary care and families and neighbourhood well-being.

There are few examples of effective health promotion in acute nursing practice (Schickler *et al.*, 2002) and so it is often taken as an add-on activity to a busy and care-oriented job. Despite this, UK national governing bodies such as the Royal College of Nursing and the Nursing and Midwifery Council have encouraged nurses to take a more health-promoting role (NMC, 2010).

Yet as Whitehead (2005) states, for the most part, nursing "*has failed to seize upon their opportunity and at best, only paid lip service to the presented opportunities. Nurses have remained firmly entrenched within the ritualised and traditional functions of limited and limiting health education practices.*" Why is this? Throughout this book we have presented the opportunities that exist for the nurse to promote health and the knowledge, skills and attitudes necessary to do so. No apology is made for rooting these in a biomedical framework since this is how most nurses work. However, the intention of this book is also to encourage a different mind-set with a much broader agenda that acknowledges the socio-political determinants of health and the necessity of the nurse contributing to the creation of supportive environments within a healthy public policy framework. In summary, there are several themes that run through this book:

- *Health* rather than health care, in particular the social and environmental influences on health and how these need to be addressed to improve health.
- *Social justice* which involves tackling inequalities in health, in particular poverty and social inclusion of individuals, families and communities.
- *Participation* in service development and delivery so patients and users are empowered to take responsibility for their own health.
- *Collaboration and partnership* between professionals, private, public and voluntary sectors and across agencies.
- *Information, research and evidence* to provide a sound base for practice.

References

Nursing and Midwifery Council (2010) *Standards for Pre-Registration Nursing Education*, NMC, London. Available at: http://standards.nmc-uk.org/PublishedDocuments/Standards%20for%20pre-registration%20nursing%20education%2016082010.pdf.

Schickler, P., James, T. and Smith, P. (2002) How do I know it's health promotion? A study of health promotion activities and awareness in student placements, *Learning in Health and Social Care*, **1**, 4, 218–228.

Whitehead, D. (2005) The culture, context and progress of health promotion in nursing. in *Health Promoting Practice: The Contribution of Nurses and Allied Health Professionals* (ed. A. Scriven), Palgrave Macmillan, Basingstoke.

14

Health promotion and people with learning disabilities

Jo Delrée

Senior Lecturer, Learning Disability Nursing, London South Bank University, London, UK

Renée Francis

Senior Lecturer, Learning Disability Nursing, London South Bank University, London, UK

Learning outcomes

By the end of this chapter, you will be able to

1. Define the role of the nurse in promoting the health of people with learning disabilities in general health care and specialist learning disability settings
2. Identify the health needs and inequalities relevant to the learning disabled population
3. Identify a range of barriers to accessing health care for people with learning disabilities
4. Discuss a range of health promotion interventions
5. Reflect on your own practice in promoting the health of people with learning disabilities

Fundamentals of Health Promotion for Nurses, Second Edition. Edited by Jane Wills.

Companion website: www.wileyfundamentalseries.com/healthpromotion

Introduction

This chapter will explore ways in which all nurses can be involved in promoting the health of people with learning disabilities. It will also discuss the health problems that people with learning disabilities commonly face. These conditions can bring people with learning disabilities into contact with a range of health and social care professionals.

The White Paper, *Valuing People: A New Strategy for Learning Disability for the 21st Century* (DH, 2001, p. 14) states that

> *learning disability includes the presence of: a significantly reduced ability to understand new or complex information, to learn new skills (impaired intelligence), with a reduced ability to cope independently (impaired social functioning);which started before adulthood, with a lasting effect on development.*

Learning disability can encompass a range of impairments that could result in someone having multiple disabilities and needing support to have all their care needs met, or mild cognitive impairments that mean that that person can live independently with minimal support. Every person with a learning disability is unique.

The *Valuing People* definition shows that learning disability is not just about someone's intellectual capacity; it is also about how they interact and manage socially. This means that health promotion activities with people with learning disabilities need to consider not only how information is presented but also the person's ability to engage:

- with professionals
- with health services they may need to access.

The nurse needs to think about how to develop a relationship with the individual and how to support them to access other services.

Scenario 14.1

Lorna is a 35-year-old British-born woman of East African descent. She has a mild learning disability. Lorna lives in flat in an inner city with her 3½-year–old son, Samuel. Lorna has no contact with Samuel's father. Lorna and Samuel's flat is quite small. It has a cramped living/dining room that is usually cluttered with Samuel's toys. There is a galley kitchen, a bedroom for Lorna and a box room for Samuel. There are damp patches in the kitchen, bathroom and lounge area since the flat above them had a leak about a year ago.

Lorna is overweight and this has worsened since Samuel was born. In the past year, Lorna has gained 1 stone (about 6.5 kg). In the past three months, Lorna has been experiencing frequent throbbing headaches, and she becomes short of breath when she takes Samuel to nursery three days a week. This scares Lorna so she tends to stay indoors more now. Lorna only has a few clothes that fit her at her current weight. She doesn't see the point of showering or putting on clean clothes when she isn't going out.

(*Continued*)

Scenario 14.1 (*Continued*)

Samuel is generally a happy boy, and Lorna has always tried to make sure that he is clean and tidy. This has seemed harder lately as Lorna struggles to find the energy to get Samuel bathed and dressed. Samuel likes watching his favourite TV shows with Lorna, especially when he has his favourite tea of pizza and chips.

So far, Samuel has been meeting his developmental milestones. He receives a 'Universal Plus' level of service from his health visitor in line with the Healthy Child Programme (DH, 2009a). This means that Samuel's Health Visitor is aware of Lorna's additional needs and is able to offer a rapid response if Lorna needs support (DH, 2011). Samuel is now due his pre-school booster vaccinations and a developmental check. Kulvinder, his Health Visitor, has sent out appointments for this, but Lorna and Samuel have not attended the clinic. They have now missed three appointments, and Kulvinder is concerned. She decides to visit Lorna and Samuel at their flat.

How could you work with Lorna to improve her and Samuel's health and well-being?

Discussion

Lorna needs support to access health appointments. This will benefit both Lorna and Samuel. Lorna's weight has been increasing, and this is affecting her bathing and possibly her blood pressure. Her increasing isolation and lack of attention to her personal hygiene could indicate the onset of depression. Lorna needs a full, holistic health assessment to help to prioritize the interventions she needs.

Activity 14.1

Think about your experiences as a patient

- Was there ever a time when you didn't understand what you were being told?
- Were you ever frightened by what you were being told or by the treatment you were receiving?
- Did you ever dislike the way that you were treated?
- What, if anything, did you do about it?
- What would have helped you in that situation?
- Now imagine how someone with a learning disability might feel in that situation. Consider whether the things that you identified as helpful might also be supportive for someone with a learning disability.

Discussion

Being in hospital can be frightening for anyone, especially if you do not understand what is happening. Like any of us, people with learning disabilities want hospital staff to take time to explain what is happening.It is also important to give people time to express their needs and feelings.

The role of the nurse in promoting the health of people with learning disabilities

In the past, people with learning disabilities lived segregated lives. Often they lived in large institutions, sometimes referred to as hospitals, which were staffed by specialist nurses. Although this was done with the best of intentions, current thinking understands that this is not the right place for people with learning disabilities (Race, 1995).

Most people with learning disabilities are no longer segregated but live in ordinary houses, on ordinary streets with a varied amount of support and in different environments depending on their needs. Staff who provide this support are often not nurses, but are social care workers with little or no training in health issues.

This has led to changes in the way that people with learning disabilities access and receive health care. Where once a General Practitioner would be employed to work within the learning disability hospital, now people with learning disabilities access the same GPs as the rest of the population. This applies across the spectrum of health services. *Valuing People* (DH, 2001) states that people with learning disabilities should be able to access the full range of ordinary health services to meet their general health needs. They should also have access to specialist health services if they have any health needs related to their specific disability or condition.

Activity 14.2

Consider the example of Lorna described in Scenario 14.1. Who would care for Lorna if she:

- Had a persistent cough?
- Fractured her arm?

Discussion

The care of people with learning disabilities is a concern for all nurses. Lorna would access her GP or Accident and Emergency in these situations.

Evidence from different reports suggests that many health professionals in mainstream health services do not understand or do not prioritize their responsibilities towards people with learning disabilities:

- Mencap's report (2007) *Death by Indifference* detailed tragic instances where people with learning disabilities had needlessly died as a result of professionals in mainstream service failing to meet their general health needs.
- *Healthcare for All* (Michael, 2008) found compelling evidence that people with learning disabilities have greater need for health care than other people, yet have worse access to health care and poorer health outcomes. It lays out clear responsibilities that must be fulfilled by all areas of the health service to meet the needs of people with learning disabilities.
- Despite this, *Valuing People Now* (DH, 2009b), an update on the 2001 White Paper, *Valuing People*, reported that access to the NHS is often poor for people with learning disabilities. Health services were found to undermine personalization, dignity and safety. It reiterates the need for the NHS to achieve full inclusion of people with learning disabilities in mainstream health services to reduce health inequalities.
- Mencap's latest report (2012) suggests that, in spite of these recommendations and requirements, little has changed in the intervening years.

In light of these failures, it is very important for nurses, whatever their field and wherever they are employed, to be equipped to work with people with learning disabilities. The NMC (2008) states that all nurses have a professional responsibility to do the following:

- Make the care of individuals their first concern, treating them as individuals and respecting their dignity.
- To work with others to protect and promote the health and well-being of those in their care.

This applies equally to any person with or without a learning disability who should happen to need care or support.

So it becomes clear that nurses in the Adult, Child and Mental Health fields must have an understanding of the needs of people with learning disabilities and are required to meet the health needs of this group in their practice.

Activity 14.3

In a specialist area it may be difficult to address the wider health issues with which a person with learning disabilities may present. How could you address this in your practice? What resources could you access?

Discussion

Many Trusts now employ Learning Disability Liaison Nurses or identify specific members of staff to be Learning Disability Champions. Community Learning Disability Teams can also provide guidance, information and often training on the health care needs of people with learning disabilities.

As well as having general health needs, shared with the general population and met by mainstream services, individuals with learning disabilities may also have more specific health needs which require specialist intervention noted in the government reports and White Papers (DH, 2001, 2009b, Michael, 2008).

The learning disability population is growing partly due to the following reasons:

- increased survival rates of pre-term babies;
- increasing rates of various conditions such as Foetal Alcohol Spectrum Disorders, Attention Deficit Hyperactivity Disorder and Autism;
- the increasing longevity of people with learning disabilities (Emerson and Hatton, 2008; RCN, 2011a).

It also means that people with learning disabilities have increasingly complex health needs, which mainstream services may not be able to meet without the support of a specialist learning disability nurse or service (RCN, 2011a, 2011b).

Activity 14.4

A middle-aged woman with a learning disability, who does not use speech to communicate, has been unwell for some time. Her support staff, who are not trained in health issues, know that something is not right, but do not know what that something is. They have accompanied her to the GP, but the GP is unable to communicate with the woman and so cannot make any diagnosis. Meanwhile the woman is increasingly unwell. What might be the role of the specialist learning disability nurse?

Discussion

- *The involvement of learning disability nurses has been shown to improve the health and well-being of people with learning disabilities, and to safeguard their rights, including the right to the best health they can achieve. (RCN,2011a; Scottish Government, 2012).*
- *Specialist communication skills combined with a background in health would enable a thorough health assessment, and so provide the GP with the information needed to attempt a diagnosis.*
- *Work holistically with the individual and her support staff, educating them in how to support this person in terms of her health and communication needs, and developing a person-centred plan of care.*
- *Recognize the need for referral to a specific service and facilitate access to it.*
- *Be a source of expert information to health care colleagues regarding issues such as consent to treatment, communication and understanding and working with any distressed and challenging behaviours.*

Priorities in health promotion and disease prevention

People with learning disabilities have many health issues in common with the general population. However, there are some important differences. These, and their causes, should be considered before entering into any health promotion work.

Causes of differences in health status for people with learning disabilities

Socio-economic factors

- Restricted access to education, good quality housing, employment and healthcare.
- Limited social networks and community involvement.
- Poverty.

Individual lifestyle factors

- Poor diet.
- Lack of exercise.
- Substance use.
- Possible high risk sexual behaviours.

Cultural factors

- Increased discrimination in all areas of life including access to health services, as shown in the reports mentioned previously.
- Exposure to abuse and crimes committed against them.
- Low uptake of health promotion or screening activities.
- Health risks and conditions associated with specific syndromes.

Activity 14.5

- Which of the above factors apply to Lorna described in Scenario 14.1
- How would these affect any decisions you make regarding working with her to promote and maintain her health?

Discussion

We know that Lorna's housing situation is poor, particularly in relation to the size of her flat and the problem with damp. Staying in her flat more often has led to her becoming more isolated and less physically active. She is finding it hard to access health appointments for herself and Samuel. It is important to work with Lorna holistically, including recognizing her cultural needs as a British woman of East African descent.

General health and life expectancy

On the whole, both adults and children with learning disabilities have poorer health than the rest of the population (Emerson *et al.*, 2012). Additionally, health screening activities targeted at this group reveal high levels of unmet physical and mental health needs (Robertson *et al.*, 2010). People with learning disabilities have a shorter life expectancy, though this is changing. This is in part due to life-limiting conditions associated with learning disability. However, the recent inquiry into premature deaths in people with learning disabilities found that the most common reasons for premature death were:

- delays or problems with diagnosis and treatment;
- problems in identifying needs and providing appropriate care to meet changing needs (Heslop *et al.*, 2013).

Cancer

People with learning disabilities die less from cancer than the rest of the population, though this seems to be changing with increased longevity and lifestyle choices which may increase cancer risk (Cancer Care Research Centre, 2008). Exceptions to this general rule are leukaemia, which is more common in children with Down's syndrome and gastro-intestinal cancer. People with learning disabilities are approximately twice as likely to die from gastro-intestinal cancer when compared with the general population. This is in part due to the high prevalence of Helicobacter Pylori in people with learning disabilities. Helicobacter Pylori is a bacterium which can live in the stomach, and it increases the risk of developing stomach cancer, gastric ulcers and oesophageal cancer (Gates and Barr, 2009).

Activity 14.6

What health promotion opportunities about cancer are there for people with learning disabilities?

Discussion

- *Primary prevention: educating people about the lifestyle factors related to gastro-intestinal cancers.*
- *Secondary health promotion: offering screening earlier than in the general population to this group, and generally being aware of the increased possibility of these cancers in order to spot early signs and limit disease progression. There is low uptake of cancer screening among people with learning disabilities, however, when screening programmes are targeted at this group, uptake can be higher than in the general population.*
- *Tertiary health promotion: individualized support to maintain well-being while living with disease, and preventing complications. Evidence suggests that these activities are not always carried out in practice (McCann and Forbat, 2007). The experience of care for people with learning disabilities who have cancer is also reported to be poorer than for the general*

(Continued)

population, with patients and their carers reporting that they were not consulted regarding their care, their pain was not well managed, and their cancer was not diagnosed in the early stages. It is clear that there is scope for health promotion activity in these areas for adult nurses, children's nurses (in the case of childhood cancers and leukaemia) and mental health nurses should the person experience any mental health problems, reactive depression, for example , as a result of their illness.

Coronary heart disease

This is a leading cause of death for people with learning disabilities, as it is within the general population (Emerson *et al.*, 2012). It is likely to increase alongside the increasing lifespan of people with learning disabilities. As such, the needs of people with learning disabilities should be considered when planning and delivering education and screening programmes in this area. Additionally, approximately half of people with Down's syndrome have a heart defect, and so will require input from cardiovascular specialists to maintain their health.

Being underweight and overweight

People with learning disabilities are more likely to be both underweight and overweight compared with the rest of the population (Beange, 2002). Although some of this is accounted for by specific conditions associated with their learning disability, lifestyle factors have a big role to play. Like many people on a low income, people with learning disabilities often have a poor diet, and they exercise less (Lennox, 2002).

Less than 10% of adults with learning disabilities in supported accommodation eat a balanced diet, with sufficient intake of fruit and vegetables. Carers generally have a poor knowledge about public health recommendations on dietary intake. Over 80% of adults with learning disabilities engage in levels of physical activity below the Department of Health's minimum recommended level, a much lower level of physical activity than the general population (53–64%). People with more severe learning disabilities and people living in more restrictive environments are at increased risk of inactivity.

Therefore, there is a need for education regarding diet and exercise, and for this to be made accessible to people with learning disabilities and their carers. There are many examples of health promotion activities which have aimed to address this issue, and could be rolled out nationally (e.g. Howe and Hancox, 2010; Jinks *et al.*, 2010).

Case study 14.1

Health check

One reason for the poorer health of people with learning disabilities is that they often have difficulty in recognizing illness, communicating their needs and using primary health care services. Since 2009, GPs have received extra money for providing annual health checks. The Cardiff Health Check form followed a tick box format with yes and no answers in response to a series of questions on the individual's health. These covered seven sections:

1. Health Promotion – information on weight, height, blood pressure, urine analysis, body mass index, cholesterol level, immunization status (tetanus, influenza, Hepatitis B) and conduct of cervical screening and mammography.
2. Chronic Illness
3. Systems Enquiry
4. Epilepsy
5. Behaviour
6. Physical Examination
7. Medication

Respiratory disease

Respiratory disease is the leading cause of death for the learning disabled population, with rates three times higher than in the general population (Emerson, *et al.*, 2012). This may be linked to specific conditions linked with learning disability. For instance, a person with cerebral palsy may aspirate food due to oral-motor dysfunction and/or postural problems, which then increases the risk of aspiration pneumonia. In instances such as this, there is a need for education and support to minimize this and therefore reduce health risks.

Asthma is more prevalent among people with learning disabilities and so should be considered by asthma clinics when planning and delivering their services. A particular need for health promotion is highlighted by the fact that people with asthma who also have a learning disability are twice as likely to smoke as their non-asthmatic peers, and women with learning disabilities and asthma are more likely to be obese (Emerson *et al.*, 2012). So colleagues in smoking cessation clinics and dietetics can also be included in promoting the health of people with learning disabilities.

Sensory impairment

People with learning disabilities are between 8 and 200 times more likely to have a visual impairment. Some 40% of people with learning disabilities have a hearing impairment (Emerson *et al.*, 2012). Mainstream services (orthoptics departments, ophthalmologists, opticians, etc.) need to be aware and prepared to meet the needs of this group. Carers of people with learning disabilities frequently fail to identify sensory impairments, so screening for this group is crucial. People with Down's syndrome are at a particularly high risk of hearing and visual impairments, and as such should be considered a target group for screening.

Mental health

People with learning disabilities experience more psychiatric disorders, and experience anxiety and depression at least as much as the general population. People with Down's syndrome are at particular risk of anxiety and depression, as are mothers with learning disabilities (Emerson *et al.*, 2012). Signs and symptoms of mental health problems may be atypical in people with learning disabilities, and often manifest themselves through behavioural change, and distressed and challenging behaviours. Unfortunately, these behaviours are often thought to be because of the person's learning disability rather than because they are experiencing distressing mental health problems, and often go undiagnosed and untreated, or poorly treated.

Good screening programmes are essential, as is collaboration between mental health and learning disability colleagues to ensure adequate support is provided to identify, treat and support those with poor mental health, and to prevent or minimize further mental illness. Mental health promotion for people with learning disability may include:

- accessible information;
- targeted employment support;
- support for people to access leisure activities;
- support around friendships.

Oral health

People with learning disabilities have poorer oral health, with more untreated decay, more missing teeth, and more problems with the alignment of their teeth. People with Down's syndrome seem to be particularly affected by poor oral health (Emerson *et al.*, 2012). Poor oral hygiene increases the risk of chest infection in people who aspirate, due to the increased bacterial growth in saliva that then enters the lungs during aspiration. Recognizing poor oral health as a possible source of pain and hence a reason for distressed behaviour is also crucial.

Examples of health promotion strategies and activities

The previous section highlighted some of the specific health needs of people with learning disabilities. A health promotion approach will be to respect their abilities and seek to empower them to make choices. Health promotion may also be viewed as those activities which seek to protect the health of people with learning disabilities such as screening. This section explores the ways that people with learning disabilities can be encouraged to adopt healthier lifestyles.

Promoting healthy lifestyles

Nurses in all areas have a responsibility to promote healthy lifestyles to people with learning disabilities. This might include advice given within the context of generic health care, or it might involve a specialist intervention by a learning disability nurse, e.g. a practice nurse giving advice on a healthy diet or ways to increase physical activity. The learning disability nurse might work directly with the individual and their carers to identify a plan for putting health promotion advice into action. A learning disability nurse might also put a specialist intervention such as a behaviour modification programme in place, where the individual is rewarded for successfully keeping to the healthy eating plan in a way that is appropriate to the individual.

Activity 14.7

Tackling obesity in people with learning disabilities

People who live in residential or supported living services often rely on paid staff to support them with buying and preparing food. Shoneye (2012) identifies several factors that may influence whether someone with a learning disability eats healthily. These include a lack of staff training in nutrition, a lack of staff cooking skills and limited budgets. She also notes that where someone also needs support with behaviour, staff may use food as a reward for appropriate behaviour.

What could the learning disability nurse do to address client obesity?

Discussion

Learning disability nurses can provide support for staff and service users by working with them to look at the barriers that prevent people from eating healthily. There may be specific chains of behaviour that lead a person to overeat and Shoneye (2012) outlines the experience of Mary who has a new alarm clock. She is having problems setting this, and it hasn't been going off at the right time. When Mary oversleeps, she skips breakfast and gets a chocolate bar and a bottle of milk shake from the shop near her bus stop. Mary gets to work late and gets told off by her boss. She feels cross about this, so on the way home she buys a bag of doughnuts that she eats in front of the telly to cheer herself up. When staff find out about the problems that Mary has been having with her alarm clock, they help her to buy one with a bigger dial that is easier to see when she sets the time for her alarm. The learning disability nurse helps Mary to think of other things that she can do if she is feeling cross, like going for a walk, drawing a picture or reading a magazine.

It is important not to make assumptions about health promotion based on a person's learning disability. It can be easy to assume that someone is, for example, overweight because of an underlying condition such as Down's syndrome. This does not mean that they would not benefit from healthy eating advice or an exercise programme. Similarly, it should not be assumed that a person with a learning disability is not sexually active and thereby exclude them from sexual health advice or cervical screening.

For health promotion activities to be successful, they also need to be sustainable. Codling and Macdonald (2008) note that sustainability can be the missing element in health promotion with people with learning disabilities. Even when people with learning disabilities understand the information they are given about healthy lifestyles, they may not apply this information to their own lives. This does not mean that attempts to change or improve the lifestyles of people with learning disabilities are a waste of time. Previous chapters have shown that health promotion is about making healthy choices easier but the obstacles to healthier choices must be considered. When working with people with learning disabilities, this will necessitate involving all the people who influence lifestyle change.

Increasing access to health services

All health services have a statutory duty under the Equality Act 2010 to make reasonable adjustments to ensure that disabled people can access their services. In this section, we will look at some of the reasonable adjustments that can be made to improve access to assessment and treatment. Sir Jonathan Michael (2008) in his report of the Independent Inquiry into Access to Healthcare for People with Learning Disabilities, identifies several reasonable adjustments that health services need to make that are outlined in Table 14.1.

Empowerment

The Mental Capacity Act 2005 provides a clear framework for involving people in their health care. Where a person has capacity to consent to a treatment decision, no one else can make that decision for them. The assumption under law is that the person has capacity unless this can be proven otherwise. For people who do not have capacity, people who are important to them can come together to decide what is in their best interest. For the purposes of the Act, best interest does not necessarily mean medical best interest.

For people to be able to make decisions about their health, they need to have information in a way they can understand. People may also have information about themselves in an accessible format. This could take the form of a hospital passport, which gives health care staff information about the person, how they communicate, their likes and dislikes, and their ongoing health needs. Additionally, people may carry a patient-held health record which gives details of basic health information, ongoing health conditions, medication and details of health reviews. Once people have routes to communicate, they can develop more sophisticated ways of empowering themselves.

Table 14.1 Tips for working with a person with a learning disability.

Tip	Suggestions for implementation
Give enough time	It can take longer for people with learning disabilities to understand information. Make sure that you have allowed enough time for the person to feel comfortable with you, take in the information, and ask questions.
Create a space to talk without distraction	Clinical and ward areas can be very busy places with different sights, sounds and smells. Taking someone to a quiet area can help them to focus on you and the information you are trying to give. This is especially important with someone who has autism, as people with autism can find it difficult to differentiate between competing stimuli in a busy environment.
Present information in a way that people can understand	This may involve using leaflets with simple language and pictures, or using DVDs, texts or computer apps to help you get your message across.
Involve carers as well as the person with learning disabilities	

Case study 14.2

Health champions

In Oxfordshire, a user-led self-advocacy group called My Life My Choice identified members to become health champions. The health champions worked towards increasing the number of annual health checks conducted with people with learning disabilities in Oxfordshire. They worked with GPs, Primary Care Trusts and the Strategic Health Authority. They provided training for staff in the GP services. They then met with their MP, who also asked questions of the PCT and SHA on their behalf. The champions made presentations, and were able to get the contracts of GP service providers changed to reflect the need to carry out health checks (Turner and Michel, 2012).

Social change

Throughout this book, we have seen that health and well-being are inextricably linked to social and cultural factors as well as personal choices and structural factors as explained by Dahlgren and Whitehead's (1991) model of health promotion (see Chapter 2).

Learning disabilities may be linked to specific health conditions. However, this is not always the case. Many people, particularly those with mild and moderate learning disabilities, have no particular physical condition, and can enjoy good health. But ill health is disproportionately over-represented in people with learning disabilities as a whole and this is due to socio-economic and cultural factors. People with learning disabilities have long been discriminated against, and excluded from mainstream society. Although this is no longer the case on paper, in reality this group continue to be excluded from the mainstream, as is demonstrated by their health status (Emerson *et al.*, 2012), and reports of quite shocking neglect while under the care of health services (Mencap, 2004, 2007, 2012). This discrimination applies not only to health services, but also cultural and social attitudes towards disability are so embedded in social institutions as to restrict the access of disabled people to living conditions that are associated with better health (e.g., better education; wealth; better quality housing; secure and rewarding employment).

On placement: checklist

- ❏ Does the setting adapt information so that it can be understood by people with learning disabilities?
- ❏ Is information available for staff, users and carers about consent to treatment, capacity and best interests?
- ❏ Are wider health needs taken into account when planning care (e.g. following the user's existing eating and drinking guidelines)?
- ❏ Is there clear information about how to make referrals to community or specialist learning disability services?

Key learning points

1. All nurses need to be aware of how to work with a person with a learning disability.
2. People with learning disabilities share many conditions in common with the general population but, in general, have poorer health than their non-disabled peers.
3. Differences in health status are, to an extent, avoidable and result from barriers people with learning disabilities face in accessing timely, appropriate and effective health care.

Chapter summary

Regardless of the branch of nursing, every nurse has a duty of care towards people with learning disabilities should they happen to need services. This chapter has emphasized that because many health care professionals currently do not understand their duty of care, or do not act appropriately, people die unnecessarily (Mencap, 2007, 2012; Michael, 2008). The chapter has also shown that many people with learning disabilities suffer poor health and are not accessing the treatments and supports that they need, and have a poor quality of life as a consequence. It is the duty of the nurse to end that discrimination.

Further reading and resources

Improving Health and Lives (IHAL) is the Learning Disabilities Observatory, a collaboration between the three organizations: Public Health England, the Centre for Disability Research at the University of Lancaster and the National Development Team for Inclusion. Its resources are available at http://www.improvinghealthandlives.org.uk/about.

References

Beange, H. (2002) Epidemiological issues, in *Physical Health of Adults with Intellectual Disabilities* (eds V. Prasher and M. Janicki), Blackwell, Oxford, pp. 1–20.

Cancer Care Research Centre (2008) *People with Cancer and an Intellectual Disability: An International Issue with Local Significance.* Available at: http://www.cancercare.stir.ac.uk/reports/Reports%20published%20before%202010/People%20with%20cancer%20and%20an%20intellectual%20disability%20%282008%29.pdf (accessed 17 May 2013).

Codling, M. and Macdonald, N. (2008) User-friendly information: does it convey what it intends? *Learning Disability Practice*, **11** (1), 12–17.

Dahlgren G. and Whitehead M. (1991) *Policies and Strategies to Promote Social Equity in Health.* Institute for Futures Studies, Stockholm.

DH (Department of Health) (2001) *Valuing People: A New Strategy for Learning Disability for the 21st Century.* Available at: http://www.archive.official-documents.co.uk/document/cm50/5086/5086.pdf (accessed 11 Jan. 2013).

DH (Department of Health) (2009a) *Healthy Child Programme: Pregnancy and the First Five Years of Life.* Available at: http://www.dh.gov.uk/prod_consum_dh/groups/dh_digitalassets/@dh/@en/@ps/documents/digitalasset/dh_118525.pdf (accessed 11 Jan. 2013).

DH (Department of Health) (2009b) *Valuing People Now: A New Three-Year Strategy for People with Learning Disabilities.* Available at: http://webarchive.nationalarchives.gov.uk/+/www.dh.gov.uk/en/Publicationsandstatistics/Publications/PublicationsPolicyandGuidance/DH_093377 (accessed 17 May 2013).

DH (Department of Health) (2011) *Health Visitor Implementation Plan 2011–2015: A Call to Action.* Available at: https://www.wp.dh.gov.uk/publications/files/2012/11/Health-visitor-implementation-plan.pdf (accessed 11 Jan. 2013).

Emerson, E., Baines, H., Allerton, L. and Welch, V. (2012) *Health Inequalities and People with Learning Disabilities in the UK: 2012.* Available at: http://www.improvinghealthandlives.org.uk/publications.php5?rid=1165.

Emerson, E. and Hatton, C. (2008) *Estimating Future Need for Adult Social Care Services for People with Learning Disabilities in England.* Available at: http://eprints.lancs.ac.uk/21049/1/CeDR_2008-6_Estimating_Future_Needs_for_Adult_Social_Care_Services_for_People_with_Learning_Disabilities_in_England.pdf (accessed 17 May 2013).

Gates, B. and Barr, O. (eds) (2009) *Oxford Handbook of Learning and Intellectual Disability Nursing.* Oxford University Press, Oxford.

Great Britain. Equality Act 2010, c.15 Available at: http://www.legislation.gov.uk/ukpga/2010/15/contents (accessed 19 February 2013).

Heslop, P., Blair, P., Fleming, P., *et al.* (2013) *Confidential Inquiry into Premature Deaths of People with Learning Disabilities (CIPOLD): Final Report.* Available at: http://www.bristol.ac.uk/cipold/fullfinalreport.pdf (accessed 17 May 2013).

Howe, P. and Hancox, L. (2010) Fit for life: promoting healthy lifestyles for adults with learning disabilities. *Nursing Times,* **106** (31): 14–15.

Jinks, A., Cotton, A. and Rylance, R. (2010) Obesity interventions for people with a learning disability: an integrative literature review. *Journal of Advanced Nursing,* **67** (3):460–471.

Lennox, N. (2002) Health promotion and disease prevention, in *Physical Health of Adults with Intellectual Disabilities* (eds V. Prasher and M. Janicki),. Blackwell, Oxford, pp. 230–251.

McCann, L.A. and Forbat, L. (2007) *Older People with Learning Disabilities Affected by Cancer: Involvement and Engagement Work to Inform a Research Agenda: Final Report. Centre for the Older Person's Agenda (COPA).* Cancer Care Research Centre, University of Stirling. Available at: http://www.qmu.ac.uk/copa/publications/documents/CancerCareFinal%20Report.pdf.

Mencap (2004) *Treat Me Right.* Available at: http://www.mencap.org.uk/sites/default/files/documents/2008-03/treat_me_right.

Mencap (2007) *Death by Indifference.* Available at: http://www.nmc-uk.org/Documents/Safeguarding/England/1/Death%20by%20Indifference.pdf (accessed 17 May 2013).

Mencap (2012) *Death by Indifference: 74 Deaths and Counting.* Available at: http://www.mencap.org.uk/sites/default/files/documents/Death%20by%20Indifference%20-%2074%20Deaths%20and%20counting.pdf (accessed 17 May 2013).

Michael, J. (2008) *Healthcare for All: The Report of the Independent Inquiry into Access for Healthcare for People with Learning Disabilities.* Available at: http://www.dh.gov.uk/prod_consum_dh/groups/dh_digitalassets/@dh/@en/documents/digitalasset/dh_106126.pdf (accessed 12 February 2013).

Nursing and Midwifery Council (2008) *The Code: Standards of Conduct, Performance and Ethics for Nurses and Midwives.* Available at: http://www.nmc-uk.org/Documents/Standards/The-code-A4-20100406.pdf (accessed 17 May 2013).

Race, D. (1995) Historical development of service provision, in *Services for People with Learning Disabilities* (ed. N. Malin), Routledge, London, pp. 46–78.

Robertson, J., Roberts, H. and Emerson, E. (2010) *Health Checks for People with Learning Disabilities: A Systematic Review of Evidence.* Available at: http://www.improvinghealthandlives.org.uk/uploads/doc/vid_7646_IHAL2010-04HealthChecksSystemticReview.pdf (accessed 17 May 2013).

Royal College of Nursing (2011a) *Learning from the Past: Setting out the Future: Developing Learning Disability Nursing in the United Kingdom.* Available at: http://www.rcn.org.uk/__data/assets/pdf_file/0007/359359/003871.pdf (accessed 17 May 2013).

Royal College of Nursing (2011b) *Meeting the Health Needs of People with Learning Disabilities: RCN Guidance for Nursing Staff.* Available at: http://www.rcn.org.uk/__data/assets/pdf_file/0004/78691/003024.pdf (accessed 17 May 2013).

Scottish Government (2012) *Strengthening the Commitment: The Report of the UK Modernising Learning Disability Nursing Review.* Available at: http://www.scotland.gov.uk/Resource/0039/00391946.pdf (accessed 17 May 2013).

Shoneye, C. (2012) Prevention and treatment of obesity in adults with learning disabilities. *Learning Disability Practice,* **15** (3), 32–36.

Turner, S. and Michel, B. (2012) Making sure service users receive health checks. *Learning Disability Practice,* **15** (5), 16–20.

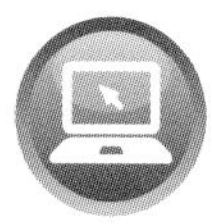

Don't forget to visit the companion website for this book: www.wileyfundamentalseries.com/healthpromotion where you can find self-assessment tests to check your progress.

15

Health promotion and people with mental health issues

Thomas J. Currid

Course Director, Mental Health Nursing, London South Bank University, London, UK

Learning outcomes

By the end of this chapter you will be able to:

1. Discuss the reciprocal relationship between mental, physical and social health
2. Discuss mental health promotion in context to policy, professional frameworks, patients and practice
3. Explain the role of the nurse in health promotion in a range of settings that mental health patients come in contact with
4. Identify and discuss possible health concerns that may be specific to patients with mental illness
5. Discuss a range of health promoting interventions that may be applicable to mental health patients

Introduction

Mental health is an integral part of daily life. Regardless of what we do each day, our emotions, thoughts and behaviours will impact on our general well-being. The current government mental health policy entitled *No Health Without Mental Health: A Cross-Government Mental Health Outcomes Strategy for People of All Ages* (DH, 2011) in part, captures the importance of mental

Fundamentals of Health Promotion for Nurses, Second Edition. Edited by Jane Wills.

Companion website: www.wileyfundamentalseries.com/healthpromotion

health across the lifespan. As the title suggests, without good mental health, it is very unlikely that a person will be physically well, regardless of their age.

Activity 15.1

- Think of a time when you were upset emotionally, a time perhaps when you felt anxious or quite sad. For example, it may have been a time when you were waiting for exam results, a relationship that had finished or even the death of a loved one.
- List the emotions you experienced (these can usually be described with one word, e.g. hopeless, angry) and the behaviours that you engaged in (actions that you took, e.g. isolated yourself).
- Now consider how you felt physically. For example, did you feel less hungry, was your stomach upset?
- Now reflect on when you have cared for someone who was physically unwell. What did you notice about their emotional mental health? Were they less happy, perhaps less talkative or even angry?

Discussion

As you may have identified, the emotions that we experience will impact on our physical well-being and how we feel physically will also impact on our mental health.

Although the terms mental health and mental illness are used interchangeably, it is important from the outset to distinguish between the two terms. In the past, mental health has been described as the absence of mental illness, an ideology which in itself is illness-orientated. This also has a negative connotation and does not focus on positive aspects such as happiness, well-being and personal fulfilment. Westerhof and Keyes (2010) have focused on two traditions of well-being. These are hedonic (psychological) and eudaimonic (social) well-being. Hedonic is characterized by feelings of happiness, satisfaction and interest in life, while eudaimonic relates to fulfilment of one's goals such as autonomy and positive relationships with others. To be mentally healthy requires a combination of both hedonic and eudaimonic experiences. The terms they use to describe these experiences are "flourishing" and "languishing".

- Flourishing is characterized by experiencing positive emotional states as well as positive outcomes (e.g. a sense of belonging).
- Languishing is considered to be a state where low levels of emotional well-being are combined with low social well-being status.

Figure 15.1 illustrates that mental health is a state of flourishing physical and emotional wellness: in which the person experiences positive feelings and thoughts, within and about themselves that enables them to actively participate, integrate and be valued by society.

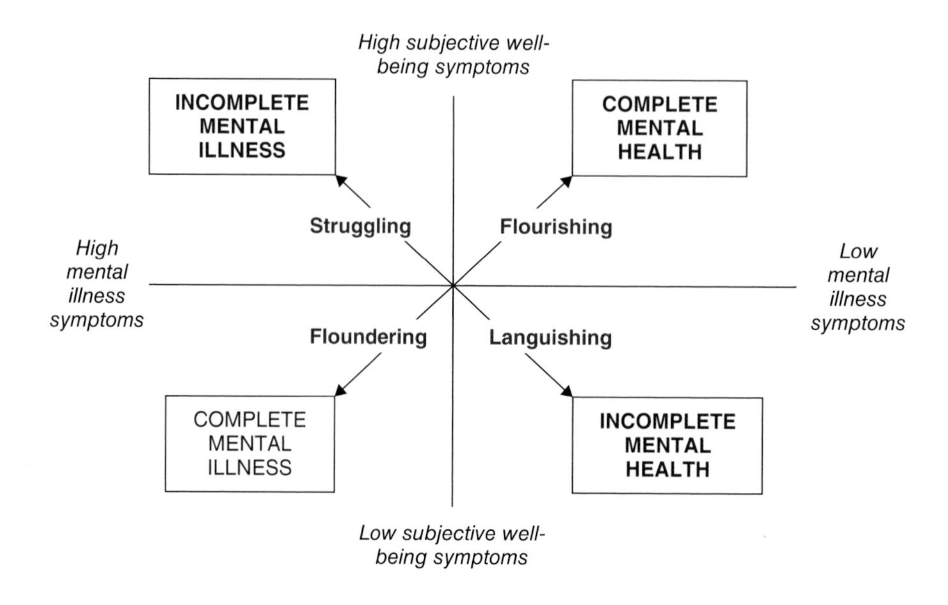

Figure 15.1 Mental well-being. Source: adapted from Keyes, 2002.

Defining mental health promotion

Mental health is as important as physical health, mental health promotion is equally important as physical health promotion. Mental health promotion contributes to and maintains our general health and well-being and is concerned with actions that enhance personal, familial, organizational and societal well-being. Mental health promotion can do the following:

- Significantly improve people`s lives.
- Prevent distress while also preventing mental and physical illness across the lifespan.
- Challenge stereotypes and discrimination against those who have a mental illness,.
- Reduce costs associated with illness and build a stronger, caring and more resilient society.

Mental illness refers to common mental disorders such as depression or anxiety and severe mental illness such as schizophrenia. Yet mental health needs or indeed mental illness are still stigmatized, discriminated against and can be seen as "abnormal". The current mental health strategy *No Health Without Mental Health* (DH, 2011) reiterates that by focusing on mental health promotion and illness prevention, we can increase individual resilience and prevent illness from perpetuating cycles through family generations.

Evidence 15.1

The benefits of mental health promotion

Mental disorder has a range of impacts and is costly to treat. Public mental health can reduce the impact and produce a range of benefits. Knapp *et al.* (2011) offer an economic case for mental health promotion and mental illness prevention, based on an analysis of 15 health promotion interventions ranging from the prevention of childhood conduct disorder to early intervention for psychosis, practical measures to reduce the number of suicides to well-being programmes provided in the workplace. They conclude that the "pay-off" for health promotion activities across the lifespan is "outstandingly good value for money". Other findings include that while interventions make a sound economic case, interventions have a strong evidence base for improving people`s lives, the community, judicial systems and the economy.

The role of mental health nursing and health promotion

While at first glance each nursing speciality may consider health promotion in context to their own area of practice, as identified in other chapters of this book, health is dependent on a range of issues and is interdependent with biological, psychological and social factors. For example, hypertension may have many contributory factors such as genetics, lifestyle and psychological issues. Though predisposing factors such as genetics may increase the likelihood of the person developing hypertension, psychological issues such as stress levels may be the precipitating triggers for the current condition. As one of the key roles of nursing is to strive to improve and promote health, mental health promotion must be inherent in all health promotion activities and should be seen as integral to well-being.

Central to mental health nursing is an understanding of the principles of the Recovery movement that commenced after the introduction of deinstitutionalization when large mental institutions were closed and patients were cared for in the community. Recognizing that many of the services that had been put in place to care for the mentally ill in the community did not meet identified needs, various groups began to challenge services and the underlying philosophies. Through concerted efforts of challenging how the mentally ill were conceptualized, the Recovery movement spread widely across the globe. Within the United Kingdom, Recovery philosophies are the cornerstone of services. Though various definitions of Recovery have been offered, there is no agreed universal definition. However, a much cited definition comes from Anthony (1993) who states that:

> *Recovery is described as a deeply personal, unique process of changing one's attitudes, values, feelings, goals, skills, and/or roles. It is a way of living a satisfying, hopeful, and contributing life even with limitations caused by illness. Recovery involves the development of new meaning and purpose in one's life as one grows beyond the catastrophic effects of mental illness.*

Activity 15.2

How is this definition different from the concept of recovery from a physical illness?

Discussion

This definition includes factors such as:

- *improved physical health;*
- *living a life that instils hope and optimism despite current illness;*
- *taking control of their lives;*
- *enabling and being able to develop, sustain and engage in activities such as employment that will offer greater quality of life. As may be seen from Table 15.1, Recovery mirrors both principles and levels of health promotion (see Chapters 1 and 3).*

Table 15.1 Recovery and health promotion principles.

Health promotion principles	Recovery principles
Empowerment	Recovery practice ensures that the individual is offered choice and control over their own lives.
Participative	Recovery involves working in partnership to ensure that the individual is involved at every step of their care.
Holistic	Recovery sees the individual as much more that the mental illness that they present with, other areas such as physical, social and spiritual health plays a key role in health and well-being.
Equitable	Recovery encourages social justice for people with mental illness and advocates for fair and equitable services and outcomes with those in other areas of health.
Intersectoral	Recovery practice involves ensuring that there is a whole systems approach by many agencies to effect the best services and outcomes.
Sustainable	Recovery includes interventions that takes account of the changing nature of the individual and therefore adopts strategies that are achievable and sustainable in the future.
Multi-strategy	
• Advocate	Recovery-orientated practitioners recognize that health is dependent on a range of factors which include: social participation, inclusion, holism and therefore advocate for these conditions to be made available to the individual.

Table 15.1 (*Continued*)

• Enable	Recovery advocates for the opportunity to have access to fair and equitable resources that will enable the individual to achieve their full potential.
• Mediate	Recovery models of practice recognize that to make Recovery a reality, services must come together and work collaboratively to ensure that they contribute services that may fall outside the remit of health services but are crucial in determining health. These include education, housing, statutory benefits, industry and media.

People with mental illness who are in recovery are those who are actively engaged in working away from the states in Figure 15.1 of Floundering (through perhaps building relationships) and Languishing (by developing a positive identity), and towards Struggling (through framing and self-managing their mental illness) and Flourishing (by developing valued social roles).

Mental health promotion is a key role for mental health nurses (MHNs) and complements all domains of mental health practice.

- *Challenging discrimination*: Patients with mental illness have experienced social injustice and therefore the role of MHNs has been central in advocating and seeking social justice for their patients. Such acts include proactively empowering, challenging discrimination and stigma and seeking equality and respect for difference. In the past, having a diagnosis of mental illness meant that one may have been prevented from many roles and activities that the general public enjoyed and considered their human right. For example, historically employers could ask about mental health status and then use it to judge suitability for a job. More recently legislation has been introduced to prevent this discriminatory practice occurring and now empowers and safeguards the rights of the individual regardless of their medical history.
- *Building a therapeutic relationship*: The essence of MHN is to seek to understand the person's distress in a non-judgemental, empathic manner based on warmth, curiosity and genuineness so that a therapeutic relationship can be formed. Although for some MHNs working in inpatient settings, the resource of time may not be as available as for those working in other environments, nevertheless, MHNs possibly have a greater amount of time to spend with their patients than other nurses.
- *Understanding unhealthy behaviours*: It is imperative to be mindful that unhealthy behaviours may in fact be the person`s way of coping or indeed a health seeking behaviour. For example, it is not uncommon for people who self-harm to say that they self-harm as a way of releasing pain (coping) and preventing them from taking more serious actions.
- *Motivational skills*: MHNs have a range of transferable skills that can be used in promoting improved health. These may include motivational enhancement techniques to increase motivation and manage anxieties and resistance to change (see Chapter 12). Throughout the change process, it is helpful to ensure that goals set are using a specific, measurable, achievable, realistic and timely (SMART) framework to ensure that they are meaningful. Discussion focused on an enriched future using hope-inspiring questions is a helpful way for also enhancing and keeping the activity in focus. Regular progress reviews are also a helpful strategy that enables the patient to see progress.

Table 15.2 provides a framework for analysing and planning the health promotion approach to working with a patient. It identifies the importance of understanding the presenting situation and the factors that are shaping it. It may help you to organize how you would work with the patient described in Scenario 15.1.

Table 15.2 Presenting situation framework for planning.

Presenting health promotion need	At first glance or from the outset what is the presenting need? Remember, often the presenting need may not actually be the need. It is likely that as you gather more in-depth information, your views may change. The initial presentation may be being used to help cope with some other underlying issue. For example, someone who drinks to excess may be doing so to cope with pain.
Predisposing factors	What are some of the past incidents/experiences/ vulnerabilities that may be contributing to this current health promotion need? For example, is it genetic, learnt/ conditioning or cultural?
Precipitating factors	What are some of the triggers or patterns of living that increase the likelihood of engaging in unhealthy behaviours? E.g. does the person drink to excess only when they have pain?
Protective factors	What are the influences that protect from greater need? What strengths, resilience factors or resources does the person have and use that protect them from more harmful health behaviours? For example why is it that the individual only drinks one bottle of wine per night and not two?
Perpetuating factors	What are the factors that keep this health promotion need on-going? Is it that the person has become so accustomed to this pattern of living that they may be unaware of other coping strategies?
Personal health promotion need development	Based on the information gleaned so far, can you identify how this need has developed?
Personal health promotion need identification	Based on all of the information that you have gathered and your enhanced understanding of the presenting issue, what have you concluded?

Scenario 15.1

Jack is a 28-year-old male who was born in Uganda and came to live in London when he was 4 years old. Jack lives with his parents. Jack`s father is a pastor in a Christian community and his mother is a secretary in a local primary school. He has one brother and two sisters. While at medical school, Jack found the subjects and commitment required for his chosen career to be very stressful and difficult to manage. In his fourth year, Jack told his parents that he was gay which created much upset and distress in the family and continues to create a strain on their relationship. This further added to his stress, Jack became ill and was diagnosed with schizophrenia. He had to leave medical school six months before he was due to qualify. Since then, Jack describes his life as a "downward spiral". He has experienced abuse because he is gay and mentally ill. He has stopped going out, does not have any friends, feels ashamed, worthless and feels hopeless. Since commencing his medication four years ago, he has noticed that his weight has increased dramatically, he is lethargic, his blood pressure has increased and recently investigations suggest that he has diabetes. He also has sickle cell anaemia which is very painful and sees the specialist nursing team at his local acute hospital for treatment. He sees his practice nurse every other week for his hypertension and his General Practitioner for a repeat prescription every month. His community mental health nurse who is also his care coordinator administers his depot injection every two weeks and provides support for him. Though Jack looks forward to his visits, he says that often the conversation that ensues between them centres on monitoring of symptoms and his illness.

- How could you work with Jack to improve his health and well-being?
- How may an area that you have identified be related to another area? What are the connections?
- Apart from MHNs, who else do you think would be instrumental in promoting his health?

Discussion

- *Presenting need. Care for Jack has focused on his immediate presenting symptoms – diabetes, sickle cell anaemia, hypertension.*
- *Predisposing factors. All physical health disorders have the propensity to contribute to mental health whether this is through pathological, psychological or social processes that people experience. Being tested for diabetes may trigger anxieties, that in turn will impact on other stressful emotional and physical illnesses. Prolonged exposure to stress hormones can be damaging and lead to other conditions such as coronary heart disease and strokes. Hypertension and psychotropic medication means Jack is at increased risk for coronary heart disease. Side effects of psychotropic medication may impact negatively on his circulatory system and can lead to iatrogenic (illness caused by other treatments) conditions.*

(Continued)

Scenario 15.1 *(Continued)*

- *Precipitating factors. In Jack`s case it may be that his sexuality conflicts with his religious beliefs and therefore negatively impacts on his emotions.*
- *Protective factors. His family, the specialist sickle cell anaemia nursing team, practice nurse, general practitioner and his community nurse. Each of these can make significant contributions in helping Jack improve his life and health particularly if a coordinated approach is taken. Within mental health services, care coordinators are appointed as the main on-going support and contact person for those who have continuing needs. Jack`s care coordinator is also his community mental health nurse (CMHN) and so he would be ideally placed to coordinate his health promotion needs as part of his care arrangements.*
- *Perpetuating factors. His mental health and physical health are inextricably linked and his psychological feelings of hopelessness and shame exacerbate his physical conditions. Together these impact on his social life and his opportunities for employment. Not going out reinforces his feeling that there is no hope and his belief he will always be abused when he goes out. Hypertension and diabetes may be connected to activity levels. Pain will impact on his emotional state, may discourage him from socializing and be significantly contributing to the "downward spiral" description that he considers, exemplifies his life.*
- *Personal health promotion needs. Self-management of diabetes. Building self-esteem and awareness and problem-solving skills to encourage him to go out and increase physical activity.*

Priorities for health promotion for people with mental health issues

- 10% of children and young people have a clinically recognized mental disorder.
- 17.6% of adults in England have at least one common mental disorder.
- 13% of women experience postnatal depression following childbirth.
- 25% of older people have depressive symptoms which require intervention: 11% have minor depression and 2% major depression.
- The risk of depression increases with age – 40% of those over 85 are affected.
- 20–25% of people with dementia have major depression.
- 40% of residents in care homes have depression, 50–80% dementia and 30% anxiety.
- 30% of people who care for an older person with dementia have depression (Royal College of Psychiatrists, 2010).

While mental health issues are likely to affect much of the population, and mental health promotion or public mental health should be a priority of all nursing, there are specific issues that affect those with severe mental illness:

- People with severe mental illness (SMI) are at increased risk of physical illness as shown in Table 15.3.

Table 15.3 Physical health and severe mental illness.

Disease category	Physical diseases with increased frequency
Bacterial infections and mycoses	Tuberculosis (+)
Viral diseases	HIV (++), hepatitis B/C (+)
Neoplasms	Obesity-related cancer (+)
Musculoskeletal diseases	Osteoporosis/decreased bone mineral density (+)
Stomatognathic diseases	Poor dental status (+)
Respiratory tract diseases	Impaired lung function (+)
Urological and male genital diseases	Sexual dysfunction (+)
Female genital diseases and pregnancy complications	Obstetric complications (++)
Cardiovascular diseases	Stroke, myocardial infarction, hypertension, other cardiac and vascular diseases (++)
Nutritional and metabolic diseases	Obesity (++), diabetes mellitus (+), metabolic syndrome (++), hyperlipidemia (++)

Notes: (++) very good evidence for increased risk, (+) good evidence for increased risk.
Source: De Hert *et al.*, 2011, Table 1, p. 53. Reproduced with permission from John Wiley & Sons Ltd.

- Rates of undiagnosed and untreated physical illnesses are higher in the SMI than the general population.
- Severe mental illness (SMI) patients may die 13–30 years earlier than the general population.
- SMI patients are more likely to smoke or be obese.

There are a number of explanations that are proposed for these risks. These include:

- side effects of medication;
- lifestyle to include dietary habits, smoking and sedentary behaviours;
- difficulty in interpreting physical signs of illness;
- poor quality of care.

There is recent recognition that the smoking and dietary behaviours of people with SMI need to be addressed. Some 40% of people with mental health disorders smoke, compared with just 20& of the general population, with the figure rising even higher among people with severe mental illness (Royal College of Psychiatrists, 2013). People with SMI also tend to be heavier smokers, smoking more than 25 cigarettes a day (McNeill, 2001). While smoking rates have declined in the UK over the past 20 years, there has been little change among those with mental disorders. Smokers with mental disorders tend to be more heavily addicted and are less likely to be successful when trying to quit than the general population. The reasons why people with SMI may have such high rates of smoking include other neurobiological, psychological, behavioural and social factors including the condoning and even active encouragement of smoking in care settings

People with SMI are also more likely to be obese. A range of factors may account for this:

- Depression may lead to reduced physical activity and increased appetite.
- The stigma associated with obesity may be a contributing factor to depression.
- Medications to manage mood, anxiety or psychoses can cause weight gain.
- Activity may be limited due to obesity or related chronic illnesses which increases the risk of depression by reducing involvement in rewarding activities.

Activity 15.3

Why is the physical health of people with SMI often neglected?

Discussion

- *Many mental health practitioners have little training in physical care.*
- *The orientation of primary care is reactive and this does not fit well with patients who may be reluctant, or unable, to seek help.*
- *When a patient with SMI reports symptoms of physical illness, their mental illness is believed to be influencing the physical symptoms that they report, known as overshadowing. Patients may be thought to be imagining symptoms.*
- *The more severely depressed the patient, the greater intensity of pain that they may feel.*
- *Short consultation times make it difficult for doctors to assess mental state and conduct a physical assessment, especially in vague or suspicious patients.*
- *When patients are accompanied by mental health staff, more emphasis may be given to psychological and social issues (Phelan et al., 2001).*

Strategies for mental health promotion

Promoting healthy lifestyles and developing personal skills

In order to encourage people with SMI to quit smoking, it is recommended that health care settings used by people with mental disorders should be completely smoke-free and that all nurses are trained in smoking cessation advice (Royal College of Psychiatrists, 2013). Smokers with mental disorders using primary and secondary care services, at all levels, should be identified and provided routinely and immediately with specialist smoking cessation behavioural support, and pharmacotherapy.

Increasing access to services

People with mental illness are as interested and concerned with their physical health as the general population. Various factors may make it difficult for them to access services or receive health promotion:

- Medication may cause tiredness.
- Lack of awareness of physical health conditions due to cognitive impairment.
- Difficulties communicating physical health complaints.
- Poor quality health care. Despite codes of professional conduct, health care practitioners may have discriminatory attitudes and stigmatize the mentally ill. This can be a barrier to them becoming involved with the mental health of their patients (Currid *et al.*, 2012) and may actually lead to them limiting the engagement with such patients.

These are all areas that nurses in other specialities (other than mental health) need to be aware of and augment their practice to maximize both engagement and access to services. NICE (2009) recommend that primary care practitioners should provide routine physical checks for people with schizophrenia, and people admitted to psychiatric wards should have their physical health routinely checked.

Case Study 15.1

Evaluation of a Well-being Support Programme

A Cochrane review of physical health monitoring for patients with SMI has concluded that there was no evidence from RCTs to support current practice (Tosh *et al.*, 2010) but many areas have adopted the model of a Well-being Support Programme (Ohlsen *et al.*, 2005). This is a health promotion initiative for people with SMI in which nurses are trained to do the following:

- ❑ Identify physical health problems.
- ❑ Promote treatment adherence.
- ❑ Encourage positive lifestyle change.
- ❑ Strengthen links between primary and secondary care.
- ❑ Provide support and advice to carers.
- ❑ Direct patients to appropriate primary and secondary care services.

The service was facilitated by a team of nurse advisors who provided Well-Being support as an adjunct to routine care. Some of the people with SMI had had no routine physical health checks for many years. The programme highlighted issues such as high blood sugar, hypertension, obesity, polypharmacy and sexual health problems which could be referred.

Empowerment

The health of people with SMI is greatly improved when their personal power is advanced. Strategies that are more likely to empower are those that enhance recovery rather than promoting an approach that suggests poor prognosis. Treatment plans should be collaborative rather than unilateral decision-making that is perceived as coercive. There are many opportunities that present where the MHN can build on protective factors for the client such as their achievements, values and hopes for the future.

Mental health is very much part of the Expert Patient Programme (DH, 2001) which seeks to use the knowledge of those living with a chronic condition to educate others (see Chapter 9). A structured training comprises:

- Recognizing and acting on symptoms.
- Learning techniques that can reduce stress.
- Using medication correctly.
- Getting the most out of health services, by using them as effectively as possible.
- Managing the distress and depression that can come with a chronic illness.
- Taking adequate physical exercise, managing relationships with professionals and family.
- Maintaining a healthy diet.
- Using community resources.

Social change

Stigma is unjust, adds to disability and is based on myth rather than fact. Though the evidence base for reducing stigma is poor, strategies to reduce stigma suggest that those with greater awareness and education about mental illness are less stigmatizing (Corrigan and Penn, 1999; Rethink, 2003). In addition, greater contact with the mentally ill provides an opportunity for people to challenge their discriminatory attitudes and change to more positive ones (Rethink, 2003; Thornicroft *et al*., 2008).

Social interventions used in health promotion activities will often depend on the needs and goals set. However, there are some specific social activities that may apply to all patients. These include: social inclusion into mainstream society so as the person feels a valued part, a good standard of accommodation and finances that facilitates a good standard of living, employment or other such activities that gives a sense of value and enables the person to realize their potential, infrastructures which provide opportunities for lifelong learning that reflects advances in education and life skills, cultural inclusion that respects the person's self-identity and relationships in context to larger communities, legal, ethical and moral duties that provide social justice and prevent the unfairness that is experienced by those with a mental illness.

On placement: checklist

- ❑ Can you identify whether the care plan includes health promotion goals, interventions and resources to aid the patient with health promotion activities?
- ❑ In the multidisciplinary team meetings, how much time or content is given to discussing, planning and reviewing health promotion activities?
- ❑ What are the main health promotion activities that you have seen in your placement areas?
- ❑ Which members of the multidisciplinary team are actively pursuing health promotion activities with the patients in your care?

Key learning points

1. It is not possible to have good physical health without good mental health.
2. Mental health promotion is an integral part of all nursing.
3. Mental health is more than simply the absence of mental illness.
4. A society needs to respect political, cultural, economic, civil rights to facilitate good mental health.
5. People with severe mental illness have physical health needs that need full attention.
6. Mental health is more than the absence of mental illness.
7. People with mental health issues are often discriminated against.
8. Effective public health interventions can enhance mental health.

Chapter summary

Mental health promotion is a complex, interesting and a varied approach that meets with the role of all nurses. It is enshrined in policy, practice, professional standards and in patients' wishes for improved services. Rather than it being an activity that is an adjunct to MHN, it is an integral part of care. It has many health, fiscal and generational benefits for the patient, the organization and wider community. In practising mental health promotion, the key is to listen and understand in a non-judgemental manner and then work in partnership using a variety of strategies that are patient centred and led.

Further reading and resources

Centre for Mental Health. Available at: http://www.centreformentalhealth.org.uk/index.aspx.

Department of Health (2011) *No Health Without Mental Health: A Cross-Government Mental Health Outcomes Strategy for People of All Ages*. DH, London. Available at: http://www.dh.gov.uk/prod_consum_dh/groups/dh_digitalassets/documents/digitalasset/dh_124058.pdf.

Friedli, L. and Parsonage, M. (2009) Promoting mental health and preventing mental illness: the economic case for investment in Wales. Available at: http://www.publicmentalhealth.org/Documents/749/Promoting%20Mental%20Health%20Report%20(English).pdf.

National Institute for Health and Clinical Excellence (2007) Public health interventions to promote positive mental health and prevent mental health disorders among adults. Evidence briefing. Available at: http://www.nice.org.uk/niceMedia/pdf/mental%20health%20EB%20FINAL%2018.01.07.pdf.

World Health Organization (2004) *Promoting Mental Health, Concepts Emerging Evidence, Practice: A Report of the World Health Organization, Department of Mental Health and Substance Abuse in Collaboration with the Victorian Health Promotion Foundation and The University of Melbourne*. http://www.who.int/mental_health/evidence/en/promoting_mhh.pdf.

World Health Organization (2013) *Health Topics, Mental Health*. Available at: : http://www.who.int/topics/mental_health/en/.

References

Anthony, W. A. (1993) Recovery from mental illness: the guiding vision of the mental health service system in the 1990s. *Psychosocial Rehabilitation Journal*, **16** (4), 11–23.

Corrigan, P.W. and Penn, D.L. (1999) Lessons from social psychology on discrediting psychiatric stigma. *American Psychology*, **54** (9), 765–776.

Currid, T.J., Turner, A., Bellefontaine, N. and Spada, M.M. (2012) Mental health issues in primary care: implementing policies in practice. *British Journal of Community Nursing*, **17** (1), 21–26.

De Hert, M., Correll, C.U., Bobes, J. *et al.* (2011) Physical illness in patients with severe mental disorders. I. Prevalence, impact of medications and disparities in health care. *World Psychiatry*, **10** (1), 52–77.

DH (Department of Health) (2001) *The Expert Patient: A New Approach to Chronic Disease Management for the 21st Century*. DH, London.

DH (Department of Health) (2011) *No Health Without Mental Health: A Cross-Government Mental Health Outcomes Strategy for People of All Ages*. DH, London. Available at: http://www.dh.gov.uk/prod_consum_dh/groups/dh_digitalassets/documents/digitalasset/dh_124058.pdf.

Keyes, C.L.M. and Lopez, S.J. (2002) Toward a science of mental health, in *Handbook of Positive Psychology* (eds C.R. Snyder and S.J. Lopez), Oxford University Press, New York, pp. 45–59.

Knapp, M., McDaid, D. and Parsonage, M. (2011) *Mental Health Promotion and Mental Illness Prevention: The Economic Case*. DH, London. Available at: http://eprints.lse.ac.uk/32311/.

Leucht, S., Burkard, T., Henderson, J. *et al.* (2007) Physical illness and schizophrenia: a review of the literature. *Acta Psychiatrica Scandinavia*, **116**, 317–333.

McNeill A. (2001) *Smoking and Mental Health: A Review of the Literature*. ASH, London.

NICE (2009) *Schizophrenia: Core Interventions in the Treatment and Management of Schizophrenia in Adults in Primary and Secondary Care*. NICE, London. Available at: http://www.nice.org.uk/nicemedia/pdf/cg82niceguideline.pdf.

Ohlsen, R.I., Peacock, G. and Smith, S. (2005) Developing a service to monitor and improve physical health in people with serious mental illness. *Journal of Psychiatric and Mental Health Nursing*, **12** (5), 614–619.

Phelan, M., Stradins, L. and Morrison, S. (2001) Physical health of people with severe mental illness can be improved if primary care and mental health professionals pay attention to it, *BMJ*, **322** (7284): 443–444.

Rethink (2003) *Reducing Stigma and Discrimination: What Works? Showcasing Examples of Best Practice of Anti-Discrimination Projects in Mental Health Conference Report, Rethink*. Available at: http://www.mmhrc.ca/sites/default/files/Stigma_best%20practices.pdf.

Royal College of Psychiatrists (2010) *No Health Without Public Mental Health*. Royal College of Psychiatrists, London. Available at: http://www.rcpsych.ac.uk/PDF/Position%20Statement%204%20website.pdf.

Royal College of Psychiatrists (2013) *Smoking and Mental Health*. Royal College of Psychiatrists, London. Available at: http://www.rcplondon.ac.uk/publications/smoking-and-mental-health.

Taylor, L., Taske, N., Swann, C. *et al.* (2007) Public health interventions to promote positive mental health and prevent mental health disorders among adults, evidence briefing, National Institute for Health and Clinical Excellence. Available at: http://www.nice.org.uk/aboutnice/whoweare/aboutthehda/hdapublications/public_health_interventions_to_promote_positive_mental_health_and_prevent_mental_health_disorders_among_adults.jsp.

Thornicroft, G., Brohan, E., Kassam, A. and Lewis-Holme, E. (2008) Reducing stigma and discrimination: candidate interventions. *International Journal of Mental Health Systems*, **2**, 3.

Tosh, R., Clifton, A., Mala, S. and Bachner, M. (2010) Physical health care monitoring for people with serious mental illness. *Cochrane Database of Systematic Reviews*, **3**:CD008298.

Westerhof, G.J. and Keyes, C.L.M. (2010) Mental illness and mental health: the two continua model across the lifespan. *Journal of Adult Development*, **17** (2), 110–119.

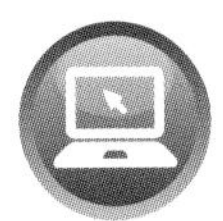

Don't forget to visit the companion website for this book: www.wileyfundamentalseries.com/healthpromotion where you can find self-assessment tests to check your progress.

16

Health promotion and older adults

Sandie Woods

Senior Lecturer, Occupational Therapy, London South Bank University, London, UK

Learning outcomes

By the end of this chapter you will be able to:

1. Discuss the impact of ageing on health and well-being and identify the health needs of older adults
2. Describe the role of the nurse in health promotion when nursing older adults
3. Outline a range of health promotion interventions

Introduction

This chapter considers the role of the adult nurse, much of whose practice will be nursing older adults:

- One in six of the UK population (over 14 million people) is currently aged 65 and over with a prediction that by 2050 it will increase to one in four (ONS, 2012).
- An estimated 4 million people (40%) aged 65+ in the United Kingdom have a limiting long-standing illness.

Fundamentals of Health Promotion for Nurses, Second Edition. Edited by Jane Wills.

Companion website: www.wileyfundamentalseries.com/healthpromotion

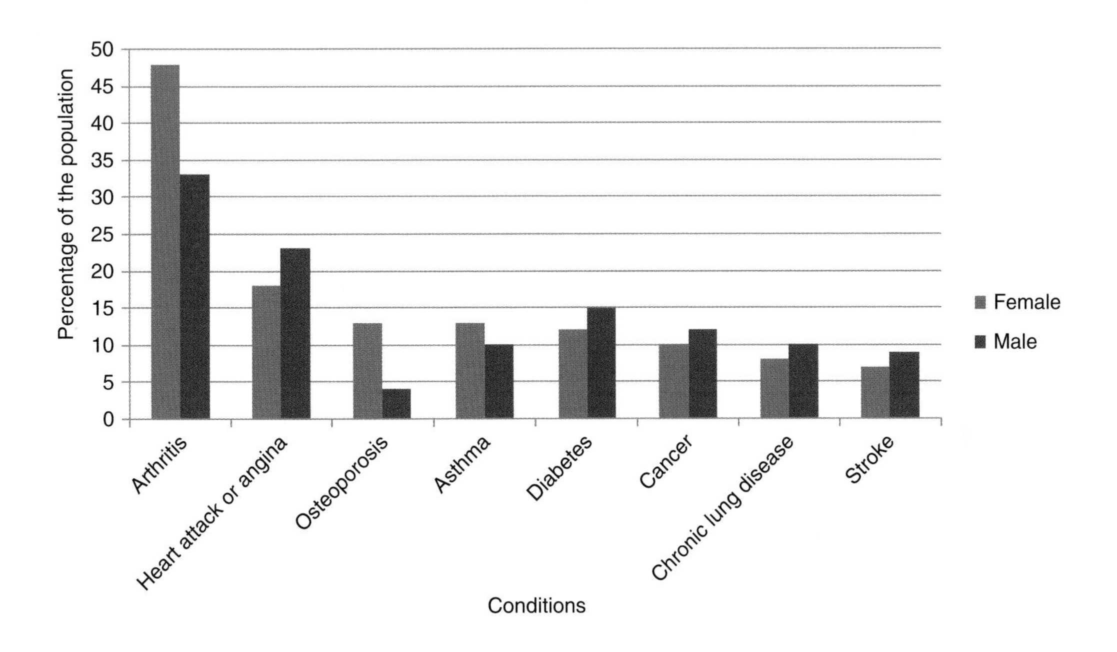

Figure 16.1 Prevalence of disease in older adults in the U.K.

- Two-thirds of people (69%) aged 85 and over in the UK have a disability or limiting long-term condition.
- Seven preventable risk factors, including smoking, high blood pressure and obesity, account for over half the disease burden in later life (Age UK, 2013a).

Figure 16.1 shows the prevalence of chronic disease among the older age group, with a representative sample of older people. For people over 65 and living in the community, osteoarthritis is the most common physical condition followed by those related to the arteries affecting predominantly the heart. Mixed anxiety and depressive disorder is the most common mental health issue in the community in older age. About a third of all people over 65 fall each year (equivalent to 3 million) with 50–70% of women having an osteoporotic fracture at some time (Age UK, 2013a). The numbers of people with dementia continue to increase.

These figures have major implications for care and the costs to the state of supporting an ageing population. Enabling people to live healthily into older age and preventing or managing illness and disability is important not only for their quality of life but also to reduce NHS costs of hospital admissions.

Older age produces a number of changes that affect health and well-being in addition to the physical ageing processes and the older the person, the more likely they are to have multiple conditions which may lead to polypharmacy or multiple prescribing. Social changes affect people in later life, including reduced income, friendship circles reducing as friends die, and difficulties with transport when no longer able to drive a car or easily access public transport.

Promoting healthy ageing is a complex arena requiring not only good information and services but also a positive approach to ageing, recognizing that people can live a healthy, safe and socially inclusive lifestyle regardless of age. Figure 16.2 illustrates those factors that can both promote and hinder well-being for the older adult (Katz *et al.*, 2011).

Health promotion is about encouraging self-efficacy where individuals can see the opportunity to improve their quality of life by preventing or delaying the onset of chronic conditions

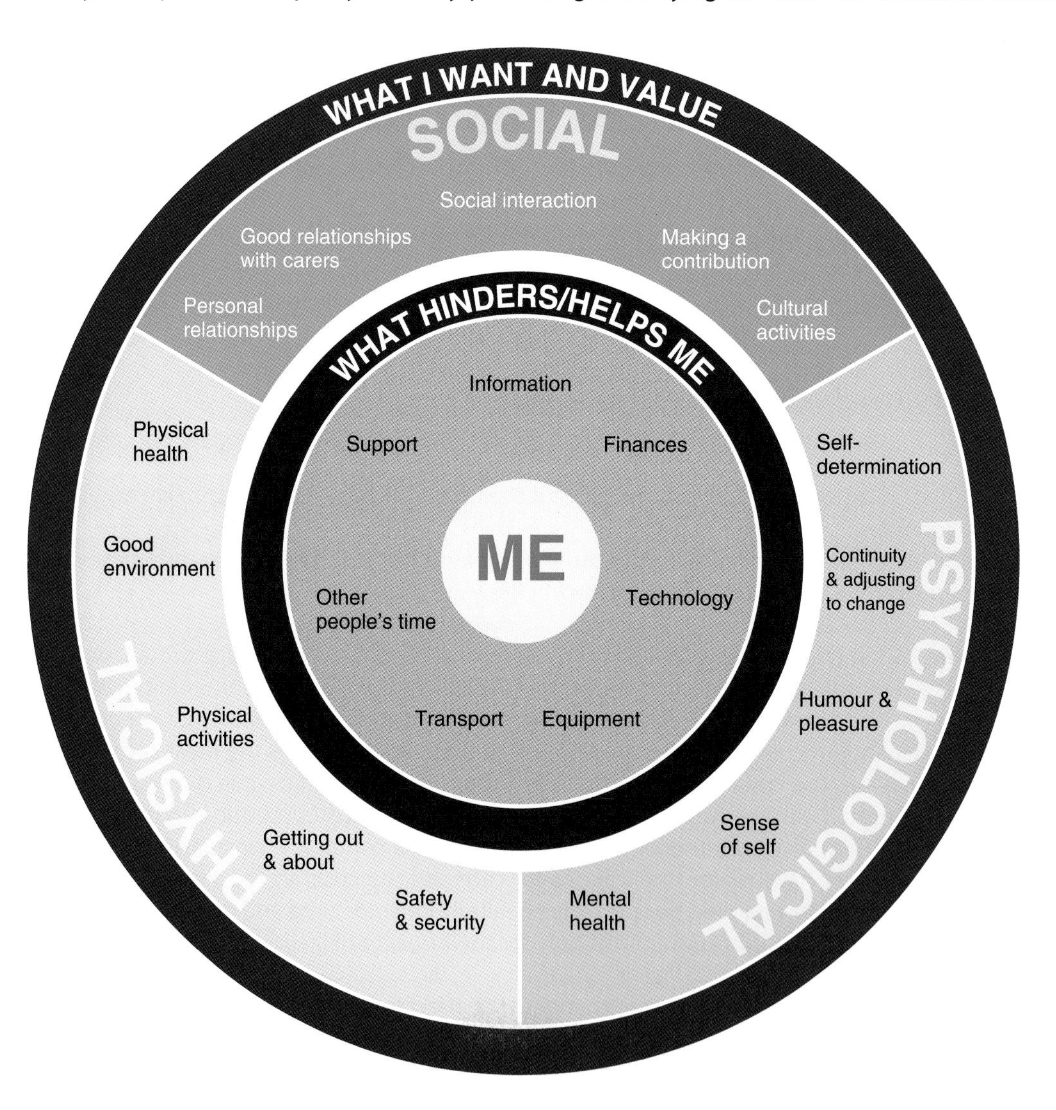

Figure 16.2 Factors that help or hinder well-being in older adults. Source: Figure 2, p.41 from *A Better Life: What Older People with High Support Needs Value* by Jeanne Katz, Caroline Holland, Sheila Peace and Emily Taylor; edited by Imogen Blood, published in 2011 by the Joseph Rowntree Foundation. Reproduced by permission of the Joseph Rowntree Foundation.

and adopting a change in behaviour and approach to health. Achieving well-being in older age involves the person having resilience, independence, health, income and wealth, having a role and having time with others (Katz *et al.*, 2011).

Health promotion may be considered in relation to physical and mental health, lifestyle, the physical environment and the social environment to enable older adults to lead active and fulfilling lives.

Activity 16.1

What are the goals of health promotion when nursing the older adult?

Discussion

These include:

- *Education and information about keeping active and eating healthily.*
- *Enabling older people to take part in activities and building social networks.*
- *Ensuring that their physical environment is safe and warm.*
- *Supporting them to quit smoking and reduce alcohol consumption.*
- *Raising awareness of opportunities for screening and immunization.*
- *Addressing health inequalities in later life, acting to improve the health of more disadvantaged social groups.*

Scenario 16.1

Millie is an 85-year-old lady who was admitted to an acute medical unit following a number of falls at home. She had sustained a fracture of the right wrist and showed signs of hypothermia on admission (confusion, disorientation, drowsy, pale, shallow breathing and slurred speech). When reading the notes you see she has a diagnosis of Vascular Dementia. You notice that her clothes appear very loose suggesting she has been losing weight. The nursing notes highlight that Millie needs assistance at meal times and she says she forgets to eat.

What health promotion priorities are evident from the case study?

Why might Millie have difficulty with eating and drinking? How will you address this?

Discussion

Priority 1: Promoting health and reducing risk

- *The physical environment needs to be safe and warm.She needs to have some social support and networks to reduce loneliness and isolation.*
- *Routine screening is important to identify the risk of malnutrition (deficiency of proteins, vitamins and minerals) and provide good nutritional care. Malnutrition has been described*

(Continued)

Scenario 16.1 (Continued)

as both a cause and consequence of disease and illness with a variety of contributing factors for example, depression, anxiety, social exclusion, poor access to transport or mobility difficulties and poverty (Malnutrition Task Force, 2013).

- *Discuss any difficulties with the team for a coordinated approach to care.*
- *Check whether there is a volunteer scheme to give support at mealtimes.*
- *Difficulty with eating and drinking: physical changes such as lack of exercise, constipation or pain can impact on the appetite and nutrition.*
- *Sufficient staff should be available to assist at mealtimes.*
- *Be vigilant to any difficulties with chewing or swallowing, and check that dentures are fitting correctly.*
- *Refer to the Speech and Language Therapist and Dietician if there are difficulties with swallowing or nutrition.*
- *Ensure the person can use the utensils and refer to the Occupational Therapist for adapted equipment if required or finger foods if preferred.*
- *Psychological changes such as depression or dementia may result in a loss of appetite, anxiety or reduced awareness of hunger or thirst (Alzheimer's Society, 2010).*
- *Social aspects such as loneliness and isolation may also result in a loss of interest in preparing food or enjoyment of meal times (Alzheimer's Society, 2013).*

Priority 2: Communication

- *Allow time to discuss the importance of a balanced diet and identify factors that may have impacted on the ability to eat and drink.*
- *Provide regular prompts and encouragement to drink and have refreshments in easy view and accessible throughout the day and at night.*
- *Ensure that the covered jugs or the drinks dispenser are easy to use and refilled with fresh water at regular intervals.*
- *Use pictures showing the amount that should be consumed per day. A guideline is 8 standard glasses per day (NPSA, 2007).*
- *Discuss favourite foods with the carers if the person is not able to express their preferences.*

Priority 3: Cognition and choice

- *Avoid distractions at mealtimes and create a calm and comfortable environment.*
- *Offer small amounts of food and drink more frequently if appetite is reduced.*
- *Take the person to see the options if they are not able to retain information or remember what they ordered.*
- *Use a range of formats (pictures and words).*
- *Keep the layout simple so that they can identify what is in front of them and give time for the person to finish each course.*
- *Check that the choices meet the requirements (ask about cultural preferences, specific dietary needs).*

Priorities for the health of older people

Growing older has been seen as a time of increasing dependency when physical health declines but this is not inevitable. The National Service Framework for Older People (DH, 2001) identifies three categories of older age:

- *Entering Older Age.* People who are nearing the end of or who have completed their paid employment and/or child rearing. This could be as young as 50 or those over 65.
- *Transitional Phase.* The transition is between a healthy active life and frailty which often occurs in the seventh or eighth decades. Degenerative conditions such as weaker muscles, loss of flexibility in joints, poor vision and hearing and loss of cognitive function may be present.
- *Frail Older People.* These people are vulnerable as a result of health problems such as stroke or dementia.

The particular health messages in relation to lifestyles are particularly relevant for older people as national health surveys such as the Scottish Health Survey (2011) reports.

Alcohol

The propensity to binge drink (at one occasion drink more than 8 units for men or 6 units for women) declines with age. Some 20% of men aged 65–74 reported drinking alcohol at levels classified as hazardous or harmful, as did more than 10% of women. Hazardous drinking was defined as a pattern of alcohol consumption associated with risks of physical and psychological harm to the individual. Harmful drinking denotes the most hazardous use of alcohol, at which damage to health is likely.

Diet

The proportion of men and women consuming five or more portions of fruit and vegetables per day reduces among those aged 75 years and over.

Activity

Levels of physical activity in England in later life are often too low to maintain health. Approximately 47% of men and 53% of women aged 65–74 year have low levels of activity (less than 30 minutes of moderate activity on less than one day a week).

Smoking

Smoking prevalence in adults decreases with increased age though 20% of those aged 50–59 still smoke.

Obesity

The prevalence of obesity is lowest among young adults and increases with age until around 65 years. In later life, muscle bulk tends to fall at the same time that adipose tissue (fat) is accumulating indicated by enlarged waists. At older ages (75 years plus) many people start losing weight.

The conclusion of a recent report into health care quality in older life highlighted that health in later life is far from fixed and there is great potential for it to be improved (Melzer *et al.*, 2012). While there have been dramatic falls in the numbers smoking since the 1960s and a corresponding fall in mortality from heart disease, the fall in smoking rates has been slow since the mid-1990s. Helping current older smokers to quit could make a positive contribution. Similarly, the dramatic rise in diabetes prevalence from around 6% in 1994 to 16% in 2009 in the 65–74 age groups can be partly attributed to a rise in obesity. The experience of more privileged groups shows that it is possible to enjoy a longer life expectancy combined with a shorter average period of disability and that there is substantial scope for improving later life health for many less privileged older people.

Another area where it is possible to improve the health of older people is by preventing hospital admissions. Older people have higher rates of hospital admission than the general population and higher rates of readmission due to complications and falls. During hospitalization, older people may experience significant functional decline which impairs their future independence and quality of life. The aim of intermediate care is to prevent unnecessary acute hospital admission or premature admission to residential care. Health promotion can support the self-management of long-term conditions (Chapter 9) and promote independence and functional ability.

Falling in older age can lead to increased anxiety and depression, reduced activity, and higher use of medication. About a third of those over 65 will fall each year and one in five of those who have a hip fracture die within three months. Yet there is a good evidence base on what works to prevent falls and that strength and balance exercise in a structured programme is effective (NICE, 2013). Evidence notwithstanding, the nurse may need to persuade an older person that they might benefit from such a programme. Chapter 12 discusses some of the reasons why a person might take protective action for their health and need to feel that they are at risk. Age UK's advice on how to communicate a falls prevention message suggests that some people:

- May not think it applies to them (they are not old or frail enough).
- May be genuinely confident (sometimes over-confident) of their capabilities and do not wish to be thought of as frail.
- Attribute any previous fall to momentary inattention or illness rather than to a persisting vulnerability.
- Accept falling as an inevitable part of ageing.

The challenge then is not to focus on risks or even potential hazards which may seem patronizing and restrictive but to stress the benefits that come from improved strength, confidence and enjoyment.

Strategies for health promotion with older adults

Developing personal skills

Communication is an essential component in nursing older adults. It should be clear concise, correct, coherent and courteous. This involves giving the individual time to explain what has occurred, how they are feeling and the impact on their health and well-being. Assessment forms and checklists may be used but there should also be opportunity for the individual to tell their story. Using a narrative approach will allow information to emerge that may not have appeared on the assessment form. Information may not be presented in a chronological order and there is a need to capture a wide range of events and interpret their meaning and significance as they emerge. The SOLAR approach (see Chapter 12) can provide a helpful tool and reminder of the components of effective communication:

Activity 16.2

What particular considerations are there in communication and health education with older adults?

Discussion

- *Sensory loss can affect communication and checking whether the person wears a hearing aid, spectacles or false teeth should be undertaken before engaging in an interview or discussion. Communication may be presented verbally and non-verbally in written form, through demonstration and by incorporating visual clues and prompts.*
- *The patient's attention, concentration and energy levels also need to be considered.*
- *Time may be needed for the person to consolidate information and opportunity for questions to be addressed at a later stage.*

Health education materials are often targeted toward elderly populations since they tend to carry the greatest burden of chronic disease. The materials may not be suitable because of the limited literacy of the population. For example, government advice on keeping warm in winter is 20 pages long!

Evidence 16.1

Health literacy and older people

A recent study investigated whether older people who have low literacy (assessed by the ability to read and comprehend the instructions in an aspirin packet) had a higher risk of mortality. The study suggests that a third of older adults in England have difficulty reading and understanding basic health-related written information, rising to half of adults over the age of 80. Poorer understanding is associated with higher mortality. This study comes at time when the prevalence of long-term conditions is rising and patients are increasingly encouraged to become responsible and active partners in their care.

In response to the survey of over 8000 adults, the Patients Association queried how patients can be expected to make informed decisions if they do not fully understand the information being given to them. They asserted that patients must be involved in the development of these information leaflets from the outset to make sure they provide relevant and clear information. *"That way, patients will be better empowered to manage their own health conditions and make the positive lifestyle choices that lead to better health and wellbeing"* (Bostock and Steptoe, 2012).

Empowering older people to take greater control over their health

Enabling older people's capacity for health and well-being to be realized may include building people's confidence or self-worth, boosting their self-esteem, developing their coping mechanisms or enhancing their personal skills in order for them to make health-related choices. A sense of control has a direct effect on improving an individual's mental and physical health.

Activity 16.3

How could your practice with older people help to build confidence?

Discussion

Working with older people may involve adapting or changing to build confidence. This may include changing the way activities are undertaken as a result of physical disability, coping with loss either as a result of health changes or loss of family and friends and possibly a change in housing or community.

- *The nurse can play a role in allowing the person to express the challenges they are facing and use a strengths approach to reinforce what the individual can do, the resources and opportunities that exist.*
- *Where signs of depression are apparent, for example, in sleeping patterns, loss of appetite or low levels of engagement or motivation, the nurse can record these changes and ensure that a referral is made for a mental health assessment.*
- *Past and present attachment has been shown to be important at all stages of life and the nurse can play a key role in identifying and highlighting the need for significant others and discuss services available such as befriending schemes and support groups.*
- *Providing information that can help the person express their views in a suitable format is important as mental capacity may diminish. This may include discussion, written information, pictures and opportunity to ask questions or clarify options.*

Self-management and expert patient programmes provide an important component of collaborative working (see Chapter 9). The knowledge, skills and experience held by patients can represent a potentially untapped and valuable resource (Fox, 2005). Informing patients of groups available and how they may assist can provide a forum for on-going support for older adults living with long-term conditions. The programmes may run within a hospital or community setting and include topics such as relaxation, symptom management, exercise, fatigue, nutrition, problem solving/action planning and communication with health care professionals

Lifestyle change

Lifestyle education remains the cornerstone of secondary prevention and has the potential to save lives and prevent any further disability. Looking after the body, eating healthily, taking exercise, foot care and falls prevention are all aspects that can be discussed and linked to self-management and reducing risk. It provides an opportunity to discuss lifestyle factors such as smoking, alcohol use and adherence to medication. It is recommended that patients at risk of recurrent stroke, for example, be assessed and given information about risk factors and lifestyle management issues (exercise, smoking, diet, weight and alcohol). Furthermore, they should be supported with possible strategies to modify their lifestyle and risk factors (Department of Health, 2007).

The Health Care Commission (2006) reported nearly half (48%) of patients said that they had not been given any information about dietary changes that might have prevented a further stroke, while 39% said they had not been given information about physical exercise. A further patient survey by the National Audit Office (2012) revealed a lack of patient awareness, with one in five respondents uninformed that lack of exercise increased their risk of stroke and only half of stroke survivors said that they were given advice on further stroke prevention when leaving hospital.

Case Study 16.1

Older people and drinking

There has been a striking rise in the rate of alcohol misuse in older people over the past two decades, with the proportion of men and women aged 65 and over drinking above safe drinking limits having risen by 40% and 100% respectively between 1990 and 2009. For men aged 75 and over, alcohol-related deaths in England have increased by 20% between 1991–1997 and 1998–2004. At least 15% of patients on the caseloads for community mental health teams for older people in London boroughs have a diagnosis of harmful use of alcohol or alcohol dependence, with a similar proportion on medical wards covering these areas.

While there are NICE guidelines for the diagnosis and assessment in general practice of harmful drinking and several screening tools as precursors to a brief intervention, the first report on substance misuse and older people (Royal College of Psychiatrists, 2011) identified that GPs were unlikely to suspect an alcohol problem and were reluctant to intervene with older patients.

The government alcohol strategy (DH, 2013) states that the Department of Health will include alcohol identification and any subsequent brief advice needed within the NHS Health Check for adults from age 40–75 from April 2013.

Screening and immunization

Early detection can reduce or prevent a condition occurring and discussing the benefits of screening programmes is an important role for the nurse. Screening for diabetes, eye conditions and bowel disorders are available through the general practitioner (GP). The health check is for any adult between the ages of 40–74 and includes height, weight, general health, blood glucose, blood pressure and cholesterol. Discussion with the nurse and GP may highlight particular risks and lead to further tests. For example, tests may be undertaken for anaemia, thyroid, heart, prostrate, osteoporosis, kidney disease and glaucoma. Some patients may be reluctant to discuss sensitive aspects such as changes in bowel function but the nursing role can facilitate the gathering of important information leading to early detection, diagnosis and treatment.

Activity 16.4

In 2010–2011 there were 9000 admissions for influenza and several hundred deaths. Although immunization is offered to all people aged 65 years and over, average immunization rates in London are only 71.4% of those over 60 (HPA, 2011).

The patient population found in hospital is much more vulnerable to the severe effects of influenza and health care workers may transmit the illness to patients even if they are mildly or sub-clinically infected.

As a nurse, you are in an ideal position to provide information for older people on the importance of vaccination, reassurance on vaccine safety and efficacy. Would you get yourself immunized?

Building social support

It is important to consider the person's function not only in the context in which you see them but also consider the community setting and home environment, local facilities and social care needs. Changes in health, lifestyle and bereavement can lead to feelings of loneliness and isolation. Age UK (2013a) reported that half of all people over 75 in the United Kingdom live alone and 7% of those aged 65 or over in the UK say they are always or often feel lonely. Mental illness, low morale, poor rehabilitation and admission to residential care have all been found to be correlated with either social isolation or loneliness or both.

Evidence 16.2

Social relationships and mortality risk

The social context in which older people live influences their health, quality of life, and well-being, as it does for other age groups. A recent review combining results from 148 studies (308849 participants) estimated that individuals reporting strong social relationships had a reduced risk of mortality (50% increase in likelihood of survival) compared with individuals lacking social support (after adjusting for important baseline socio-demographic and health-related confounders). These findings suggest that the influence of social relationships on the risk of death is comparable with well-established risk factors for mortality such as smoking (Holt-Lunstad *et al.*, 2010).

Guiding patients to services or sources of information is an important role. Contact with the Patient Advice and Liaison Services (PALS) can be a good starting point. There are many schemes available, for example, befriending, online support, day services and community group programmes that can provide not only company and social engagement but may also address a specific aspects of health promotion such as walking groups.

Evidence 16.3

Effectiveness of one-to-one support

There is a lack of evidence regarding the effectiveness of services providing one-to-one support to reduce loneliness and social isolation among older people, in improving their health and quality of life. In particular, the impact of interventions, for example, befriending services for older people such as telephone befriending and other forms of low-level support, has been the subject of considerable debates. Recent evaluations of assistive technology suggest that low-level technology such as telephone support can help older people to stay socially connected and reduce their feelings of loneliness. One review found that the relationship established with their befriender was crucial to the quality of life of the older person as well as the maintenance of their emotional and physical health. The service was described as a lifeline, and many participants believed that not having access to it would make them increasingly lonely and socially isolated, which could lead to long-term ill-health (Cattan *et al.*, 2009).

Supporting carers

Consideration needs to be given to the carers of older adults. Carers may be family, friends or neighbours. Older couples may find themselves caring for each other and children in their seventies may be caring for their parents over many years.

Some 1:8 adults are carers (6.4 million) with a predicted increase to 9 million by 2037(Carers UK, 2012) and 2.3 million people gave up work to care for an elderly parent, disabled or seriously ill loved one. The Department of Health (2010, p. 12) acknowledge that

> *There is a good evidence base on the problems that may be associated with caring responsibilities including mental and physical health problems, social isolation and lowered social functioning, and increased mortality as a result of mental or emotional distress, especially in more elderly carers.*

Work can be affected as a result of caring with a high proportion having to quit work or reduce working hours. This can lead to financial hardship in the short and long term and impact on the carer's health and well-being. People who provide higher levels of care are twice as likely to be permanently sick or disabled. Therefore, supporting carers to remain physically and mentally well has been set as a priority by national and local governments (DH, 2012).

Scenario 16.2

Mrs Pathos is 78 years old. She moved from Cyprus to England 40 years ago and lives in a terraced house in London. Her husband passed away two years ago and her son died a year ago. Her daughter Maria works full-time and visits at weekends. Mrs Pathos has osteoarthritis (OA) affecting both her hip joints, and type 2 diabetes. Over the last five years she has experienced increased pain, stiffness and reduced range of movement. She recently fell, when hanging out her washing. She experiences pain when climbing the stairs to reach the toilet and as a result she has reduced her fluid intake. She had a urinary tract infection and her diabetes is no longer within the recommended guidelines. She takes medication for her OA and diabetes. Mrs Pathos sleeps poorly, has lost her appetite and has lost a lot of weight. She is finding it difficult to carry out personal and domestic activities of daily living. She is tearful and has stopped visiting friends. Maria has recently been doing more of the household duties and getting the shopping. She feels very tired, and is finding it difficult to cope.

Describe the action you would take to promote the health and well-being of Mrs Pathos in relation to:

- physical health
- mental health
- social care needs.

Discussion

Table 16.1 summarizes some of the health needs of this patient and some actions that should be considered

Table 16.1 Meeting the health needs of the older adult.

Health and well-being	Needs	Action
Physical health	Osteoarthritis Diabetes Falls Pain Weight loss Fatigue Urinary tract infection	Communication Assessment Screening Investigation Information Treatment options Collaborative working
Mental health	Depression Bereavement and loss Insomnia	Communication Assessment Information Support Collaborative working

(Continued)

Scenario 16.2 *(Continued)*

Table 16.1 *(Continued)*

Social care	Loneliness Isolation Care support	Communication Assessment Investigation Information Collaborative working

On placement: checklist

- ❑ Were the patient's social circumstances recorded, e.g. who was in the household, fuel, social contacts, carers?
- ❑ Were the patient's mobility, oral health, lifestyle risks recorded?
- ❑ What strategies did you observe that were used to enable better communication?
- ❑ How did you ensure that care was personalized and the patient able to take control?
- ❑ Was there opportunity for the patient to ask questions?
- ❑ Did you or other staff speak to relatives or family members?
- ❑ Was the evironment confidential and free from distractions?
- ❑ Did you provide information about procedures and gain consent?
- ❑ Did you discuss goals and plans with the patient?
- ❑ Did you discuss goals and plans with the team?
- ❑ Did you document your actions and interventions clearly and concisely?
- ❑ Did you provide opportunities to discuss health issues or concerns?
- ❑ Did you provide information about services and resources available to promote health and well-being?

Key learning points

1. Many patients in primary and acute care will be older adults over the age of 60.
2. Many will be living with one or more long-term conditions.
3. The aim of health promotion is to help older people to manage their condition, live healthily and independently with quality of life to prevent future diseases.
4. For the frail elderly, a priority will be to meet physical care needs, ensuring safety asnd secirity, and having social contact, including being valued and respected.

Chapter summary

Older adults, defined here as those at least 65 years of age, are more likely to suffer from chronic illness and impairments in function and are more likely to take multiple medicines. It is very easy for the nurse to overlook the potential for health promotion while dealing with these immediate concerns. Primary prevention is aimed at preventing disease before it occurs and may focus on lifestyle advice to keep mobile and eat healthily or the benefits of flu immunization. Secondary prevention detects disease before it is usually found and includes screening, which is part of the GP contract. The agenda for later life (Age UK, 2013b) highlights the importance of challenging negative attitudes about later life, recognizing the contributions older people make and also the need to plan for later life. Health and care services need to recognize that health can be modified in older age and tackling risk factors such as high blood pressure, smoking and obesity can make a difference. Older people should have the opportunity and support to optimize their health and well-being through equitable access to prevention, treatment and rehabilitation delivered with dignity and compassion (Age UK, 2013b). Prevention and public health require collaborative working to address health and social care needs, improve later life and promote positive ageing.

Further reading and resources

Age UK provides resources for professionals including statistics and evidence reviews on health and well-being. Available at: http://www.ageuk.org.uk/professional-resources-home/knowledge-hub-evidence-statistics/evidence-reviews/.

The British Heart Foundation also has professional resources on issues such as falls prevention. Available at: http://www.bhfactive.org.uk/userfiles/Documents/FallsPreventionGuide2013.pdf.

The Cochrane Library has brought together evidence reviews on what works to keep older people physically active. Available at: http://www.thecochranelibrary.com/details/collection/2043267/Physical-activity-and-exercise-for-health-and-well-being-of-older-people.html.

NICE guidance exists on what works to promote mental well-being of older people. Available at: http://guidance.nice.org.uk/PH16.

Joseph Rowntree Foundation have a research and policy programme to improve the lives of older people that includes health care, housing and welfare. Available at: http://www.jrf.org.uk/work/workarea/better-life.

References

Age UK (2013a) *Later Life in the United Kingdom*. Age UK, London. Available at: http://www.ageuk.org.uk/Documents/EN-GB/Factsheets/Later_Life_UK_factsheet.pdf?dtrk=true.

Age UK (2013b) *Agenda for Later Life 2013: Improving Later Life in Tough Times*. Age UK, London.

Alzheimer's Society (2010) *Factsheet: Eating and Drinking*. Alzheimer's Society, London. Available at: http://www.alzheimers.org.uk/site/scripts/documents_info.php?documentID=149.

Alzheimer's Society (2013) *Dementia 2013: The Hidden Voice of Loneliness*. Alzheimer's Society, London. Available at: http://www.alzheimers.org.uk/dementia2013.

Bostock, S. and Steptoe, A. (2012) Association between low functional health literacy and mortality in older adults: longitudinal cohort study, *British Medical Journal*, **344**, e1602.

Carers UK (2012) *Statistics and Facts about Carers*. Available at: http://www.carersuk.org/newsroom/stats-and-facts.

Cattan, M., Kime, N. and Bagnal,l A-M. (2009) *Low Level Support for Socially Isolated Older People: An Evaluation of Telephone Befriending*, Age UK, Leeds.

Department of Health (2001) *National Service Framework for Older People*. DH, London.

Department of Health (2007) *National Stroke Strategy*. DH, London.

Department of Health (2010) *Carers and Personalisation: Improving Outcomes*. DH, London.

Department of Health (2012) *Health and Social Care Act*. TSO, London.

Department of Health (2013) *Reducing Harmful Drinking*. DH, London.

English Longitudinal Study of Ageing (2012) *The Dynamics of Ageing: Evidence from the English Longitudinal Study of Ageing 2002–2010 (Wave 5)*. Institute of Fiscal Studies, London.

Fox, J. (2005) The role of the expert patient in the management of chronic illness. *British Journal of Nursing*, **14** (1), 25–28.

Health Care Commission (2006) *Caring for People After They Have Had a Stroke. A Follow Up Survey of Patients*. Health Care Commission, London.

Health Protection Agency (2011) *Surveillance of Influenza and Other Respiratory Viruses in the UK, 2010–2011Rreport*, HPA, London.

Holt-Lunstad, J., Smith, T.B. and Layton, J.B. (2010) Social relationships and mortality risk: a meta-analytic review. *Public Library of Science - Medicine*, **7**, e1000316.

Katz, J., Holland, C., Peace, S. and Taylor, E. and Blood, I. (2011) *A Better Life: What older People with High Support Needs Value.* Joseph Rowntree Foundation, York.

Malnutrition Task Force (2013) *Prevention and Early Intervention of Malnutrition in Later Life: Best Practice Principles and Implementation Guide*. Malnutrition Task Force, London.

Melzer, D., Tavakoly, B., Winder, R. *et al.* (2012) *Health Care Quality for an Active Later Life: Improving Quality of Prevention and Treatment Through Information - England 2005 to 2012. A Report from the Peninsula College of Medicine and Dentistry Ageing Research Group for Age UK*. PCMD/University of Exeter, Exeter, UK. Available at: https://wombat.pcmd.ac.uk/document_manager/documents/files/epidemiology/Health_Care_Quality_for_an_Active_Later_Life_2012.pdf.

National Audit Office (2012) *Progress in Improving Stroke Care*. NAO, London.

National Patient Safety Agency (2007) *Water for Health: Hydration Best Practice Toolkit for Hospitals and Healthcare*, NPSA, London.

NICE (2013) *Falls: The Assessment and Prevention of Falls in Older People. CG161*, NICE, London. Available at: http://www.nice.org.uk/CG161.

ONS (Office for National Statistics) (2012) *Focus on Older People- Population Ageing in the UK and Europe*, ONS, South Wales. Available at: http://www.ons.gov.uk/ons/dcp171776_258607.pdf.

RCN (Royal College of Psychiatrists) (2011) *Our Invisible Addicts: First Report of the Older Persons' Substance Misuse Working Group of the Royal College of Psychiatrists*. RCPsych, London. Available at: http://www.rcpsych.ac.uk/files/pdfversion/cr165.pdf.

Scottish Health Survey (2011) *Topic Report on Older People's Health from the Scottish Health Survey Series*. Available at: http://www.scotland.gov.uk/Publications/2011/11/24083430/49.

Social Care Institute for Excellence (2009) *Nutritional Care and Older People*, SCIE, London. Available at: http://www.scie.org.uk/publications/ataglance/ataglance03.asp.

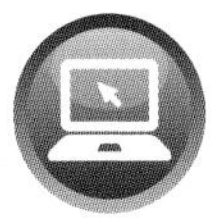

Don't forget to visit the companion website for this book: www.wileyfundamentalseries.com/healthpromotion where you can find self-assessment tests to check your progress.

17

Health promotion and nursing in the community

Sandra Horner

Senior Lecturer, Specialist Community Public Health Nursing, London South Bank University, London, UK

Maxine Jameson

Senior Lecturer, Specialist Community Public Health Nursing, London South Bank University, London, UK

Learning outcomes

By the end of this chapter you will be able to:

1. Define the role of the community nurse in health promotion
2. Have an understanding of nursing teams and roles in the community
3. Discuss community engagement and community development in the context of nursing practice
4. Develop strategies to encourage populations to take greater control over their health
5. Reflect on your own practice in promoting health in the community

Introduction

Primary care is the first point of contact for most people and is delivered by a wide range of independent contractors including GPs, dentists, pharmacists and optometrists. Clinical

Fundamentals of Health Promotion for Nurses, Second Edition. Edited by Jane Wills.

Companion website: www.wileyfundamentalseries.com/healthpromotion

commissioning groups (CCGs) and Local Area Teams (LATs) work to ensure that health and social care needs of local populations are met. Registered nurses are employed by the NHS in a variety of roles to improve health of communities, families and individuals in the community and encourage self-management of long-term conditions (see Chapter 9). *Liberating the Talents* (DH, 2002) identified three core functions for community nurses:

- first contact care: acute assessment, diagnosis, care treatment and referral;
- chronic disease management, continuing care and rehabilitation;
- public health: health protection and promotion programmes that improve health and reduce inequalities.

These functions are inter-related and influenced by each other. However, taking a public health approach and planning work around the needs of a specific population are an essential starting point for all nurses working within a community setting. This chapter introduces the principles of community-based health promotion work, including health needs assessment, patient and public involvement and community development. It challenges nursing students to consider whether they can move from a more expert-led, authoritarian role to one that encourages patients and the public to be more involved in the determinants of health – personally and in their community.

Defining community

Nurses work with communities and patients who are members of many communities and they need to understand communities and how to work with them. They also need to identify how to assess the needs of these communities. In order to gain a full understanding of what this means, it is necessary to define "community", which is not an easy thing to do.

Community can be defined in many ways; it is most commonly defined as a collective body of individuals identified by geography, common interests, concerns, characteristics or values (World Health Organization, 1998). In recent years, the definition of community from a social perspective has evolved from a structural focus of geographic boundaries to a focus on people interacting in social units and sharing common interests. The community in which people live and work is critical to health promotion and prevention; culture also is a large contributor to the character of a community.

Activity 17.1

Discuss a community you are familiar with, what defines that community?

Discussion

You may have mentioned an area that you live in, a group you belong to, or a characteristic of your identity such as your ethnicity or gender. Community is a group of people who have something in common.

These communities may share beliefs about their health and ill health and the ways in which they make health decisions. For example, the Mens Health Forum (www.menshealthforum.org.uk) exists to ensure that health services and policy take account of the specific experiences and needs of men and boys. Yet communities and groups are not necessarily homogeneous – though Black and minority ethnic groups have higher than average health and social care needs, there is a substantial variation in the health status of ethnic groups. It is important for the nurse to recognize difference and diversity but at the same time avoid stereotyping especially on the basis of supposed cultural differences. One way to avoid this is to work with groups and communities to identify their needs.

The concept of social inclusion/exclusion is used as a way of focusing on populations that do not make use of opportunities to participate in society, such as migrants or older people who may be marginalized, harder to reach, or excluded from mainstream services. These vulnerable or excluded groups may be seen as "communities" and targeted for particular services.

Activity 17.2

Consider a "community" or population group whose health needs are prioritized, e.g. teenage mothers, people living with HIV, farmworkers. Why are these groups targeted for particular interventions or services?

Discussion

An ethical rationale argues that targeting the most vulnerable and marginalized is needed to supplement a universal service if the needs of all population groups are to be met equally. An economic rationale argues that it is more cost-effective to provide resources to meet needs effectively rather than spend resources later to address the multiple social effects (e.g., acute and chronic ill health) resulting from a failure to meet needs. A scientific rationale rests on a notion of risk. Epidemiological evidence identifies population groups on the basis of their behavioural risk factors, environmental risk conditions, their health outcomes (i.e., ill health or premature death), or ease of access to care and services (Naidoo and Wills, 2010).

Defining community nursing

Some nurses work *in* communities in primary care. These nursing roles are varied as shown in Table 17.1 and include posts such as:

- health visitor
- practice nurse
- school nurse
- district nurse.

Table 17.1 The role of community nurses.

	Health visitor	School nurse	District nurse	Practice nurse
Posts	Staff nurse Nursery Nurse	Staff nurse Youth worker	Staff nurse or Community Nurse Specialist	Staff nurse
Focus	Under-5s	5–19 age group	Adults Sick/chronic illness Hospital discharge	Population
Setting	Community	School	Community	Health centre or general practice
Typical health promotion activity	Supporting new mothers Running health promotion programmes, e.g. breastfeeding, weaning, parenting Safeguarding children at risk Community development activities	Contribute to school health promotion programmes, e.g. sex education Advise young people on health issues such as diet, smoking, drugs Conduct health interviews Support parents and teachers Contribute to immunization and screening programmes such as the National Child Measurement Programme for obesity	Advice on healthy eating Mobility assessment and falls prevention Risk assessment for medication, drinking Linking to community support and social networks Support for carers	Opportunistic health education, e.g. during new patient medicals Advise on the management of long-term conditions Contribute to immunization and screening programmes e.g. Health checks Smoking cessation

The work of nurses in the community encompasses the promotion of health, healing, growth and development, as well as the prevention and treatment of disease, illness, injury and disability. Community-based nurses, and the health care assistants who work with them, enable people to achieve, maintain or recover independence where possible, minimizing distress and promoting quality of life (Sines *et al.*, 2013). They may work with specific population groups such as families or schoolchildren or they may help those with long-term conditions to better manage that condition and avoid hospital stays. The roles vary from providing one-to-one clinical care to the activities that a health visitor might do in working in the community such as running a support group or attending safeguarding meetings. Many of these roles have changed in the past decade and have moved towards a public health role with more of a population focus and an expectation of working in collaboration with local agencies, local communities and local authorities.

Nursing in the community is different from nursing in acute settings in several ways:

- The complexity of working with people over whom you have no authority.
- The uncertainty of the home environment, where the nurse is a guest with no right to enter or remain.
- The nurse–client relationship is very different in the community with frequently long relationships that allow for the development of a therapeutic and trusting bond between client and community nurse.
- The nurse provides a small amount of care, health maintenance and health promotion activities in comparison to patients and carers.
- In homes the nurse has to be observant, not just of the patient or client, but also of the carers, the other relatives and the setting in which they live. Observation of whether the family has the basic needs to live such as heating, food, running water, warm clothes is part of our duty of care.
- In the acute care setting, nursing staff make decisions around client care while in the home the client and family are encouraged to participate more in decision-making, with goals usually being more long-term outcomes.
- The nurse needs to assess whether anyone is in danger or at risk whether from domestic or elder abuse or injury or from medication abuse.

Priorities for health promotion in the community

Nurses who work in the community are regarded as public health workers and numerous policy documents signal this key aspect to their role (WHO, 2000; DH, 2004; RCN, 2007). The main priorities for all community nurses are to do the following:

- Influence healthy behaviours.
- Target vulnerable populations to improve health outcomes and access services.
- Promote social capital through building networks in communities.

Each community nursing role has different opportunities for health promotion. A new vision for district nursing published by the Queen's Nursing Institute in (QNI, 2013) highlights the opportunities that district nurses have to "make every contact count" in promoting healthier lifestyles because of the following factors:

- Accessibility (largest number of primary health care employees seeing 2.75 million people each year).
- Acceptability (referrals include chronic illness, terminal illness, incontinence, wound management, diabetes).

Several research studies have found, however, that their public health work is often confined to opportunistic health education (Whitehead, 2000).

Scenario 17.1

Alice is 60; she has heart failure, poorly controlled type 2 diabetes and extensive pressure ulcers and leg ulcers. She has attended accident and emergency department four times in the last month and each time had taken her own discharge before getting treatment. Alice lives with her son who works long hours and she has daughter with a young family who lives nearby, both have been struggling to cope with their mother's deteriorating condition. Alice is not known to any other services and is isolated and vulnerable.

- ❑ What are Alice's health promotion needs?

Discussion

The district nurse needs to encourage Alice to manage her diabetes medication and to be more mobile. The National Institute for Health and Clinical Excellence (NICE) (2009) suggests that between one-third and one-half of all medications prescribed for individuals with long-term conditions are not used in the intended manner. Communication and support are vital components in managing Alice's diabetes.

A systematic review of evidence of effective interventions to reduce isolation and loneliness in older people (Cattan et al., 2005) has found that one-to-one support, in the form of befriending, home visiting and carer support, is one of the most frequently provided activities to alleviate loneliness, and older people respond favourably to such support especially when the client and provider belong to the same generation, have common interests, and share a common culture and social background. Social activation programmes in sheltered accommodation and bereavement support for recently widowed older people have been found to reduce loneliness.

The long-standing role and purpose of health visiting have been to focus on families with young children. Early child development is vital in setting the stage for the child's future (adult) health. It is recognized as a key social determinant of health and health inequalities (see Chapter 2) and a critical period for intervention. There is also strong evidence to demonstrate that supporting new parents (particularly mothers) leads to improved health, social and educational outcomes for children (Marmot *et al.*, 2010). Following the death of Peter Connelly ("Baby P"), health visitors have been identified as central to the identification and protection of children known as safeguarding.

Case study 17.1

Safeguarding

Community nurses are constantly assessing the community in which they work and promoting harmony within the homes they visit as this is obviously conducive to health and well-being. However, abuse of human beings does occur, particular those who are vulnerable, they are usually at either end of the age range, that is children and older people but not always. Abuse of children is well recognized (Laming, 2009) and it is a community nurse's role to promote good parenting, providing children and adults with at least adequate self-esteem and social capital which can be tapped into when needed.

Elder abuse is an attack on any older individual's civil or human rights by another (Welsh Assembly, 2000). A community nurse may have encouraged independence, self-caring and mobility in her patient, but find evidence of financial, sexual or physical abuse for example. She or he needs to always be alert to the risks to her susceptible clients (www.elderabuse.org.uk).

Domestic abuse meaning intimate partner violence, is often hidden from professionals like community nurses for a considerable time before trust is established enough to disclose or there is a major incident which precipitates the vulnerable partner fleeing, often with the children (www.womensaid.org.uk). The health promotion role here for the community nurse has to be about capacity building within the family and the immediate community. If there are young children, then the health visitor may have asked direct questions about domestic violence around the time of birth, giving the mother opportunity to ask for support to build her self-esteem/resilience and empower her to leave if she would feel safer to do so. If this is not the case, then other means can be sought to safely offer support (if covertly) to this family. Cultural and religious issues need to be borne in mind here too. Some women will find it more difficult to leave even the most desperate, dangerous situations due to cultural beliefs.

Part of the work of the health visitor is in ensuring the development of the child in the family. The Healthy Child Programme (DH, 2009a, 2009b) provides the framework for an early intervention strategy for children from 0–19. The priorities are:

- 0–5 years : nutrition, active play and obesity prevention; immunization; personal, social and emotional development; speech, language and communication; and injury prevention.
- 5–19: prevention and early intervention; safeguarding; health and development reviews; screening programmes; immunization programmes; signposting services; environments that promote health; support for parents and carers (including those whose children have additional health needs).

Families receive different levels of intervention – the Universal Plus level, for example, includes a rapid response when families need specialist help. The Family Nurse Partnership (FNP) is an intensive, structured, home visiting programme which is offered to first-time parents under the age of 20 until the child is 2 years old. The early evaluation (http://www.iscfsi.bbk.ac.uk/projects/files/third_year.pdf) suggests good outcomes in relation to breastfeeding, use of contraception, positive parenting, and return to education.

The role of the school nurse in the community is to support children and young people to achieve the best possible health, stay safe and achieve as they grow up. This involves:

- reviewing health at key stages and supporting the development of children's personal health guides
- providing general information, advice and support about health issues such as diet and nutrition, physical activity, emotional well-being, puberty, smoking and sexual health and about where to get further help and advice.

Although stretched as a workforce across schools in all the home countries of the UK, the contribution of school nurses is valued by young people who appreciate their clinical knowledge and the confidentiality afforded to them. In particular, young people expressed a preference for a nurse, rather than a teacher, when it comes to discussing the sensitive issues covered in Sex and Relationships Education (SRE) and Personal, Social, Health and Economics (PSHE) Education sessions (Thomas Coram Research Unit, 2009).

Case study 17.2

The National Child Measurement Programme

The National Child Measurement Programme (NCMP) is one element of the government's *Healthy Weight, Healthy Lives* strategy (DH, 2008). It aims to gather population level data to analyse trends in childhood obesity, inform local planning and engage with families regarding healthy lifestyles and weight issues. Routine feedback of NCMP results informs parents if their child's weight is unhealthy. School nurses are instrumental in weighing and measuring reception and Year-6 aged children for the NCMP on an annual basis. They are also the first point of contact for parents who are concerned about their child's weight.

Implementing policy initiatives such as the NMCP has implications for practice. Several surveys of school nurses have found that the targets for weighing and measuring set for PCTs had an influence on school nurses' ability to deliver other parts of the government's obesity strategy. A study commissioned by the DH on the role of nurses in schools (Chase *et al.*, 2010) likewise concluded that the NCMP took up a substantial amount of the time of school nurses working in primary schools and detracted from the proactive health promotion and prevention work that they could otherwise be doing.

For the community nurse, supporting people in the community means understanding and addressing the social context in which people live and the political, social and economic factors that influence behaviour, together with the ability to identify and address community priorities through community engagement. The community nurse needs to be involved in all aspects of health not just focus on medical issues. Issues such as housing and fuel poverty all affect health, it is not enough for the community nurse to support clients with asthma when they live in damp housing that constantly exacerbates their condition. Community nurses need to be able to empower clients and support them to make changes in their lives that will help them to improve their living conditions. Nurses in the community need to work with other professionals and non-professionals to promote health, working, for example, with schools to look at school meals and exercise, working with the police to ensure public parks are safe and inviting, working with housing departments to ensure families have dry, warm homes.

Scenario 17.2

Jane and Michael live on a low-rise estate in the Midlands. They share their 3-bedroomed flat with their two children, Tamsin, aged 11, and Flora, aged 2. Also Jane's grannie who brought her up has recently come to live with them. She is 70 now and a heavy smoker. Michael's son from a previous relationship, Dan, who is nearly 16, likes to stay at weekends. Jane works three nights a week as a barmaid in the local pub while Michael looks after the children. Michael is a warehouseman working shifts. He does not really get on with Jane's grannie and there is some friction.

- Dan: enjoys his weekends with his Dad's family. What might be a threat to this enjoyment? Are there any health promotion issues to be considered for a young person in this age group?
- Tamsin: Is in Year 6 and is hoping to get a place with her friends at the local comprehensive but is anxious because places are sought after. She resents her great-grannie because she now has to share a room with Flora. Suffers from mild asthma. What are the health threats here? Who might the team collaborate with to promote the health of this child/family?
- Flora: will be mostly at home with Jane and grannie. Her development has been normal to this point. What health promotion strategy could be used to keep Flora healthy and avoid the effects of e.g. secondary smoke?
- Grannie: How can her health status be assessed?
- Michael: What help might you offer him/identify him as needing?
- Jane: What are her health promotion needs?

Discussion

- *Dan, aged 15: The threats to his enjoyment of family life might be overcrowding in the flat and friction between his Dad and step-great-grannie. He is soon eligible for a DPT booster (diphtheria, tetanus and pertussis) and could be advised about this preventive strategy. Sexual health awareness could also be promoted. This young man will be developing independence so lifestyle issues are relevant such as healthy diet, sleep patterns and avoiding risky behaviours such as substance misuse. He may have questions about bodily changes if he is comfortable asking or the nurse may act as a referral agent.*

- *Tamsin, aged 11: Her relationship with her school friends will be very important. The cigarette smoke from Grannie may be exacerbating the asthma. The asthma needs to remain stable and the School Nurse can support Jane to help with this. Referral can be made to the transition team in school making them aware of Tamsin's anxiety about moving school. Collaborative work can then be put in place.*
- *Flora, aged 2: Appears to thrive. The health visitor could suggest that great-grannie smoke outside the flat and change clothes before handling Flora.*
- *Grannie: The health visitor might assess whether great-grannie is ready to give up smoking or at least cut down and use motivational interviewing techniques (see Chapter 12).*
- *Michael: May appreciate talking to the school nurse about the frustrations he feels juggling the needs of all his children including overcrowded housing, possibly leading to a referral to Housing based on health grounds.*

Strategies for health promotion in the community

Health promotion places an emphasis on empowerment and people taking control over their health. Aspects of this are about increasing information to enable people to make choices but it also includes improvements in a person's self-efficacy or ability to do something and their self-esteem. Other characteristics concern group dynamics and refer to improved abilities to support and network in a community, sometimes known as capacity building. Community development (CD) is one approach to developing communities which is based on the idea that people in communities already know what the issues and problems are and how to solve them. The CD approach can assist communities to undertake projects in planned and structured ways, acknowledging the skills and knowledge of local people.

The following scenario illustrates the key features of health promotion practice and community involvement in health issues.

Scenario 17.3

Helen is a community nurse working in primary care in a large urban area in the UK. Her work involves providing educational opportunities for expectant and new mothers to ensure that they have the knowledge and skills necessary to give their children a healthy start in life. Many of these parents are considered "at-risk" because they live on a housing estate in a deprived area where they face barriers to good health such as low income, social isolation and limited employment skills.

Participants meet every week. At the end of each class, participants identify the topics they want addressed at the next session. In response to their information needs, Helen covers

(*Continued*)

Scenario 17.3 (*Continued*)

topics such as the birthing process, breastfeeding, healthy eating during and after pregnancy, smoking, drugs, alcohol, healthy child development, making baby food, and parenting skills. To ensure that participants have adequate resources to meet their nutritional needs, Healthy Start (food and milk) vouchers are provided. The programme also provides access to childcare so participants can attend the classes.

While the women were satisfied with the classes, there was a growing concern that other important health issues in the community were not being addressed. Over time, discussions held during the classes focused on other barriers to health faced by participants and their families, such as a lack of recreation facilities for young children and a shortage of affordable day care spaces. While many of the women expressed their need to get a job and support their families once their children were old enough, they were concerned that barriers such as a lack of proficiency in English and a lack of job training programmes in the community would limit their ability to do so.

In response to the needs expressed by participants, Helen contacted several community service agencies in the neighbourhood. She collaborated with the other agencies to organize a community-wide forum at one of the community centres. This event resulted in the formation of an inter-sectoral committee made up of agency representatives and community residents.

Over the next two years, the committee pursued activities in response to the needs and priorities identified by community members. These included:

- one of the Sure Start programmes providing parents with access to computers so they could develop résumés and upgrade their computer skills;
- a successful proposal for funding which allowed a local day care centre to offer free half-day "play-days" twice a week for children aged 2–4 years;
- residents successfully lobbying the council to clean and up-grade playground facilities in two housing estates;
- the local library expanding its story-telling programme to include local language stories every week;
- the committee organizing fun days as a social event for community residents during the summer;
- Helen's agency setting up an education and support group for new fathers.

What features of health promotion are evident in Helen's practice?

Adapted from: Ontario Health Promotion Resource System (2005).

Discussion

The scenario highlights:

- *a holistic view of health that went beyond the physical health status of new and expectant mothers and children to encompass the social and mental dimensions of health and well-being;*
- *a focus on participatory approaches that entailed the direct involvement of community members in planning and implementing activities in response to their shared health concerns;*
- *a focus on the determinants of health through activities addressing the social, economic and environmental factors contributing to health such as employment, recreation, social support, literacy skills, healthy child development and access to childcare;*
- *building on existing strengths and assets by making use of existing community resources and facilities wherever possible and building on the capacity of community residents;*
- *using multiple, complementary strategies including health education, self help/mutual aid, organizational change, community mobilization and advocacy.*

Community nurses, with their considerable knowledge and unique roles within the local communities they serve, have long been identified as being in an ideal position to be at the forefront of initiatives to tackle healthy lifestyles (CPHVA, 1999; DH, 2011a, 2011b). Their everyday experience of home visiting and their long-term knowledge of individuals, families and networks built up over time mean they possess an abundance of knowledge about the health and social needs of both individuals and their communities and about how those needs can be met. As public health nurses move into the newly formed public health teams within local government there will be increased opportunities for greater engagement with the communities in which they work and perhaps more opportunities for community development work which has never been prominent in the demanding caseloads of community nurses despite its potential : health visitors, for example, facilitated a radical transformation on estates in Redruth and Falmouth in Cornwall in the 1990s through this approach (Stutely, 2002).

On placement: checklist

- What particular effects of health inequality and poverty have you noticed on community visits?
- What examples are there of building capacity in individuals and developing lifeskills and ability to engage with mainstream services?
- Did you observe opportunistic health promotion about healthy eating, physical activity or substance use?
- What examples are there of signposting or referral to other agencies?
- How do community groups help to build knowledge and skills?
- What examples did you observe of inter-agency working?

Key learning points

1. Nurses are seen as acceptable to the public and part of the community and so have a legitimate health-promoting role in the community.
2. Nurses have extensive knowledge of the communities that they serve and their needs and have a long-term relationship with individuals and can tailor health messages to individuals and communities.
3. Nurses in the community are known as public health nurses.

Chapter summary

Community nursing is about building relationships with an individual or a family. The impact of the work of the community nurse on the overall community can be difficult to measure because the effects are so far-reaching. When a person's health and social needs are met, he or she is more likely to behave in ways that will promote his or her overall health. This chapter discussed the role of nurses in the community, the differences between nursing in hospitals and clients homes and the concept of community.

Further reading and resources

Whether intending to become a public health nurse or not, these two resource packs given an insight into the work of school nurse and health visitor. Although over ten years old, the principles are still relevant.

School Nurse Practice Development Resource Pack (2006). Available at:
http://webarchive.nationalarchives.gov.uk/20130107105354/http://www.dh.gov.uk/prod_consum_dh/groups/dh_digitalassets/@dh/@en/documents/digitalasset/dh_4132070.pdf.

Health Visitor Development Resource pack (2001). Available at: http://webarchive.nationalarchives.gov.uk/20130107105354/http://www.dh.gov.uk/prod_consum_dh/groups/dh_digitalassets/@dh/@en/documents/digitalasset/dh_4058110.pdf.

Sines, D. *et al.* (2013) *Community Health Care Nursing*, 5th edn. Wiley, Chichester.
A useful introduction to all aspects of the community nurse role.

References

Cattan, M., White, M., Bond, J. and Learmouth, A. (2005) Preventing social isolation and loneliness among older people: a systematic review of health promotion interventions. *Ageing & Society*, **25**, 41–67.

Chase, E., Warwick, I., Hollingworth, K., *et al.* (2010) *Promoting the Health of Children and Young People Through Schools: The Role of the Nurse. Final Research Report*. Department of Health, London.

Community Practitioners and Health Visitors Association (CPHVA) (1999) *Joined up Working: Community Development in Primary Care*. CPHVA, London.

DH (Department of Health) (2002) *Liberating the Public Health Talents of Community Practitioners and Health Visitors*. DH, London.

DH (Department of Health) (2004) *Choosing Health: Making Healthy Choices Easier*. DH, London. Available at: http://webarchive.nationalarchives.gov.uk/+/dh.gov.uk/en/publicationsandstatistics/publications/publicationspolicyandguidance/dh_4094550.

DH (Department of Health) (2008) *Healthy Weight, Healthy Lives*. Available at: http://webarchive.nationalarchives.gov.uk/20100407220245/http:/www.dh.gov.uk/prod_consum_dh/groups/dh_digitalassets/documents/digitalasset/dh_084024.pdf.

DH (Department of Health) (2009a) *Healthy Child Programme: Pregnancy and the First 5 Years of Life*. Available at: https://www.gov.uk/government/publications/healthy-child-programme-pregnancy-and-the-first-5-years-of-life.

DH (Department of Health) (2009b) *Healthy Child Programme from 5–19*. Available at: http://webarchive.nationalarchives.gov.uk/+/www.dh.gov.uk/en/publicationsandstatistics/publications/publicationspolicyandguidance/dh_107566.

DH (Department of Health) (2011a) *Health Visitor Implementation Plan 2011–2015: Call to Action*. DH, London.

DH (Department of Health) (2011b) *Getting It Right for Children, Young People and Families: Maximising the Contribution of the School Nursing Team: Vision and Call to Action*. DH, London.

DH (Department of Health) (2012) *Getting It Right for Children Families and Young People*. DH, London. Available at: http://www.dh.gov.uk/prod_consum_dh/groups/dh_digitalassets/@dh/@en/documents/digitalasset/dh_133352.pdf.

Laming, Lord (2009) *The Protection of Children in England: A Progress Report*. London: TSO. Available at http://dera.ioe.ac.uk/8646/1/12_03_09_children.pdf.

Marmot, M. *et al.* (2010) *Fair Society, Healthy Lives: Strategic Review of Health Inequalities in England Post-2010*. DH, London. Available at: http://www.instituteofhealthequity.org/projects/fair-society-healthy-lives-the-marmot-review.

Naidoo, J. and Wills, J. (2010). *Developing Practice for Public Health and Health Promotion*. Baillière Tindall, London.

National Institute for Health and Clinical Excellence (2009) *Medicines Adherence: Involving Patients in Decisions about Prescribed Medicines and Supporting Adherence*. Clinical guideline 76. National Collaborating Centre for Primary Care, London.

Queens Nursing Institute (2013) *A New Vision for District Nursing*. Available at: http://www.qni.org.uk/docs/2020_Vision.pdf.

RCN (Royal College of Nursing) (2007) *Nurses as Partners in Delivering Public Health*. London: RCN.

Sines, D., Aldridge-Bent, S., Fanning, A., Farrelly, P., Potter, K. and Wright, J. (eds) (2013) *Community Health Care Nursing* 5th edn. Wiley, Chichester.

Stutely, H. (2002) The Beacon Project: a community-based health improvement project. *The British Journal of General Practice*, **52** (Suppl.), S44.

Thomas Coram Research Unit (2009) *Promoting the Health and Wellbeing of Children and Young People Through Schools: The Role of the Nurse*. Institute of Education, University of London, London.

Welsh Assembly (2000) *In Safe Hands: Implementing Adult Protection Procedures in Wales* National Assembly for Wales, Cardiff.

Whitehead, D. (2000) The role of community-based nurses in health promotion. *British Journal of Community Nursing*, **5** (12), 604–609.

WHO (World Health Organization) (1998) *Health Promotion Glossary*. WHO, Geneva.

WHO (World Health Organization) (2000) *Munich Declaration: Nurses and Midwives: A Force for Health 2000*. Available at: www.euro.who.int/AboutWHO/Policy/20010828_4

Don't forget to visit the companion website for this book: www.wileyfundamentalseries.com/healthpromotion where you can find self-assessment tests to check your progress.

18

Children's nursing and health promotion

Jane Wills

Professor, Health Promotion, London South Bank University, London, UK

Matt Lester

Senior Lecturer, Child Nursing, London South Bank University, London, UK

Learning outcomes

By the end of this chapter you will be able to:

1. Describe the role of the nurse in health promotion when nursing children
2. Outline the priorities for children's health
3. Outline approaches and strategies to facilitate healthier lifestyles including health education, health information, individual, group and peer education

Introduction

Children's nurses care for children and young people, from birth to mid-to-late teens, and in exceptional circumstances in their young twenties, in a wide range of health care and community settings. They care for those who are sick or injured or have life-limiting illnesses and work with them to promote healthy behaviours and prevent ill health. They have been instrumental in promoting the welfare of children in hospital and ensuring that children who need nursing are treated with respect as equal members of society and have information to enable them to

Fundamentals of Health Promotion for Nurses, Second Edition. Edited by Jane Wills.

Companion website: www.wileyfundamentalseries.com/healthpromotion

take greater control over their health according to their age. They also seek to protect children from abuse and neglect, and work in partnership with other agencies to promote child safety.

Activity 18.1

What does health mean for the children's nurse?

Discussion

Defining health is not always easy. Some argue that health is to be free from disease or illness, others say to be healthy allows individuals to lead and independent life (see Chapter 1). So the children's nurse needs to take into consideration the child's age, their development, both cognitive and physical, any chronic illness they may have or any disability, when considering what health means in relation to a child. At one end of the spectrum there may be a child, fit and well, reaching all developmental milestones at the expected times, and towards the other end is a child who has a profound developmental delay, unable to speak, unsure if they can see, hear or understand, who requires a ventilator and tracheostomy to breathe, a gastrostomy tube to be fed and 24-hour care. Yet each of these child's parents may regard their child as healthy and flourishing within their own potential.

As the nurse's primary focus is to assist the child or young person and their family to prevent or manage the physiological, physical, social, psychological and spiritual effects of a health problem or condition and its treatment, the role encompasses health promotion and health education (RCN, 1991). However, there is little to support the nurse in this role and it is rarely seen as a discrete area of practice. For example, the desired outcomes when nursing a sick child relate to the following:

- successful disease management and reduced hospitalizations (secondary prevention, see Chapter 1);
- improved knowledge through health education;
- improved health outcomes such as reduced risk of developing a condition and improved general health (primary prevention, see Chapter 1);
- parental education and parental support (health education) which can empower the parent to cope with a sick child and also to recognize when a child is becoming unwell.

A national consultation in 2003 that preceded the publication of a government Green Paper on children, "Every Child Matters" (DfE, 2003) identified five outcomes as key to well-being in childhood:

- *being healthy*: to enjoy good physical and mental health and living a healthy lifestyle;
- *staying safe*: being protected from harm and neglect
- *enjoying and achieving*: getting the most out of life and developing the skills for adulthood;

- *making a positive contribution*: being involved with the community and society and not engaging in anti-social or offending behaviour;
- *economic well-being*: not being prevented by economic disadvantage from achieving their full potential in life.

Chapter 3 explored different models of health promotion. Using the seven domains of Tannahill's model, it is possible to identify the focus for the children's nurse:

1. preventative health services, such as developmental checks to monitor a child's growth or immunization programmes;
2. preventative health education to have a positive influence on a healthy lifestyle, such as exercise and play activities;
3. preventative health protection, such as the legal requirement for a child to be in an appropriate seat or booster seat;
4. health education for preventative health protection which is seeking to persuade policymakers for greater protection such as lobbying for a ban on smoking in cars or campaigning to provide better school meals;
5. positive health education, to reinforce the benefits of exercise;
6. positive health protection aims to make it easier to adopt healthier choices such as healthier food in hospitals or making hospitals completely smoke-free sites;
7. health education aimed at positive health promotion such as food labelling.

A scoping review of the contribution of nurses, midwives and health visitors to child health (While *et al.*, 2005) identified the problems of distinguishing the health promotion contribution. While it was evident across the integrated domains of health promotion (education, protection and preventive), health education remains the dominant mode. Health education methods were seen as:

1. therapeutic communication (developing a supportive relationship);
2. individual and group health education interventions;
3. peer group initiatives (facilitating young people to support each other in developing health promoting behaviours);
4. preventative treatment (such as the mass immunization programme);
5. helping young people access health information using methods such as open access health clinics.

Figure 18.1 illustrates the scope and levels of health promotion. Midwives, health visitors and school nurses all have a key role to play in promoting children's health in the early years and at school in the community (see Chapter 17), children's nursing is a specialty within nursing which, it is argued, is not simply general nursing at a special age period. Part of children's nurse training focuses on care of the hospitalized child which includes advanced clinical procedures and the use of technology. Advice and support in the home may be by health visitors or the community children's nurse. Paediatric community nursing services enable treatment at home, thereby avoiding hospital admission but services vary across England.

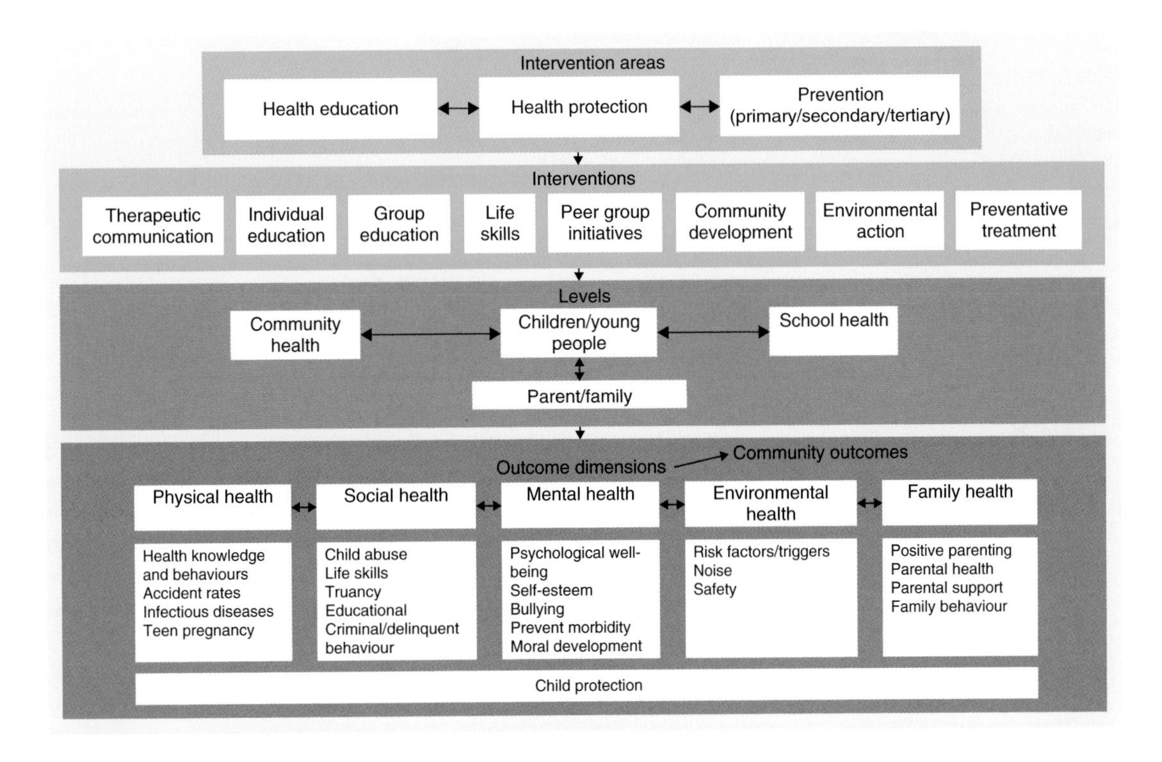

Figure 18.1 The contribution of health promotion. Source: While *et al.*, 2005, Figure 4, p. 70. Reproduced with permission of the National Co-ordinating Centre for NHS Service Delivery and Organisation.

Priorities in health promotion for children

The central importance of the children's nurse is shown by the following figures on the number of children who use health care services:

- There are more than 1.7 million admissions to hospital of children aged 14 and under (including babies born in hospital) each year.
- There are around 3 million attendances in A&E of children up to 16, and 4.5 million outpatient appointments each year.
- Around 1 in 10 consultations in GP practices each year are for children aged 14 and under.
- Over 100000 children and young people aged up to 18 years received some form of care from child and adolescent mental health services each year.

Activity 18.2

What would you say were the three main priorities for health promotion for children?

Discussion

UK policy highlights overweight and obesity, improving access to treatment, reducing accidental injuries, increasing immunizations against childhood diseases, safeguarding children and mental health promotion.

Child Health Profiles provide a snapshot of child health and well-being for each local authority in England using key health indicators, which enables comparison locally, regionally and nationally (available at the Child and Maternal Health Observatory website: www.chimat.org.uk). The profiles concentrate on different indicators, e.g. infant death, teenage pregnancy, dental health, immunization, obesity, smoking in pregnancy, breastfeeding.

England has one of the highest mortality rates in Europe for those aged 0–14 (see figure 18.2).

- Death rates for illnesses that rely heavily on primary care services (e.g. asthma, meningococcal disease, pneumonia) are higher in the UK and the UK has the worst asthma mortality rate among 0-14-year-olds among eight European nations and was fourth worst out of 15 for pneumonia deaths.
- Survival rates for childhood cancer are lower.

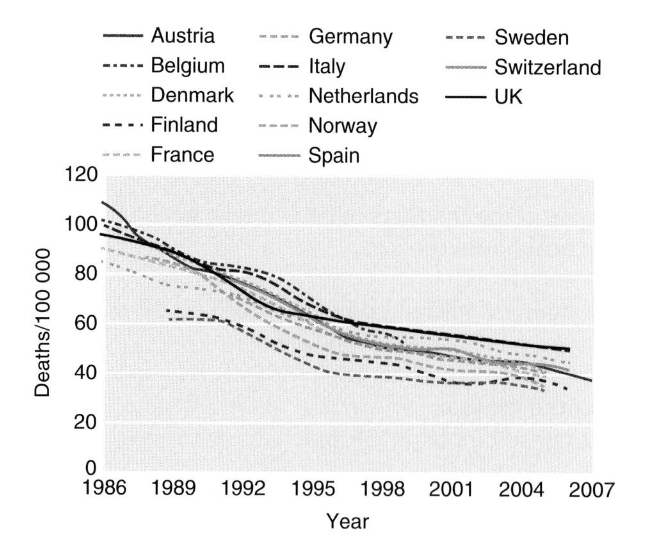

Figure 18.2 Infant mortality in Europe. Source: Wolfe *et al.*, 2011. Reproduced with permission from the *British Medical Journal*.

- Diabetic control markers in children are significantly worse than in other countries with comparable information.
- More than 1 in 5 children are overweight or obese by age 3.

Activity 18.3

Consider the following information on breastfeeding from the Infant Feeding Survey and identify the main priorities for child health interventions.

- The initial breastfeeding rate in 2010 was highest in England at 83% (compared with 74% in Scotland, 71% in Wales, and 64% in Northern Ireland). Exclusive breastfeeding at six weeks was 24% in England and 22% in Scotland, compared to 17% in Wales and 13% in Northern Ireland.
- Across the UK, at three months, the number of mothers breastfeeding exclusively was 17% (up from 13% in 2005) and at four months, it was 12% (up from 7% in 2005). However, exclusive breastfeeding at six months remains at around 1%.
- Rates of "any breastfeeding" showed a rise. At six weeks, the number of women breastfeeding at all was 48% in 2005 and 55% in 2010, while at six months they were 25% in 2005 and 34% in 2010.
- The survey also found that mothers are introducing solids later, with a significant fall in the number introducing solids by four months from 51% in 2005 to 30% in 2010.
- Breastfeeding was most common among mothers who were: aged 30 or over, from minority ethnic groups, who had left education aged over 18, in managerial and professional occupations and living in the least deprived areas.

Discussion

A priority is to get mothers to breastfeed for longer and to support them to do so as many give up within two weeks. Breastfeeding should be promoted to younger women and those in areas of disadvantage. Education on later weaning is also a priority.

In addition, the UK has currently the highest birth rate in 40 years, which adds further weight to the case for addressing key child health and well-being challenges.

What happens to children before they are born and in their early years can affect their health and opportunities later in life. For example, babies that are breastfed have less chance of getting infections or of becoming obese and therefore developing type 2 diabetes and other illnesses when they get older. The Marmot Review (2010) showed clearly that those who grow up in a safe environment, with good education and have a healthy relationship with their parents are more likely to do better as they go through life.

The UK has marked inequalities in child health and the gap between the most and the least disadvantaged children has widened in the last decade. According to Roberts (2012), children born into poverty are more likely than their better-off neighbours:

- to die in the first year of life;
- to be born small, to be born early, or both;
- to be bottle fed;
- to die or be seriously injured in a childhood accident;
- to smoke and have a parent who smokes;
- to become overweight or obese;
- to have or father children before they are ready to;
- to parent alone;
- to die younger.

Mortality, breastfeeding and accidental death in childhood and other health-related factors all form a gradient from the poorest doing worst to the least poor tending to do best.

Children's health has been a government priority for more than a decade in an attempt to reduce health and social inequalities, as a consequence of some high profile child abuse cases and in recognition of changes in health care delivery which gives a much stronger voice to patients, including children, in decision-making. The developments of child health promotion that focus on child health promotion, children's services and child protection are outlined in Table 18.1.

Table 18.1 Some key policy developments in child health promotion.

1999	Sure Start children's centres for children up to the age of 5 introduced
2002	*Preventing Accidental Injury: Priorities for Action* published by the Department of Health
2004	"National Service Framework for Children, Young People and Maternity Services"
	Choosing Health: Making Healthy Choices Easier, a White Paper on health promotion published by the Department of Health
	Every Child Matters: Change for Children that sets out new services and emphasis on children published by the Department for Education
	The Children's Act passed
	"Getting it Right for Every Child", the Scottish government review of the country's child protection and youth justice system. Getting it Right for Every Child is now the name of the Scottish government's overall approach to supporting children and young people
2007	The Children's Plan published

2008	Healthy Child Programme launched by the Department of Health that sets out a health development programme for every child from 0–19
2009	"Healthy Lives, Brighter Futures: A Strategy for Children and Young People's Health" launched and in Northern Ireland, "Healthy Child, Healthy Future: A Framework for Universal Child Health".
	The Protection of Children in England: A Progress Report (the Laming Report) published
2010	The Munro Review of child protection in England published and final report, *A child-centred system* published in 2011
	Professor Sir Ian Kennedy's report *Getting it Right for Children and Young People* finds that NHS services are patchy and much greater integration is needed and children should be at the centre of service delivery
	Healthy Lives, Healthy People, a `White Paper, is published by the DH which sets out the Healthy Child Programme, the role of health visitors and the Family Nurse Partnership
2012	The Children and Young People's Health Outcomes Forum report sets new quality standards and clinical indicators
2013	"Working together to Safeguard Children" sets out the core requirements for services

The Healthy Child Programme (HCP) is the universal clinical and public health programme for children and families from pregnancy to 19 years of age. The HCP, led by health visitors and their teams, offers every child a schedule of health and development reviews, screening tests, immunizations, health promotion guidance and support for parents tailored to their needs, with additional support when needed and at key times.

The service is built on a principle of "progressive universalism" – a universal service is offered to every family and the progressive services are for children and families with additional needs and risks. Table 18.2 shows the range of preventive and early intervention services for different levels of risk, need and protective factors for newborns. The priorities are to address:

- Breastfeeding initiation and prevalence at 6–8 weeks after birth.
- Child development at 2–2½ years.
- Excess weight in 4–5-year-olds.
- Hospital admissions caused by unintentional and deliberate injuries in under-5s.
- Access to non-cancer screening programmes.
- Population vaccination coverage.
- Infant mortality.
- Tooth decay in children aged 5.
- Improving the wider determinants of health school readiness.

Table 18.2 Progressive universal service for newborns as part of the Child Health Promotion Programme.

New baby review by 14 days	
Universal	**Progressive**
• Infant feeding • Promoting sensitive parenting • Promoting development • Assessing maternal mental health • SIDS • Keeping safe	• Babies with health or developmental problems or abnormalities, including prematurity and low birthweight • Parents who smoke • Children at risk of obesity • Parental relationships • Maternal depression

Strategies for health promotion with children

Health surveillance

Child health surveillance and screening have been central to monitoring children's health and development and are regarded as a key part of secondary prevention. *Health for All Children* (Hall, 1989) established the tests and procedures carried out by health care professionals on children in the first few years of life which focus on primary prevention as well as identifying health problems. The Hall Reports became fundamental to the development of child health services. The fourth edition of *Health for All Children* (Hall and Elliman, 2006), commonly known as Hall 4, included recommendations for a streamlined surveillance programme, with even greater emphasis on health promotion and primary prevention.

Activity 18.4

You are working as a Children's Community Nurse in a GP surgery. Part of your role is to screen new patients after they have registered with the GP. Today you meet a mother and her 4-year-old son who have recently both registered. The child has a history of atopic eczema. Consider what aspects of the child development and well-being would need to be assessed by the nurse.

Discussion

The nurse will measure the child's height and weight (and plot it on the growth charts in the child's Red Book [the Personal Child Health Record (PCHR)] if they have brought it with them.) This will allow the practice nurse to see if the child is growing at a steady rate or are they showing signs of malnutrition if their rate of growing in both height and weight have slowed down. If the family have moved regularly over the past 5 years, the nurse may want to ask about what GPs they have been registered with. If the family have moved after only a short period of time in one house, did they register with a GP? It may be possible that the child has missed some developmental checks. The nurse may discuss any missed immunizations and discuss with the mother if there was any reason why they were not given on time. If it was simply because the family were moving house, which can be appreciated as key life moment and it was forgotten, then the nurse may make arrangements for the immunizations to be given.

In relation to the child's eczema, the nurse will conduct a holistic assessment that considers (NICE, 2007):

- *Diet and allergies: Are there known food allergies or other allergies such as hay fever? Is the child receiving adequate nutrition? Are there other known allergies that exacerbate the eczema? Does the child need a referral to a dietitian?*
- *Social assessment: Who does the child live with and in what kind of housing? Is the school /nursery understanding and helpful?*
- *Psychological assessment: How does living with eczema affect the child, siblings and carers? Is the child subjected to teasing or bullying? Are there concerns about the child's mood or behaviour such as withdrawal, self-consciousness, anxiety, or dependence?*

Improving access to information

Patient-centred care includes empowering the patient to take control over their health through the provision of clear and accessible information and the involvement of the patient in decision-making about their care. The Children's National Service Framework (DH, 2003) highlights the need for children and parents to be given the support and information they need to understand and cope with illness or injury. This forms the basis for family-centred care that children's nurses deliver.

Children and young people who have chronic health conditions or need operations do not always have access to the high-quality, child-friendly information that is matched with their age, circumstances and is relevant to them at key points, such as at diagnosis, starting school, changing school, growing up with the condition, lifestyle issues and the transition to adult care. For example, the government announced in March 2012 that pupils in schools in England should have better access to their school nurses and should be able to text them to make an appointment (DH, 2012).

In hospitals and clinics, children need to be informed and involved in decision-making about:

- the care they receive;
- medicines they may need to continue at home (liquid vs. tablet);
- specific instructions to ensure optimum effect (such as when to ingest);
- how to explain their condition to others.

A report on health information for children and young people (Williams *et al.*, 2011) highlights the range of information that is available from commercially produced publications, the internet and telephone services but not all of these are quality-assured or tailored to the child's needs.

Activity 18.5

Figure 18.3 is an example of information produced for children about epilepsy. What is the message of this leaflet?

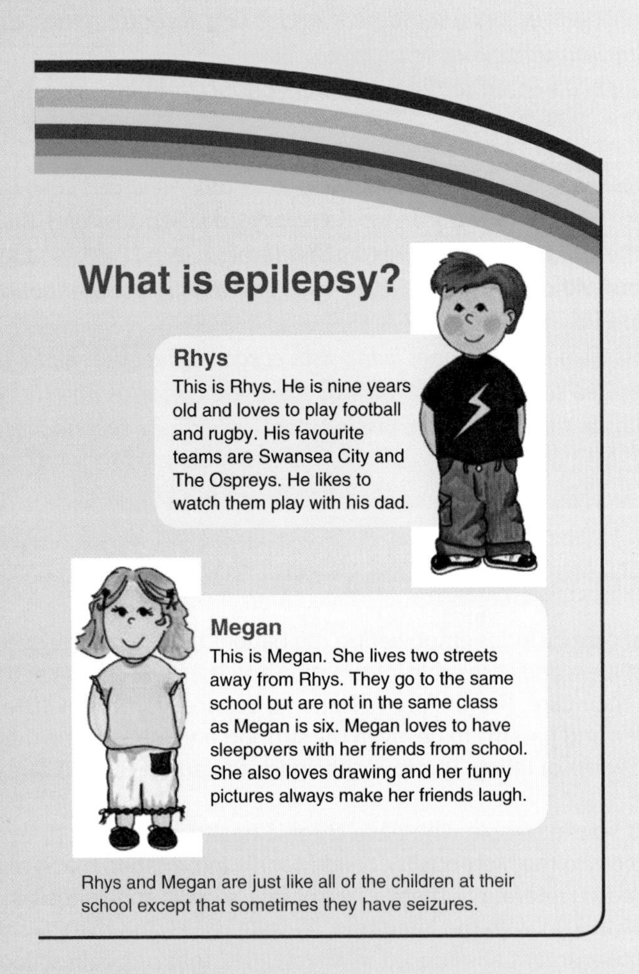

Figure 18.3 Information for children on epilepsy. Source: Children's Epilepsy Service, Swansea NHS Trust. Reproduced with permission from Abertawe Bro Morgannwg University Health Board.

Discussion

The message of this leaflet is intended as an empowering one – that the child or young person living with the illness may live a "normal" life. It aims to counter the negative social views of epileptic seizures by describing them as constituting a "minor" difference between a child with epilepsy and those who do not (e.g. "Rhys and Megan are just like all of the other children at their school except that sometimes they have seizures"). The leaflet also suggests that a child with epilepsy is just like a "normal" boy or girl (e.g. Rhys "loves to play football and rugby"; Megan "loves to have sleepovers with her friends from school"). As the Child Health Information project identifies, this is an example of information that presents a message that the child can aim "for a very definite ideal, a clear model of childhood" (Williams et al., 2011, p. 81).

The health information needs of a child living with a condition change as they grow up. For example, a child of 7 who is newly diagnosed with diabetes may have only a limited understanding of the causes of their condition and their main priority may be to be accepted among their peers and to feel safe at school, their teachers knowing what to do should the child become hypoglycaemic and their emergency glucose supply being in an accessible place. In later teenage years, the young person needs to know how to manage their diet as their lifestyle becomes less regular and also know the impact of alcohol consumption on their diabetes.

Case study 18.1

HELP – Harmonising Education about Leukaemia for Parents

Acute lymphoblastic leukaemia (ALL) is the most commonly diagnosed childhood cancer, with up to 400 children diagnosed every year in the UK. When a child is diagnosed with leukaemia, their parents worry a great deal about how to look after their child and how to talk to them about their illness and their treatment. While older children often communicate directly with health professionals, children aged 4–11 years rely primarily on their parents as their main source of information and parents must first understand the complex issues and then translate them for the child and other family members.

HELP – Harmonising Education about Leukaemia for Parents is a web-based system developed at Great Ormond Street Children's Hospital in London that provides easy access to information about acute lymphoblastic leukaemia (ALL). It is designed to supplement the information provided by the child's doctors and nurses.

Preventing non-accidental injuries and safeguarding

Following every serious case of child maltreatment or neglect there is considerable consternation that greater progress has not been made to prevent such occurrences. Over the past three decades reviews and enquiries across the UK, have often identified the same issues – among them, poor communication and information sharing between professionals and agencies, inadequate training and support for staff, and a failure to listen to children. The names, Victoria Climbé, Baby Peter, Shannon Matthews, Holly Wells, Jessica Chapman and more recently Daniel Pelka may be familiar.

The terms child abuse and child maltreatment have been replaced with the terms child protection and safeguarding children. This has been done as children are vulnerable and the first two terms suggest that abuse has happened. The new terminology sets out to remind us that there are vulnerable children and they need to protected. Nurses are in a very good position to deal with these situations as their roles in health surveillance, monitoring and health promotion. This makes them very approachable and less stigmatizing than social services. In March 2012 there were 42850 children in England alone who were the subject of a Child Protection Plan, 11% (4850) of whom were aged under one year (or 13% (5730) including unborn children) and mostly for an initial category of neglect (DfE, 2012).

Activity 18.6

What types of abuse might you see as a nurse?

Discussion

Types of abuse can be physical abuse such as hitting, biting, and burning. It may be neglect with a parent failing to meet the child's basic care needs, or failing to provide adequate supervision resulting in a child opening a front door and stepping out into a road.

It may be sexual abuse with either physical or non-physical actions. The child exploitation and online protection centre (http://ceop.police.uk) have a number of resources available to children, parents, carers and teachers on the subject of online safety and have reported 184 cases of children in the UK being blackmailed into performing sex acts in front of a web camera in the last two years.

It may be emotional abuse with the child being made to feel worthless, intimidated or allowing a child to see and/or hear the maltreatment of others. This may be domestic violence between the child's parents. The child may be forced to participate or the child may sustain physical injuries from the abusive parent as they try to protect their other parent (NSPCC, 2007).

Promoting healthy lifestyles

There are many ways in which a child in hospital or living with a condition that requires nursing care or support may also need education in order to lead a healthier life.

Obesity

Obesity for example, is a major national priority for children. NICE (2006) identifies the following as potential reasons for early childhood obesity:

- eating behaviour;
- comorbidities, e.g. type 2 diabetes, hypertension, cardiovascular disease, osteoarthritis;
- lifestyle, including diet and physical activity;

- family history of obesity;
- psychosocial distress.

Children in hospital, for example, should be encouraged to eat a healthy diet though the setting may not make this easy. Saxena *et al.* (2013) published the results of a study that looked at trends of hospital admissions between 2000 and 2009 with a focus on obesity as either a primary diagnosis and comorbidity or bariatric surgery procedures in England. It demonstrated that in 2000 there were 872 admissions in these categories, however, in 2009 the figure had jumped to nearly five times the number of admissions. It also showed that these admissions were predominantly girls with 56.2% of the admissions.

Case study 18.2

Food in hospital

Action on Salt, a campaign group (www.actiononsalt.org.uk) analysed the nutritional content of 451 main meals, snacks and desserts served to children in hospitals in England in 2010 and found that:

- Almost half the main meals, 85 of 189, contained so much salt or saturated fat that they would be deemed too unhealthy to be offered to school pupils.
- High levels of both salt and saturated fat meant that 30% of all the 451 dishes would be classed "red" under the traffic-light food labelling system used by some major supermarkets.
- A lasagne had 3.2 grams of salt.

Oral care

Tooth brushing is a common activity that is performed daily by most people. Oral hygiene often becomes secondary to the medical problems of children who are hospitalized. Unless a child has an obvious high risk for oral health problems, such as oral mucositis associated with cancer treatments, oral care often loses priority with the nursing staff. Many hospitalized children receive medications that may contain artificial sweeteners or sugar substitutes. Parents may also give their child in hospital more sweets as a way of helping the child to feel better, or to help the feelings of guilt that the parent may have themselves for their child being in hospital. The National Oral Health Plan for Wales identified 9600 children in Wales having teeth extracted between 2010–2011 (Welsh Government, 2013) and a separate study over the same time period undertaken by Cardiff University School of Dentistry and Public Health Wales (Public Health Wales, 2013) identified 41% of 5-year-olds with dental decay.

Child and adolescent mental health

In 2004, 1 in 10 children between the ages of 5–16 were identified as having a clinically diagnosable mental health disorder with rates higher for boys than girls and varying with ethnicity being highest in black children and lowest in Indian children. The most common mental health conditions for children and young people are emotional disorders (depression, anxiety and obsessions), hyperactivity (inattention and over-activity), and conduct disorders (awkward, troublesome, aggressive and antisocial behaviour). Some 28% of children aged between 11–16 with an emotional disorder had reported that they had attempted to self-harm or to kill themselves (ONS, 2005). Children in the care system and children in young offenders institutes are some of the most vulnerable children and are susceptible to multiple mental health problems (DfE, 2013).

The long-term consequences of mental health problems in childhood are considerable. At 33 years, children who had conduct disorder are more likely to be on benefits, unemployed or homeless, to have been a teenage parent, and to suffer poorer health than their peers (Collishaw, 2004).

Health promotion in child mental health aims to allow a child to develop appropriate coping mechanisms, respond within normal limits when under stress, continue to learn and play so that attainments are appropriate for their age and cognitive ability.

Examples of mental health promoting factors include:

- levels of self-esteem and emotional resilience;
- sociability;
- family warmth and affection;
- being loved and feeling secure;
- living in a stable home environment;
- social support systems and positive peer relationships;
- good communication skills;
- a good sense of humour.

There is evidence that it is possible to enhance these protective factors. As poor parenting is associated with conduct disorder, anxiety and depression, and low self-esteem, interventions that target certain risk and protective factors (e.g. parenting) may be more effective than others. The Child and Maternal Health Observatory summarizes some of the evidence on what works for those who commission services as shown in Figure 18.4.

Children and exercise

Exercise is also a consideration for hospitalized children and children in the community. A recent study found that only half of 7-year-old boys achieve the recommended levels of physical activity of an hour a day and only a third of girls achieve this (Griffiths *et al.*, 2013). The Change4Life campaign is aimed at encouraging people of all ages to lead healthier, more active lives with an "Eat well, move more, live longer" message. Using apps and email messages, it encourages children at the start of the school year to take several small steps that will help lead to a permanent improvement in their health. This includes breaking down the perhaps daunting task of being active for at least 60 minutes into 10-minute chunks, plus suggestions for games to tempt children away from their screen.

NICE Guidelines for Mental Health and Behavioural Conditions
Details of all the clinical guidelines, published or in development, including guidelines relating to treatment and care of children and young people and the promotion of wellbeing in schools.

CAMHS Evidence Based Practice Unit (EBPU)
The CAMHS EBPU aims to develop and disseminate information about the latest research on helping children and young people with emotional and behavioural difficulties, and their families.

No Health Without Mental Health: Delivering improved outcomes in mental health (Department of Health, 2011)
Published alongside the mental health strategy this sets out six shared objectives to improve mental health outcomes and the evidence base which underpins them.

How to Use NICE Guidance to Commission High Quality Services (NICE, 2009)
Explains how NICE guidance supports the commissioning of high quality services, and describes how the guidance can be used throughout the commissioning cycle.

Knowing Where To Look: How to find the evidence you need (CSIP, 2008)
Best practice guidance to assist in planning or providing services; useful for decision-making around commissioning services. Published in conjunction with YoungMinds and the CAMHS EBPU.

TaMHS: Using the evidence to inform your approach (Department for Children, Schools and Families, 2008)
An overview of the evidence on school-based mental health interventions which commissioners may find useful. Developed for the Targeted Mental Health in Schools (TaMHS) programme.

The Evidence Base to Guide Development of Tier 4 CAMHS (Department of Health, 2009)
Summary paper on developments including inreach, outreach and community-based services; plus the supporting evidence base. Commissioned by the NCSS Tier 4 Advisory Group.

Improving the Emotional and Behavioural Health of Looked After Children and Young People(Centre for Excellence and Outcomes in Children and Young People's Services, 2010)
Systematic review focusing on proven interventions such as enhanced foster care, as well as the general lessons to be drawn from Multisystemic Therapy and mentoring. The importance of relationships and the role of professionals are also considered.

Improving Access to Psychological Therapies (IAPT): Children and young people programme
The initial phase of IAPT concentrated on developing better access to evidence-based psychological therapies for adults of working age with mild to moderate depression. From 2011-12 this is extended to include a three year programme to ensure that children and young people have better access to talking therapies.

Multisystemic Therapy
Information from the National Mental Health Development Unit on how Multisystemic Therapy can significantly cut reoffending in troubled and aggressive young people.

Figure 18.4 What works to promote mental health for children. Source: National CAMHS Support Service 2011, p. 13. Reproduced under the Open Government Licence.

Case study 18.3

Exercise and cystic fibrosis

A programme at Great Ormond Street Hospital (GOSH) offers physiotherapy, dietary support and personal training sessions to children with cystic fibrosis (CF). The 12-month Frequent Flyer Programme aimed to reduce the need for children and young people with CF to be admitted to hospital. A child with CF may spend two to three weeks in hospital every few months for antibiotic treatment. The pilot programme resulted in a 21% reduction in the total number of days spent receiving intravenous (IV) antibiotic treatment at GOSH, from 619 days in the preceding year to 478 in the pilot year. Added to this was a 20% reduction in home IV antibiotic treatment from 304 to 243 days. The patients also showed a significant increase in their exercise capacity. Exercise capacity has been previously shown to help to maintain or increase lung function in the longer term. Children who could not maintain steady growth as a result of exercising more, were prescribed additional calorie supplements to meet their higher energy needs (http://blog.gosh.org/research/cystic-fibrosis/#sthash.OXrQSOB3.dpuf).

The role of the children's nurse in health promotion

On admission to hospital the child needs to be assessed by a nurse and a doctor. The nurse will obtain information relating to the health of the child, both currently and prior to admission. This will provide a snapshot of the child's health. Should a problem relating to the child's health be identified, it will be documented and incorporated into their care plan during their stay. The nurse will provide the child and family with information about their illness or condition, often in the form of a leaflet. The leaflets often come in two basic formats. The first for parents, and the second written for children in easy to understand terms. Again they may be written for younger children and take the form of a colouring book, or for the older child an activity book. The nurse may well refer the child to another health care professional, such as a physiotherapist, dietician or pharmacist. At the start of the admission the nurse will also begin the process of discharge planning. In order for a child to be safely discharged home, a number of criteria will need to be met. While not an obvious task of health promotion, the process of discharging a child home will need a number considerations.

Activity 18.7

James is 13-year-old boy who was admitted to the children's ward last week via Accident and Emergency after being knocked off his bike on his ride to school. He was not wearing a crash helmet and suffered a broken tibia. He also had multiple lacerations to his arms. He was very lucky and did not have any serious head injury. James is due to be discharged home in 5 days' time.

- What health promotion areas need to be addressed before James can be discharged home?

Discussion

James will be going home with a leg in a plaster cast that goes from just below his knee to the tips of his toes. James also has a number of dressings on his arms from the lacerations that are still healing. James is still finding his leg painful and is taking regular analgesics.

Examples of health promotion topics to cover with him and his family could be:

- *care of a plaster cast;*
- *wound care and dressing changes for his arms;*
- *mobility issues to ensure minimal muscle wastage while the cast is on;*
- *hygiene issues such as washing and dressing;*
- *knowledge of medications to ensure his pain is managed safely at home;*
- *road safety in relation to wearing a crash helmet.*

On placement: checklist

- How would you rate the quality of face-to-face communication to children about their condition on placement?
- Were patient information materials available? Were these tailored appropriately for children of different ages?
- What factors are included in the initial assessment, e.g. housing and family composition?
- Are parents informed about medication including storage and dosage?
- Did any health education take place on hygiene issues such as hand washing skills if a child or family have had frequent infections, oral care if a child has tooth decay?
- Do you think the practice you observed on placement was able to empower the child and family? What happens if the child becomes unwell in the future?
- Have the child and family been given the necessary information and skills to deal with situations in the future?

Key learning points

1. Children's nursing includes both primary prevention (promoting good general health) and secondary prevention by helping the child and parent/carer to manage the physiological, physical, social, psychological and spiritual effects of a health problem.
2. Child health population profiles show the UK does particularly badly in relation to the prevention and management of respiratory problems, oral health, diabetes and obesity.
3. Health education for child and parent about their condition will be a key role.

Chapter summary

While children and young people are cared for by children's nurses, all nurses and health professionals will come into contact with children. It is the duty of all nurses to be mindful of the children of families they come into contact with and to ensure a referral to the correct member of staff if a health issue is identified. In this chapter, we have seen that health promotion with children must involve the rest of the family and may centre on health education about a condition. Core skills in communication will be essential in health promotion with children as it will be necessary to explain and listen to concerns of both the child and family. At the same time, nursing a sick child can provide opportunities to promote health as illness or an accident can become a big wake-up call for the child and family and encourage change.

Further reading and resources

Department of Health (2013) *Improving Children and Young People's Health Outcomes: a system wide response*. DH, London.

The Child and Maternity Health Observatory provides profiles and data on many aspects of child health. Available at: www.chimat.org.uk.

The Royal College of Paediatrics and Child Health provides updates and resources on aspects of child health promotio. Available at: http://www.rcpch.ac.uk.

Moyse, K. (ed.) (2009) *Promoting Health in Children and Young People*. Blackwell, Oxford.
This is an introductory text on many aspects of child health.

References

Childrens Epilepsy Service, Swansea NHS Trust (2006) *So... What Is Epilepsy?* Swansea NHS Trust.

Collishaw, S., Maughan, B., Goodman, R. and Pickles, A. (2004) Time trends in adolescent mental health. *Journal of Child Psychology and Psychiatry*, **45** (8), 1350–1362.

Department for Education (2012) *Characteristics of Children in Need*. Department for Education, London.

Department for Education (2013) *Statutory Guidance on Promoting the Health and Well-being of Looked After Children*, DfE, London.

Department for Education and Skills (2003) *Every Child Matters*, DES, London.

DH (Department of Health) (2003) *Children's National Service Framework*. DH, London.

DH (Department of Health) (2008) *The Child Health Promotion Programme*. DH, London.

DH (Department of Health) (2012) *Getting It Right for Children, Young People and Families: Maximising the Contribution of the School Nursing Team: Vision and Call to Action*. Available at: https://www.gov.uk/government/uploads/system/uploads/attachment_data/file/216464/dh_133352.pdf.

Green, H., McGinnity, A., Meltzer, H., Ford, T. and Goodman, R. (2004) *Mental Health of Children and Young People in Great Britain*. Office of National Statistics, London. Available at: https://catalogue.ic.nhs.uk/publications/mental-health/surveys/ment-heal-chil-youn-peop-gb-2004/ment-heal-chil-youn-peop-gb-2004-rep1.pdf.

Griffiths, L., Cortina-Borja, M., Sera, F., *et al.* (2013) How active are our children? Findings from the Millennium Cohort Study. *BMJ Open*, **3**, e002893 doi:10.1136/bmjopen-2013-002893.

Hall, D.M.B. (1989) *Health for All Children: A Programme for Child Health Surveillance: The Report of the Joint Working Party on Child Health Surveillance*. Oxford University Press, Oxford.

Hall, D. and Elliman, D. (2006) *Health for All Children*, 4th edn. Oxford University Press, Oxford.

National CAMHS Support Service (2011) *Better Mental Health Outcomes for Children and Young People*: A Resource Directory for Commissioners. National CAMHS Support Service, London.

NICE (2006a) *Obesity Guidance on the Prevention, Identification, Assessment and Management of Overweight and Obesity in Adults and Children*. Available at: http://guidance.nice.org.uk/CG43/NICEGuidance/pdf/English.

NICE (2006b) *Promoting Children's Social and Emotional Wellbeing in Primary School.* Available at: http://www.nice.org.uk/nicemedia/pdf/ph012guidance.pdf.

NICE (2007) *Management of Atopic Eczema in Children from Birth Up to the Age of 12 Years*. CG 57. Available at: http://guidance.nice.org.uk/CG57.

NSPCC (2007) *Worried About a Child? How You Can Protect Children from Abuse*. Available at: http://www.nspcc.org.uk/help-and-advice/for-parents-and-carers/guides-for-parents/worried-about-a-child/worried-about-a-child-english-pdf_wdf90895.pdf.

ONS (Office of National Statistics) (2005) *Mental Health of Children and Young People in Great Britain 2004*. Available at: https://catalogue.ic.nhs.uk/publications/mental-health/surveys/ment-heal-chil-youn-peop-gb-2004/ment-heal-chil-youn-peop-gb-2004-rep1.pdf.

Public Health Wales (2013) *Picture of Oral Health*. Available at: 2012 http://www.cardiff.ac.uk/dentl/resources/A%20Picture%20of%20Oral%20Health%20-%20School%20Year%201%20-%202011-12.pdf.

RCN (1991) *Children and Young People's Nursing: A Philosophy of Care*. Available at: http://www.rcn.org.uk/__data/assets/pdf_file/0003/78573/002012.pdf.

Roberts, H. (2012) *What Works to Reduce Inequalities in Child Health*, 2nd edn. Policy Press, Bristol.

Saxena, S., Jones Nielson, J., Laverty, A. *et al.* (2013) *Rising Obesity-Related Hospital Admissions among Children and Young People in England: National Time Trends*. Plosone open. Available at: ttp://www.plosone.org/article/info%3Adoi%2F10.1371%2Fjournal.pone.0065764.

Welsh Government (2013) *A National Oral Health Plan: Something to Smile About*. Available at: http://wales.gov.uk/docs/phhs/publications/130318oralhealthplanen.pdf.

While, A., Forbes, A., Ullman, R. and Murgatroyd, B. (2005) *The Contribution of Nurses, Midwives and Health Visitors to Child Health and Child Health Services: A Scoping Review. Report for the National Co-ordinating Centre for NHS Service Delivery and Organisation R&D (NCCSDO)*. Kings College London, London. Available at: http://www.netscc.ac.uk/hsdr/files/project/SDO_ES_08-1305-068_V01.pdf

Williams, A., Noyes, J., Chandler-Oatts, J., *et al.* (2011) *Children's Health Information Matters: Researching the Practice of and Requirements for Age Appropriate Health Information for Children and Young People. Final Report*. NIHR Service Delivery and Organisation Programme. Available at: http://www.nets.nihr.ac.uk/__data/assets/pdf_file/0017/64322/FR-08-1718-145.pdf.

Wolfe, I., Cass, H., Thompson, M.J. *et al.* (2011) Improving child health services in the UK: insights from Europe and their implications for the NHS reforms. *British Medical Journal*, **342**, d1277.

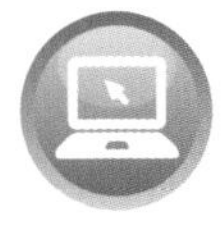

Don't forget to visit the companion website for this book: www.wileyfundamentalseries.com/healthpromotion where you can find self-assessment tests to check your progress.

Index

Fundamentals of Health Promotion for Nurses, Second Edition. Edited by Jane Wills.

Companion website: www.wileyfundamentalseries.com/healthpromotion